T0329665

# PERILOUS MEDICINE

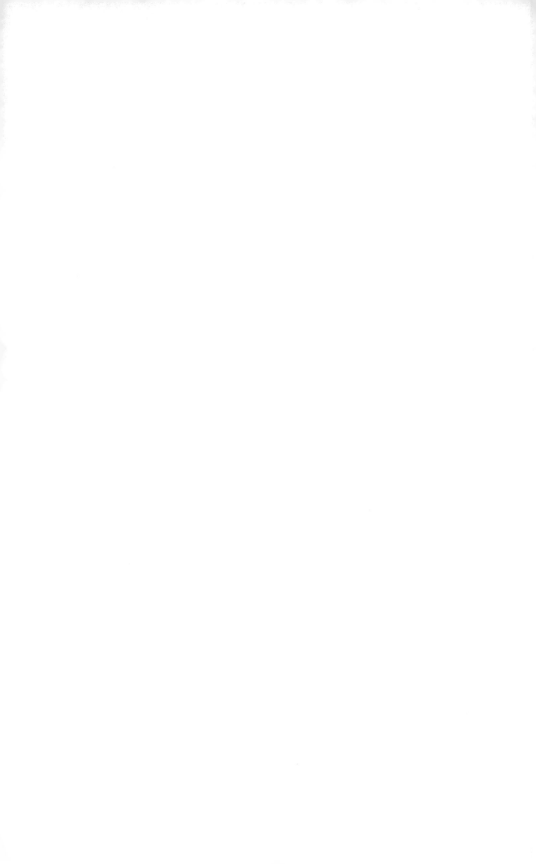

LEONARD RUBENSTEIN

# PERILOUS MEDICINE

The Struggle to Protect Health Care
from the Violence of War

Columbia University Press / New York

Columbia University Press
*Publishers Since 1893*
New York    Chichester, West Sussex
cup.columbia.edu
Copyright © 2021 Columbia University Press
All rights reserved

Library of Congress Cataloging-in-Publication Data
Names: Rubenstein, Leonard S., author.
Title: Perilous medicine : the struggle to protect health care from the
violence of war / Leonard Rubenstein.
Description: New York : Columbia University Press, 2021. |
Includes bibliographical references and index.
Identifiers: LCCN 2020056451 (print) | LCCN 2020056452 (ebook) |
ISBN 9780231192460 (hardback) | ISBN 9780231549820 (ebook)
Subjects: LCSH: War—Medical aspects. | War—Protection of civilians. |
Civilian war casualties.
Classification: LCC RA646 .R83 2021 (print) | LCC RA646 (ebook) |
DDC 362.1—dc23
LC record available at https://lccn.loc.gov/2020056451
LC ebook record available at https://lccn.loc.gov/2020056452

Cover design: Julia Kushnirsky
Cover image: AP Photo/Al-Hadji Kudra Maliro

*To the memory of Dr. H. Jack Geiger,*

*pioneer in human rights and health,*

*mentor and source of inspiration.*

*Of that many-threaded drama [of the Civil War], with its sudden and strange surprises, its confounding of prophecies, its moments of despair, the dread of foreign interference, the interminable campaigns, the bloody battles, the mighty and cumbrous and green armies, the drafts and bounties—the immense money expenditure, like a heavy pouring constant rain—with, over the whole land, the last three years of the struggle, an unending universal mourning-wail of women, parents, orphans—the marrow of the tragedy concentrated in those Hospitals . . . forming the Untold and Unwritten History of the War.*

—Walt Whitman, *Memoranda During the War*

# CONTENTS

CONTENTS

# ACKNOWLEDGMENTS

W HILE IT IS customary to save an acknowledgment for one's partner until the end, I part with convention because my wife,
Margaret Lorber, supported me in writing this book from
beginning to end. She was my constant adviser, a tough editor of every
draft—gentle in her incisive critiques—and cheerleader throughout. This
book would not have been possible without her wisdom and love.

My great thanks go to the hundreds of health workers and humanitarians who have shared their experience of working in war and political conflict over the past two decades despite knowing that doing so was not
likely to offer them greater security. I am awed by their dedication to the
people they serve. Four of them, Khassan Baiev, Markus Geisser, Luan
Jaha, and Şebnem Fincancı, who I had known as many as twenty years
ago, agreed to speak to me again as I was writing this book, offering even
more detail about their lives and thoughtfully reflecting on their experiences. I am also grateful to my many colleagues and former colleagues at
Physicians for Human Rights and Johns Hopkins who participated in
human rights investigations and research projects described here, and to
the students whose energy and indefatigable work contributed so much to
them.

I especially thank the extraordinary research help from my former student and dedicated nurse Sarah Woznick, who conducted interviews in the Central African Republic and shared her knowledge from many years of working in conflict-affected countries for MSF. I also appreciated the willingness of Michael Barnett, Rohini Haar, and Trevor Keck to read through an entire draft, and their graciousness in pointing out errors, offering suggestions for improvement, and encouraging me to keep at it.

Others who had detailed knowledge of a country or topic took the time to fill in gaps, track down an elusive fact, correct mistakes, or provide new insights about a chapter. They included Abudar Alganadi, Tayseer Alkarim, Francois Bellon, Lt. Col. Daniel Beaudoin (retired), Alexander Breitegger, Bill Davis, Will Cragin, Matt DeCamp, Mohammad Darwish, Anne Decobert, Nancy Ebb, Colette Gadenne, Tom Geoghegan, Vince Iacopino, Ashley Jackson, Khalil Fahim, Mohamad Katoub, Larry Lewis, Gen. Louis Lillywhite (retired), Rob Malley, Luke Mogelson, Racha Mouawieh, Nuriya Oswald, Stephen Pomper, Diana Rayes, Paul Spiegel, Zaher Sahloul, Rohan Talbot, Sandrine Tiller, and Paul Wise.

I am indebted to the International Committee of the Red Cross, which has strict rules regarding outsiders who wish to tell the stories of their work, for permitting me to tell the story of Markus Geisser in Afghanistan. Sebastien Carliez, Mary Werntz, Maciej Polkowski, Juan-Pedro Schaerer, Reto Stocker, Jerome Meyer, and Fiona Terry all kindly reviewed the chapter for accuracy and to ensure that I didn't inadvertently reveal confidences. I thank Médecins Sans Frontières for its willingness to permit interviews with its staff in the Central African Republic.

My work on this problem began when I was executive director of Physicians for Human Rights. There I was mentored by its founders, board members, and activists, who were pioneers in the field of human rights, revealing abuses against health care in war when no one was paying much attention. They include Charlie Clements, Jim Cobey, Carola Eisenberg, H. Jack Geiger, Bob Lawrence, Jennifer Leaning, and Ron Waldman. Susannah Sirkin, my longtime colleague on the staff at PHR, is not only an indefatigable human rights defender but a good friend who always has reminded me why we were doing this work.

Many other colleagues helped shape my understanding of the issues over the years and provided insights that I absorbed so thoroughly that I often don't remember from whom I gained them. They include Elizbeth Adams, Joe Amon, Carol Bales, Karl Blanchet, Alexandra Boivin, Rudi Coninx, Larissa Fast, Norbert Goldfield, Maria Guevara, Amy Hagopian, Samer Jabbour, Ambassador Jimmy Kolker, Joanne Liu, Diederik Lohman, Maurice Middleburg, Jason Mills, Steve Morrison, Roisin Read, Hazem Rihawi, Stephanie Rinaldi, Les Roberts, Annie Sparrow, Bertrand Taithe, Ahmad Tarakji, Adriaan van Es, and Christina Wille. I am fortunate to work with wonderful colleagues (and former colleagues) at the Center for Public Health and Human Rights, and the Center for Humanitarian Health at the Johns Hopkins Bloomberg School of Public Health: Stef Baral, Chris Beyrer, Gilbert Burnham, Michele Decker, Courtland Robinson, Sheree Schwartz, Sonal Singh, Mija Ververs, and Andrea Wirtz tolerated my obsession with the subject and taught me a lot. I am grateful, too, to Mohammad Darwish, Sandra Hsu Hnin Mon, and Natalya Kostandova for their translations.

Thanks, too, to Donna McKay, executive director of Physicians for Human Rights, for permission to use copyrighted material from its reports and releases, including *Endless Brutality: War Crimes in Chechnya*, copyright © 2001 Physicians for Human Rights, *Perilous Medicine, The Legacy of Conflict on Health in Kosovo*, copyright © 2009 Physicians for Human Rights and "Raqqa Offensive Has Destroyed the City's Health Care System," copyright © 2017, Physicians for Human Rights. I also appreciate permission to use the following copyrighted material: "Checkpoints," *Boston Review*, copyright © 2012 Oded Na'aman; "On the Frontlines of Eastern Burma's Chronic Conflict: Listening to the Voices of Local Health Workers," *Social Science and Medicine*, copyright © 2014 Elsevier; "Providing Health Care Under ISIS: A Qualitative Analysis of Healthcare Workers Experiences in Mosul, Iraq Between June 2014 and June 2017," *Global Public Health* copyright © 2019 Taylor and Francis 2019. Some of the interviews discussed in this book were originally conducted in connection with research I carried out at the Johns Hopkins Bloomberg School of Public Health. I thank the school's Institutional

Review Board for permitting me to use portions of the interviews for this book.

Many people provided financial support for the research for this book. I am especially grateful for the generosity of Kathy and Ed Ludwig, Conrad Fischer, and Kelly Kellogg for their major significant support for the research for this book. I deeply appreciate the support I received from Nan Aron and Bernie Arons, Fred Baurer and Sharon Pollack, Andrea Capachietti, Greg Carr, Marshall Dinowitz, Nancy Ebb and Gary Ford, Claire Engers and David Silberman, Irene Frary, Norbert Goldfield, Elaine and Dave Leaverton, and Thalassa Scholl.

Finally, I cannot sufficiently convey my gratitude to journalist, writer, and friend Marianne Szegedy-Maszak, who encouraged me to write the book, guided me in figuring out how to structure it and convey its stories, and edited multiple drafts. Caelyn Cobb, my editor at Columbia University Press, was willing to take a chance on the book and bring it to the finish line.

# ABBREVIATIONS

| | |
|---|---|
| DRC | Democratic Republic of the Congo |
| ICRC | International Committee of the Red Cross |
| IDF | Israel Defense Forces |
| ISAF | International Security Assistance Force (Afghanistan) |
| JIAT | Joint Incident Assessment Team (Saudi Arabia) |
| KNLA | Karen National Liberation Army |
| MINUSCA | United Nations Multidimensional Integrated Stabilization Mission in the Central African Republic |
| MONUSCO | Mission de l'Organisation des Nations Unies pour la stabilisation en République démocratique du Congo (UN Organization Stabilization Mission in the Democratic Republic of the Congo) |
| MSF | Médecins Sans Frontières (Doctors Without Borders) |
| NGO | Nongovernmental Organization |
| PHR | Physicians for Human Rights |
| PKK | Kurdistan Workers' Party (Turkey) |
| PRCS | Palestine Red Crescent Society |
| UNAMA | United Nations Assistance Mission in Afghanistan |

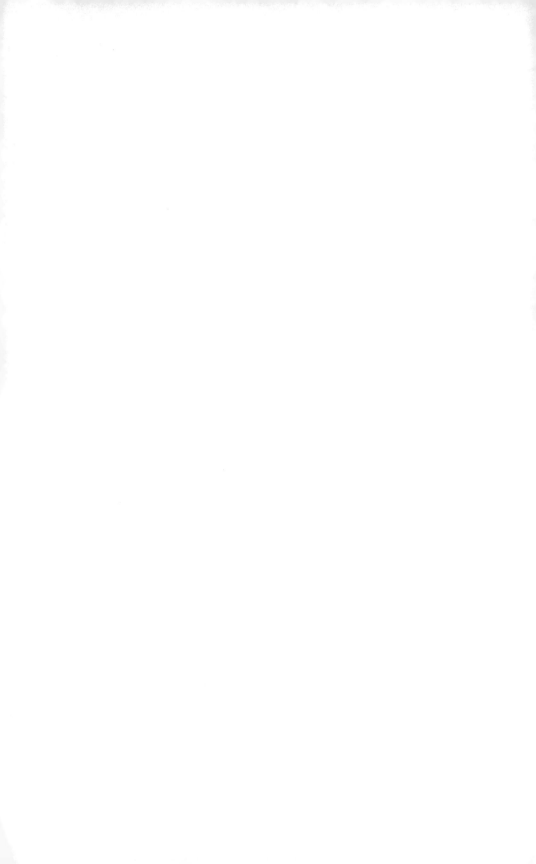

# PERILOUS MEDICINE

# INTRODUCTION

## When the Hospital Is a Battlefield

O N THE MORNING of May 26, 1992, a month into the war in Bosnia, Serbian forces loyal to Yugoslavia's president, Slobodan Milosevic, shelled Sarajevo, Bosnia's capital. Dr. Esma Zecevic, chief pediatrician at the country's main referral center for pediatrics, saw that the Serbian forces were very close to the hospital and worried about the safety of the staff and patients. A Bosnian territorial defense commander told her that it was unlikely that the Serbian forces would directly bombard the hospital. Yet by 4 o'clock in the afternoon, she wrote, "We realized that our hospital was being directly bombarded. We simply could not believe this at first."[1] She and her colleagues decided they had to evacuate.

There were seventeen premature infants in incubators in the neonatal wards. "Each of us carried two or three babies and ran to the basement of the Obstetric and Gynecological Hospital. Bullets and shells fell all around us as we ran carrying the children," she wrote.[2] Thirty-three older children had to be moved as well. Five minutes after the staff got all the children out, a shell hit the neonatal unit, destroying the incubators and incinerating the unit. Soon afterward, the Obstetric and Gynecological Hospital was shelled and the floors above them began to collapse. They spent a frightening night without light, supplemental oxygen, or water. In the morning trucks and cars evacuated the group to Kosevo Hospital, a few kilometers away, as snipers fired at the convoy. As a result of the lack of oxygen, warmth, and incubators, nine of the babies died.

Kosevo Hospital, part of a large medical complex, was regularly shelled. By 1993, the UN reported that the complex had been hit 170 times, destroying large parts of the buildings and putting at further risk the thousands of Sarajevans who had already suffered war-related injuries from the relentless shelling of the city. The staff managed to keep the hospital open despite shortages of fuel for generators, medical supplies, painkillers and antibiotics, and broken central heating that caused its water pipes to freeze during the long winter. They sterilized instruments using a wood-burning stove, but had few options for preventing patients from succumbing to hypothermia. As staff moved through the building, they had to be vigilant to stay away from corridors near windows to avoid sniper attacks. Bombardments eased in 1994, but the hospital still lacked water or heat. Food ran low, too, leading to the anomaly of malnutrition inside a hospital. Dr. Zecevic said, "We often feel on the edge. We come to work every day exhausted. We have received no salaries since the beginning of 1994."[3] Later, she herself was seriously wounded when a shell entered her home and penetrated her chest. She returned to work two months later. A few months before the war ended in September 1995, snipers killed two patients in the hospital, and shelling killed two other patients. Two staff members in front of the hospital, who were carrying water to it, were also killed by shelling.

I learned of these horrors in the spring of 1996, when I started a new job as executive director of Physicians for Human Rights (PHR) after having spent most of my career working on civil rights issues in the United States. The story of the attacks on Kosevo Hospital was contained in a just-completed report written by my predecessor, Eric Stover, and a team of investigators who recounted assaults on health care during the war in Bosnia and Croatia in former Yugoslavia.[4] As I read the report, I was stunned by its wrenching accounts of people wounded in the almost constant shelling of the city, and of caregivers trying desperately to save them while they and their hospitals were under attack. I learned, too, that in 1993 the UN had awarded a human rights prize to the Kosevo Hospital staff in recognition of their courage in the face of the barrage. By then, five members of the staff had already been killed and only half of prewar medical staff remained on duty. Through 1994, the UN estimated that 35 to 50 percent of health facilities in Bosnia had been damaged by shelling, which resulted in severely limited medical services for people when they most needed them.

Before taking the job, I had known from the news about the savagery of the war, the concentration camps, the widespread rapes, and other atrocities, but little about attacks on hospitals, patients, and health workers, nor the history of the norms and laws that prohibited them. It didn't take much sophisticated understanding, though, to appreciate that the conduct of the Serbian forces mocked the laws of war contained in the Geneva Conventions and the principle of humanity—the requirement to avoid unnecessary suffering—that underlies them. I soon learned that the original rule, dating back to 1864, is the prohibition on attacking the wounded and the sick, and on assaulting or punishing military or civilian health workers who offer them care, or inflicting violence on hospitals or ambulances.[5] In each revision and expansion of the original Convention in the many years since, the protections of the wounded and sick grew broader and stronger, extending from the initial concern with wounded soldiers to civilians, from conflicts between nations to civil wars, from targeted attacks to indiscriminate ones. Every member of the United Nations has ratified the four modern Geneva Conventions of 1949, and about 170 governments have ratified additional provisions, called protocols, adopted in 1977. The health-care provisions of the conventions and protocols have become so universally recognized that most are binding on all combatants—including nonstate armed groups—in all circumstances of armed conflict. Moreover, in situations of political violence short of war, international human rights law, also well accepted throughout the world, offers similar protections for the wounded, the sick, and their caregivers.

Two of my new colleagues at PHR, Susannah Sirkin and Barbara Ayotte, thought it best to release the report in Sarajevo, where reporters were covering the implementation of the agreement signed in late 1995 that ended the war. I agreed to go, but it was with some trepidation that

I traveled to Bosnia that June. I had never seen a war-torn country. It helped that I was accompanied on the trip by PHR's forensic program director, the late Dr. Robert Kirschner, a pathologist from Chicago whose swashbuckling manner belied his careful, pioneering work in conducting medical examinations and autopsies that revealed evidence of war crimes. Even though the war had been over for eight months, the Sarajevo airport remained closed to commercial flights, so we had to drive there from Zagreb, Croatia. As we crossed into Bosnia, the road revealed one village after another where nothing was left but the shells of destroyed houses. As we approached the city, we were greeted by ubiquitous blue plastic sheeting that still covered blown-out windows of buildings, the large Holiday Inn and Kosevo Hospital among them. Buildings everywhere were sprinkled with the pock marks of artillery shells.

In Sarajevo, I also met Bill Haglund, PHR's forensic anthropologist, who had assembled a team to investigate mass graves on behalf of the International Criminal Tribunal for the former Yugoslavia. This was the first international criminal court established to investigate war crimes in the fifty years since the Nuremberg tribunal after the Second World War. As recounted in Stover's report, one of the graves contained the remains of more than two hundred people murdered after being removed from a hospital in Vukovar, Croatia in 1991. The men responsible for that massacre were later prosecuted, the first—and to date last—time that perpetrators of an attack on a hospital and patients were subject to prosecution for war crimes. Bill had a custom that demonstrated his care—he always wore a tie when working at the sites, out of respect for the dead. Bill's teams exhumed mass graves spread around the town of Srebrenica in Bosnia, which contained bodies of as many as eight thousand Bosnian men and boys murdered outside the town in 1995. Years later, their work contributed to the criminal prosecutions of Radovan Karadžić, the president of the breakaway Serb state in Bosnia, and General Ratko Mladić, whose forces committed the Srebrenica massacre. Both were convicted of genocide and crimes against humanity. Yugoslav President Slobodan Milošević, also accused, died in his cell before a verdict was rendered.

About a dozen reporters attended our press conference, but the report received little coverage. The lack of attention was my first lesson among many to follow, that assaults on health care in war were widespread, but unless an event was as spectacular as the Vukovar mass killings, addressing them was not a global health, diplomatic, or human rights priority. No serious thinking, much less strategy, to prevent attacks and end impunity was evident among international institutions concerned with global health or human rights. Humanitarian organizations offering health care did what they could to secure facilities, but had little support. Even when the assaults did gain some notice, nothing was done. In 1993, the World Health Assembly, the governing body of the World Health Organization (WHO), adopted a brief resolution condemning attacks on hospitals, calling on combatants to obey the law.[6] But it did not require the WHO to take concrete actions other than a vague call to advocate for protection, liaise with other UN agencies, and write a follow-up report. Two years later, the called-for report recited a litany of violations: combatants damaged and looted three provincial hospitals and fifty health posts in Burundi; massively destroyed health services in Rwanda; inflicted mortar and heavy gunfire on health facilities and kidnapped health workers in Somalia; and carried out missile attacks on medical facilities in Yemen.

The follow-up report noted pointedly that "one of the grimmest features of the conflict in former Yugoslavia is the deliberate attack on health personnel and health care institutions." It said that a "vigorous response from the international community is essential," one that should include strong advocacy, and a common approach within the UN system to respond to violations.[7] Its recommendations went nowhere. Six years later, the World Health Assembly adopted yet another resolution, this time noting the bombing of hospitals in Chechnya and Sri Lanka, the burning of clinics in Kosovo, and attacks on medical staff in Colombia, the occupied Palestinian territory, and elsewhere. The resolution stated that the assembly was "deeply disturbed by recent reports of increasing attacks on medical personnel, establishments and units during armed conflicts" and "alarmed" by the consequences of the attacks on civilian populations.[8] Its response, though, was even more empty than the generalities of the 1994 resolution, omitting a call for monitoring or a subsequent report. Officials at the WHO later told me that the issue was considered too controversial for an organization controlled by member states.

In the years after that first trip to Sarajevo, I participated in human rights investigations and, when I left PHR and came to Johns Hopkins in 2009, academic research, concerning violence against health care in Afghanistan, Bosnia, the Central African Republic, Chechnya, Israel, Kosovo, Liberia, Myanmar, the occupied Palestinian territory, Syria, and Turkey. I heard the anguished stories of health workers who had been arrested, assaulted, shot at, and bombed in the hospitals where they worked; of patients attacked in their beds; of clinics looted or forced to shut down under threat; of emergency responders frantically trying to persuade indifferent soldiers to allow patients in dire need to get through checkpoints.

We don't even know with any precision how many attacks have taken place in wars and situations of political violence over the last twenty-five years. Even in the last few years, as efforts to document attacks on health care have proliferated, ascertaining the number of attacks remains difficult, as many incidents go unreported and methods of documentation vary. We do know that, from 2016–2020, more than four thousand acts of violence in conflict against health care led to a health worker killed every three days and a facility damaged or destroyed every other day.[9] This figure is likely to be significantly understated. Many incidents are not recorded because systems for reporting remain fairly primitive. Blockages of the passage of the wounded and sick at checkpoints, violent hospital intrusions, and threats that lead to the closure of health facilities are rarely reported. Collection of data is generally restricted to situations of armed conflict and UN-designated emergencies, thus excluding attacks on health care in countries where political or gang violence short of armed conflict predominates.

The assaults often create havoc far beyond the deaths and injuries in the moment. After a year of Bosnia's war, the staff of a hospital in the town of Srebrenica, though only occasionally subjected to shelling, felt so exhausted, stressed, and deprived of resources that "the structured and formal trappings of medical practice" simply disappeared.[10] These conditions, in turn, lead many doctors and nurses—often those with the most experience—to flee. Those who remain are often fearful for their lives, their families, and their futures. They frequently feel conflicted about subjecting their families to worries about the risks they are taking. With resources for appropriate care scarce, many of them also feel profound distress because they can't meet their ethical obligations to provide the care their patients need and deserve. Where hospitals are hit, they have to shut down or suspend operations, crippling health systems' capacity to provide care when patient needs are greatest.

The long-lasting, indirect effects, though difficult to measure and so rarely assessed, are enormous.[11] Over the past thirty years, an estimated 29 million civilians have died in armed conflict from communicable, maternal, neonatal, and nutritional diseases, as well as noncommunicable diseases and injuries.[12] We don't know how many deaths are a product of the destruction of health capacity. We do know people in need either cannot access care or stop seeking it out of fear that the hospital or clinic is a dangerous place. In Afghanistan, the UN's humanitarian agency reported that in 2019 approximately 24,000 hours of health-care delivery were lost, and 41,000 consultations missed due to the forced closure and destruction of health facilities.[13] In northwest Syria, more than eighty airstrikes against hospitals in the Idlib and Aleppo Governates in 2019 and early 2020 left only half the health facilities functioning. As a result, the World Health Organization estimated that over a four-week period, more than 133,000 medical outpatient consultations would not take place, 11,000 trauma patients would not receive treatment, and 1,500 major surgeries would not be performed as they normally would in the region.[14] Attacks often force a realignment of priorities in health care as the need to try to save the lives of people with traumatic injuries catastrophically force hospitals to reduce services for chronic illness and maternal and child care.[15]

Insecurity in Pakistan, where more than seventy attacks on vaccinators have been committed, pushed back by years, perhaps decades, the realization of the comprehensive global plan to eradicate polio from the planet.[16] The violence also impairs the ability of officials to address health crises caused by war. Saudi Arabia's air attacks on hospitals and water systems in parts of Yemen led to the largest outbreak of cholera the world has ever seen, more than one million cases.[17] Containment of the 2018 Ebola outbreak in the Democratic Republic of the Congo was repeatedly set back by hundreds of attacks on clinics and health workers. The deterioration of health systems by violence in war created havoc when COVID-19 spread in 2020.

During my years at Physicians for Human Rights, I was also struck by the paradox of global indifference to the problem. During the early 2000s, global health was moving to the center of the international agenda. New drugs became available to treat HIV/AIDS and governments vastly increased spending, saving the lives of millions of people and preventing new infections. Large investments in improving health, especially in poor countries, dramatically reduced the number of children who die before age five. Donors helped ministries of health in low-income countries develop effective systems to advance the health of their people. The idea of health security as an element of national security became fashionable. People living in war zones, though, were largely left out of this progress. They still died young and pointlessly from preventable or treatable conditions, in part a consequence of the violence inflicted on health infrastructure and staff. As Physicians for Human Rights and a few other human rights groups cranked out reports documenting attacks on health care in wars and situations of political violence, we gained little traction in bringing attention to the problem, understanding the dynamics of attacks, gaining commitments to prevent them, or ending impunity. Until very recently, attacks were not tracked and strategies toward greater security largely absent. Even research on the problem was rare, as 90 percent of studies on violence against health care concern interpersonal violence in routine health settings, as compared to 5 percent on the assaults in war that destroy so many lives and compromise the health of millions of people.[18]

To the extent any attention was paid, it was concentrated on the more visible violence against civilians and on humanitarian aid workers in wars. Political scientists have employed sophisticated statistical methods to explore the likely sources of violence against civilians, particularly those committed by nonstate armed groups in civil wars. Yet, as I discuss in chapter 7, the reasons for violence against health care and attacks on civilians generally may often differ. Studies, conferences, reports, and a small shelf of books have shared experiences and offered recommendations to improve aid workers' safety. The strategies focused mostly on adjusting their own operations, increasing knowledge of the security environment, improving attitudes toward and relationships with communities, acquiring skills in negotiating with armed actors, ensuring a neutral stance in the conflict, and adopting more sophisticated risk management and security procedures.[19] These strategies are valuable and necessary to reduce risk in the field. They are usually designed, however, from the viewpoint of potential victims, not from the perspective of changing the political calculations of attackers. Moreover, the vast majority of nurses, doctors, pharmacists, emergency responders, and community health workers in wars are not associated with international aid groups, but are employed instead by ministries of health, sectarian health organizations and NGO hospitals and clinics, or are in private practice. In 2020, Humanitarian Outcomes, which collects information on attacks on aid workers, searched its database to determine the number of attacks it recorded on humanitarian organizations' health programs, transports, and facilities from 1997 to 2019. It found 423 incidents over the 2 decades.[20] That figure is less than half the number of attacks on all health workers and facilities in conflicts in 2019 alone.[21] These local health workers and providers frequently lack the resources for sophisticated security management and the leverage needed to influence combatants. Yet they are especially vulnerable, since they are often members of the very ethnic, religious, or national groups under assault or affiliated with a government that is the enemy of the attackers.

Only in the last decade did violence against health care in war finally begin to receive global attention. UN bodies adopted resolutions and recommendations demanding concrete steps by governments, military forces, and global institutions to increase the protection of health care and end impunity. The World Health Organization began tracking attacks on health-care personnel and facilities in war zones. Academics and think tanks conducted research to increase knowledge about the dynamics of the violence and its impact. Yet the fervor did not lead to action by governments, militaries, and the UN to prevent attacks and end impunity for them. The attention the problem received did not bring about amelioration of the violence. Instead, it seemed that it was increasing or becoming a new normal. The persistence of violence against health care in conflict zones, especially in the face of increased knowledge and unfulfilled commitments about what should be done to stop it, raises urgent sets of questions: What is driving these attacks? Has the nature of contemporary warfare, most often involving state forces facing a plethora of armed groups, often in urban areas, led to an increase in attacks? Are the values of humanity and human dignity that underlie the laws of war eroding? What can be done to persuade, induce, or compel combatants to adhere to the laws protecting health care from violence? What are the impediments to implementing the required steps?

This book is my effort to answer these questions. I begin with history. Chapter 1 reviews the origins and evolution of norms and laws on the subject in the 150 years after the adoption of the first Geneva Convention in 1864. It opens with the competing visions of two seminal figures of the laws of war relating to the protection of health care, Francis Lieber and Henri Dunant. In an amazing historical coincidence, in the 1860s, they independently developed theories about the moral basis for military conduct toward the wounded and the sick in war. Extraordinarily, each succeeded in converting their theories into law and policy. Lieber, fascinated by the morality and purposes of war, drew up a code of conduct for the Union Army during the American Civil War. Dunant's vision grew out of a war that pitted Napoleon III in France against other European states. With a handful of colleagues, he managed to secure adoption of the first international treaty to protect the wounded and sick on the battlefield and their rescuers and caregivers from harm.

Chapter 1 particularly explores the evolution of the law of war in addressing the tension between Dunant's embrace of the principle of humanity—the imperative to reduce unnecessary human suffering—and Lieber's idea that it is moral to use brutal means to end a just war quickly.

The primacy of humanity in Dunant's thinking ultimately prevailed in the law, but chapter 1 considers how Lieber's thinking has remained influential in the conduct of military forces and rationalized and created a logic for widespread noncompliance with the Geneva Conventions' requirements to protect and respect health care in war. The chapter also explores how Lieber's approach had calamitous consequences for health care in long postponing the laws' attention to the indiscriminate use of new technologies of war, especially air power. The chapter finally turns to how the principle of human dignity, the fulcrum on which human rights law turns, became influential in the laws of war and shaped government obligations to protect health-care workers in times of political violence.

The centerpiece of the book consists of thirteen case studies covering the last quarter century that I believe illuminate the drivers of attacks on health-care workers, patients, and facilities. The case studies focus not so much on the motivations of the actors, which are so difficult to determine, but on the logic or apparent purposes (sometimes multiple ones) of the perpetrators, with the aim of developing a framework for understanding the violence. Throughout the book, I rely heavily on the stories of health workers who experienced the violence, and often the trauma and despair that accompanied it, most of whom I met while engaged in human rights investigations or conducting academic research. In each conflict, I focus intensively on the conduct of one or a few of the combatants to illustrate a particular kind of logic in the violence inflicted. As a result, most of the case studies touch only briefly on the conduct of other combatants, such as the Houthis in Yemen, Hamas in Gaza, and government security forces in the Central African Republic.

The case studies also consider whether countervailing policies and pressures, internal or external to the combatants, did or could have ameliorated or ended the violence. They look at questions such as the extent to which international norms are fully embraced, fairly interpreted, and implemented through domestic law, military doctrine, training, operations, and the discipline of fighting forces. As part of that exploration, the case studies address whether tactics in the field are consistent with fighting force's or political commitments to health-care security. The case studies additionally look at whether effective domestic or international investigations of violations were undertaken, and if so, whether perpetrators were held to account. Finally, they consider whether pressure to secure compliance on entities that breach the law was or could have been effectively exerted by domestic entities or by UN institutions and governments not directly involved in the conflict through the leverage potentially available to them through political, diplomatic, economic, military (including leverage from providing military support), investigative, and judicial channels.

Chapters 2 through 6 consider state militaries' infliction of violence on health care and chapter 7 addresses the conduct of nonstate armed groups (referred to throughout the book as armed groups) in five conflicts. Chapters 2 and 3 address resistance to the underpinnings and texts of the laws of war since Dunant's time that require that all wounded and sick people, by virtue of their humanity, receive care without distinction based on affiliation, identity, or beliefs. Correspondingly, their caregivers cannot be punished for offering health care. In chapter 2, I explore the ethics and morality of the requirement of impartiality in care through the lens of conflicts in Chechnya and Afghanistan and consider why combatants find the provision of health care for enemies to be illogical and even paradoxical. I next turn to Myanmar, where entire communities were perceived as enemies, which in turn led to the targeting of medics who provided care to them. Chapter 3 addresses a recent variation on this theme, the new policy stance and legal regime that holds that individuals deemed to be terrorists are unworthy of health care and the act of providing it to them is properly criminalized. Chapter 3's first two sections review the precursors of this development by recounting the persecution and prosecution of doctors in Turkey and Kosovo in the 1990s for providing care to alleged terrorists. At the time, the United States government vocally supported the doctors. The next section shows how, after the attacks of 9/11, the United States as well as other countries reversed that posture, adopting and enforcing counterterrorism laws that follow the same logic as the tormenters of health workers in Turkey and Kosovo.

Chapter 4 addresses the logic of targeting hospitals and health care workers as a military strategy. It focuses on the most egregious case, Syria.

Its first section recounts the conduct of the regime of President Bashar al-Assad in arresting and torturing health workers who treated protestors. I then turn to the relentless bombing and shelling of hospitals, ambulances, and first responders by Assad and his ally, Russia. The third section reviews how the UN and the Obama administration stood by, appalled, condemning the horrors but too politically paralyzed to take steps to stop the killing.

I then turn, in chapter 5, to the reckless air campaign employed by Saudi Arabia and its partner, the United Arab Emirates, in Yemen that included the bombing of dozens of hospitals. The indiscriminate nature of the airstrikes appears to have lacked a strategic purpose. Instead, political and military leaders of the Saudi-led coalition lacked the commitment to engage in the careful and rigorous procedures needed to distinguish military targets from hospitals and other civilian structures and to avoid attacks that cause disproportionate harm to civilians. Their conduct suggests they considered it too inconvenient to adhere to the rules and were more interested in feigning compliance than achieving it. The chapter then reviews how international institutions capitulated before this conduct even when their own investigations revealed evidence of war crimes, and how the United States and the United Kingdom, which were in a strong position to force a change in Saudi conduct by virtue of their military support for the war, declined to stop selling weapons or invoke other sources of leverage they had.

Chapter 6 turns to the problem of obstruction of access to care for the wounded and the sick, both in combat and during chronic conflict. It traces the policies and practices of Israel over two decades on medical evacuation during active fighting and the passage of ambulances through occupied territory. It addresses how tensions between the passage of medical transport and prevention of terrorism can be straightforwardly resolved, and indeed how, for a time, Israel enacted reforms to facilitate medical evacuation safely for all. The chapter also shows the need for commitment to safe and expeditious passage, and how reforms evaporated when political postures changed and pressures for compliance diminished.

In chapter 7, I review the conduct of nonstate armed groups in the proliferating and often chaotic civil wars that predominate today. The chapter examines five conflicts: Liberia, Afghanistan, the Central African Republic, the Islamic State in Syria and Iraq, and the Democratic Republic of the Congo. In the first four, I look at the influences on the groups' conduct exerted by political and military objectives, organizational structures, ideology, recruitment practices, and the health-care needs of its fighters and the populations they sought to influence. In the Democratic Republic of the Congo, I explore the relationship between governance and violence against health-care workers and facilities in connection with the Ebola outbreak of 2018 in its eastern provinces. As in other chapters, I look at how internal and external pressures affected, or might affect, their behavior toward health-care workers and infrastructure.

Finally, in chapter 8, I look back at the case studies and propose a framework for understanding the violence. I identify five common logics in the attacks, though with the caveat identified by Fabrice Weissman, the director of MSF's internal think tank, that context is critical. Weissman warned against "heterogenous events in a wide range of volatile settings being lumped together into a single aggregation in the hope of detecting statistically significant trends, probabilities and risk factors."[22] Chapter 7 then address two major challenges in countering the logic behind this violence, the contemporary threats to the norms of respect for and protection of health care and the fraught global and domestic politics that have impeded the implementation of now-widely embraced strategies domestically and internationally for reducing the violence and ending impunity.

I conclude with a potential path forward. We know that, given the human propensity for cruelty, especially in war, this violence will never entirely cease, any more than war itself and the atrocities that too often accompany it will end. Bringing humanity to the midst of war is always a struggle, as it requires restraint by fighters who are trained and motivated to engage in lethal violence to achieve their objectives. Trends in contemporary warfare pose obstacles to the work of prevention of and accountability for this violence. Internal conflicts now predominate, often involving multiple armed groups. Jihadist groups celebrate and publicize atrocities they commit. Fighting in urban areas, where health facilities are often located, puts health care at greater risk. Advanced air power is available to militaries whose commitment to the rules is shaky at best. Powerful states increasingly rely on proxy and partner forces to avoid use of their own troops while taking no responsibility for the conduct of their partners. Compliance on the basis of reciprocal adherence—I will treat your wounded and sick well if you do the same for mine—is no longer the powerful motivator it once was, as in so many wars one side shows no respect for the Geneva Conventions. The counterterrorism paradigm that challenges the norms of the Geneva Conventions and human rights law is ascendant.

Given these developments and the numbing frequency of this form of violence, a fair degree of cynicism has set in. A narrative has taken hold that the rules are either obsolete or incapable of being realized. To preview my conclusion, I view the problem differently: too few strategies that could prevent the assaults have been tried. It is not the inevitability of massive assaults on health care that allows the violence to continue, but the abdication of responsibility by those in a position to prevent and end impunity for them. The record today is one of lassitude and evasion of responsibility, along with an unacknowledged chipping away at norms, which together exact incalculable costs on people caught up in war and those who, because they can't leave or choose to stay, care for them.

I believe we have an obligation to seek to reverse that trend, for the values at stake, for the wounded and sick people who suffer, and for the health workers who attend to them. Over the years, in dozens and dozens of encounters, I have come away feeling awe for the doctors, nurses, and emergency medical workers who continue to serve their patients not just in the chaos and violence of war, but where they themselves were targets. They have told me vivid and often tragic stories about carrying on while they faced enormous physical and psychological burdens. None of the doctors, nurses, medics, pharmacists, lab technicians, dentists, and others consider themselves heroic, though of course they are. Their personal experiences, and their often-wrenching encounters with people who are wounded or sick, recounted in the pages that follow, demonstrate, more than any report or statistic possibly can, the true measure of what is at stake.

# 1

## PROTECTION OF HEALTH CARE IN WAR

---

### A Brief History

W AR," SAID THE Prussian-born soldier, scholar, and writer Francis Lieber, brings "moral electricity," that is "vital to the moral progress of virtuous nations."[1] In the 1850s, from his adopted American perch, he wrote that for democratic governments, "freedom is a goddess who cannot afford to sheathe her sword forever" against barbarism and injustice.[2] Across the ocean, around the very same time, Henri Dunant, a Swiss businessman, witnessed the battle of Solferino in 1859 as wounded soldiers died of thirst in the heat, leading him to believe that suffering, not heroism, progress, or justice, is the real story of war. He wrote that war "kills not only the body but also too often the soul. It humiliates, corrupts, withers, demeans. Cloaked in the most deceptive appearances, it is the source of a thousand degrading, cruel and bestial things."[3] From these equally passionate, but wildly divergent perspectives, Lieber and Dunant each became pioneers in laws defining the moral boundaries of the conduct of war, including obligations of combatants toward the wounded and the sick. Their common ground and the tension between their approaches remain with us today.

For centuries, philosophers wrestled with questions of the justice of going to war but paid less attention to the moral constraints on conducting it. By the eighteenth century, though, both philosophers and military leaders, including George Washington, looked more closely at questions of morally acceptable behavior by combatants in war. Are there limits to the violence soldiers could inflict on the enemy? What are their obligations to avoid harm to civilians? Is it acceptable to torture captured prisoners? How does the principle of humanity, reflecting the value of alleviating human suffering, align with taking the actions needed to win a war? Enlightenment thinkers pressed the view that all combatants should observe rules designed to limit the destructiveness of war, no matter how just their cause. In the 1830s, the most famous theorist of war, Carl von Clausewitz, opposed that view, urging that the moral end of war is achieving a swift victory. Clausewitz's position left no room for restraint, mercy, or concerns about humanity. He therefore justified total brutality, or whatever level of it is needed to quickly prevail.

As influential as Clausewitz's writing on the conduct of war was, however, Lieber and Dunant soon eclipsed it. Perhaps not coincidentally, they were writing at a time when the industrial revolution brought technological advances in ballistics and increased the precision, range, and lethal power of rifles and cannons, raising new concerns about war's destructiveness.[4] In 1863, the U.S. War Department appointed Lieber to a board to write a code to regulate the behavior of Union soldiers in the Civil War. Though the only civilian on the board, he did most of the drafting. Ever since, the order has been known as the Lieber Code, and it exerts significant influence even today. The very same year, Dunant pressed for an international treaty on protection of health care in war, which became the original Geneva Convention, adopted a year later. In the years since, the convention evolved into four treaties and two additional protocols that constitute the centerpieces of the law governing the conduct of war, now known as international humanitarian law.

## FRANCIS LIEBER: MILITARY NECESSITY AND THE LIMITS OF PROTECTION

Born in 1798, Francis Lieber always wanted to be a warrior. During his boyhood, Prussia was allied with Napoleon, but after 1806, it switched sides. At the age of fifteen, after witnessing Napoleon's troops march into Berlin, Lieber attempted to assassinate him. Lieber subsequently enlisted with Prussian forces fighting Napoleon. In the lead-up to the battle of Waterloo, Lieber fought hard and witnessed the blood and suffering of war, including seeing his fellow soldiers killed or dying. French troops shot him in the head and neck, and he was left for dead.[5] Local peasants searched his pockets and took his valuables.[6] Somehow Lieber survived. The experience, far from convincing him of the futility or horror of war, reinforced his belief in its glory, and what one historian calls "a source of moral regeneration" in the service of great causes.[7] Lieber continued to fight, including in a war for Greek independence against the Turks.

Once his soldiering days were over, Lieber became a political reformer and was arrested on suspicion of subversion. Even with a doctorate in mathematics, his reputation made him unemployable and subject to police harassment, so in 1827, Lieber left the country for London. There he managed to meet and befriend leading philosophers of the day, including Jeremy Bentham and John Stuart Mill. Lieber eventually made his way to the United States, settling in Boston, where he edited the *Encyclopedia Britannica* and established himself as a leading public intellectual. He exchanged ideas with Henry Wadsworth Longfellow, dined with Andrew Jackson, and conversed with Supreme Court justice Joseph Story.[8] Having worked as a research assistant to Alexis de Tocqueville, who was studying prisons in the United States, Lieber became a prison reformer and became so respected for his work that South Carolina, where he later moved, named a prison after him.[9]

Lieber taught at the University of South Carolina for two decades. Even before his arrival there, his association with northern intellectuals and writings on political philosophy and social reform made colleagues there suspicious about his views on slavery. To prove his southern bona fides, he announced he was not an abolitionist and acquired slaves. Yet seeing slavery close-up, Lieber became ever more appalled by what he called this "nasty, dirty, selfish institution."[10] Attuned to the dangers of expressing his views in the most proslavery state in the Union, he never spoke of his doubts publicly, costing him friendships with anti-slavery advocates in the north, including Charles Sumner, the leading Radical Republican senator. Even so, he was denied the presidency of the University of South Carolina because he was considered insufficiently devoted to the cause of slavery.[11] After his second rejection from the post, and ever more disgusted by slavery, he left for Columbia University in 1857 to teach history and a new field he called political science, the first scholar to use that term.

By then, Lieber had become preoccupied by the law of war, writing articles and papers on prisoners of war and other contentious topics that gained wide attention from scholars and the general public. During the Mexican War of 1846–48, he argued that soldiers had individual moral responsibility for their conduct, an idea we now take for granted, but which was then a breakthrough. He also developed an overarching view of war that linked what traditionally were thought to be two separate moral dimensions: *jus ad bellum*, whether going to war is just, and *jus in bello*, permissible conduct in war. Lieber came to believe that war is necessary to secure national interests and a "requisite of civilized existence that men live in political, continuous societies" and advance human progress.[12] Securing national purpose and preserving freedom and justice might require war, and he took a consequentialist moral stance about what actions are permitted in a just war, that is, judging actions by their results, not by their inherent nature. From this foundation, Lieber argued that brutal acts are moral if they more quickly bring a just war to an end. He believed that the infliction of suffering, even on those not engaged in fighting, is not inherently wrong, as it can advance the legitimate goals of a just war. Lieber nevertheless called for some restraints on conduct in war, usually because, in his view, they did not advance the war's just aims. Thus, he found gratuitous cruelty to civilians, prisoners, or wounded sol-diers, always wrong because it did nothing to advance the war's purposes.[13] He saw the legitimacy of other conduct as situational, depending on whether it advances the cause.

When the Civil War came, Lieber was firmly on the side of the Union, viewing a war to end slavery as just. His own sons, who grew up in South Carolina, were split. Two of them signed up to fight for the Union. One of them, Hamilton, bravely led his company in the cold and snow against a larger Confederate force and fought on even after being shot, contributing to one of the first major Union victories, at Fort Donelson, in 1862. Hamilton's arm had to be amputated.[14] Learning of his son's injury, Lieber searched one hospital after another until he found him. His other son, Oscar, joined the Confederacy and died painfully in battle. Even as deeply and personally aggrieved as he was by the death of one son and severe injury to the other, Lieber never changed his mind about the need for the war. On the contrary, he urged the use of massive force against the Confederacy.

In 1862, Lieber befriended General Henry Halleck, then in charge of Union Army forces in Missouri. Halleck was unsure how he should deal with pro-Confederate guerrillas in his sector. Could guerrillas be legitimately killed as a combatant, or should they be arrested as civilians and imprisoned? Did guerrillas' failure to wear a uniform make any difference in how they should be classified and treated? In making that decision, did it matter if someone reported through a clear command structure? Another concern was how prisoners in Union custody should be treated. Halleck asked Lieber to help develop rules addressing these and other perplexing questions. Lieber dived into the task. After he produced a report on the status of guerrillas under the laws of war, Halleck ordered that five thousand copies be printed. Lincoln, also bedeviled by these and other legal questions arising during the war, eventually commissioned Lieber and four Union officers to write a code of conduct for the entire Union Army. Within a few months the work was done, almost all of it by Lieber. In the summer of 1863, shortly before the battle of Gettysburg, Lincoln issued General Order 100, consisting of 157 articles, to regulate soldiers' conduct in the war.[15] It was the first-ever codification of the rules of war.

Among its many provisions, the code addressed the question of on whom suffering can be imposed in war and under what circumstances. It recognized that infliction of suffering was germane to determining acceptable conduct, as "men who take up arms against one another in public war do not cease on this account to be moral beings" (Article 15). Following Lieber's philosophy, though, the code did not consider preventing or alleviating suffering an end in itself.[16] It reflected, rather, Lieber's belief that a just war sometimes warranted savage measures to achieve its objective. To operationalize the idea, he applied the now-familiar, but then-novel concept of military necessity, which the code defined as "those measures which are indispensable for securing the ends of war, and which are lawful according to the modern law and usages of war" (Article 14).[17]

The code applied the principle of military necessity to harm inflicted on civilians. It recognized "the distinction between the private individual belonging to a hostile country and the hostile country itself, with its men in arms" (Article 22). It nevertheless considered the inhabitants loyal to the other side as an "enemy" subject to the "hardships of war" (Article 21). Unarmed citizens are to be spared "in person, property and honor," but only "as much as the exigencies of war admit" (Article 22). Thus, though the code outlawed "useless destruction," it broadly permitted "all destruction of property, and obstruction of the ways and channels of traffic, travel, or communication, and of all withholding of sustenance or means of life from the enemy" (Article 15). For the same reasons, it permitted sieges and considered starving the hostile belligerent, "armed or unarmed," permissible because its objective was "the speedier subjugation of the enemy" (Article 17). It prohibited the torture and mistreatment of prisoners, and the rape, wounding, maiming, or killing of civilians as retaliation for abuses by the other side (Article 16) because they amounted to no more than gratuitous cruelty and did nothing to advance the ends of war. Despite its otherwise strict rules for humane treatment of prisoners, though, it allowed that, in some circumstances, prisoners could be subjected to retaliatory measures (Article 58). Such measures, though, could not be employed for mere revenge (Articles 27, 28). As historian John Fabian Witt has put it, "In Lieber's hands, military necessity was both a broad limit on war's violence and a robust license to destroy."[18]

Lieber's code took a similar approach to medical care of the sick and wounded. During the Civil War, wounded soldiers were sometimes grossly abused. Confederate forces especially targeted Black soldiers.[19] After the Confederate Army defeated Union forces at the battle of Fort Pillow in 1864, they murdered wounded Union soldiers. A doctor working in a hospital reported that all but two of his patients were slaughtered. In the battle of Saltville, the same year, a military surgeon watched with horror as Confederate soldiers seized and killed wounded black soldiers. Another incident was later recounted by Walt Whitman. The poet spent part of the Civil War visiting more than eighty thousand sick and wounded soldiers in six hundred Union hospitals, sitting with them, comforting them, offering them small gifts, and empathizing with them. In his accounts of his experience during the war, he recalled an incident where Confederate cavalry attacked a convoy of ambulances carrying sixty wounded soldiers:

> No sooner had our men surrender'd, the rebels instantly commenced robbing the train, and murdering the prisoners, even the wounded. . . . Among the wounded officers in the ambulances were one, a Lieutenant of regulars, and another of higher rank. These two were dragg'd out on the ground on their backs, and were now surrounded by the guerrillas, a demoniac crowd, each member of which was stabbing them in different parts of the body. . . . The [other] wounded had all been dragg'd . . . out of their wagons, some had been effectually dispatched, and their bodies lying there lifeless and bloody. Others, not yet dead, but horribly mutilated, were moaning or groaning.[20]

Lieber was likely aware of abuses that predated these incidents and the drafting of the code. From his perspective, they served no legitimate military purpose, amounting to gratuitous outrages. Thus, like its prohibition on torturing prisoners, the code said, "Whoever intentionally inflicts additional wounds on an enemy already wholly disabled, or kills such an enemy, or who orders or encourages soldiers to do so, shall suffer death" (Article 71). The provision was consistent with the philosophy of the code, as harming a wounded enemy served no military purpose. Similarly, he saw no reason for the army to decline care for soldiers it captured. The code required that "Every captured wounded enemy shall be medically treated, according to the ability of the medical staff" (Article 79). The code was silent, though, on whether a civilian doctor could be punished for offering treatment to a wounded soldier not in custody. All other obligations toward the wounded and sick were contingent upon the limitations of military necessity. The code urged that hospitals should be secured against all avoidable injury but were protected only as much as "the contingencies and the necessities of the fight will permit" (Article 116). The "necessities of the fight" gave ample room to deny care to the wounded and destroy the hospitals where they were housed. Indiscriminate attacks in civilian areas were also permitted because Lieber asserted that individuals living in a hostile country who were "loyal to the enemy" could be considered enemies and therefore subject to war's hardships.

The conduct of the Union Army in the Civil War both illustrated and challenged the code's attempt to achieve the balance Lieber's code sought. He viewed military necessity broadly to allow its invocation to justify the destruction of housing, commercial establishments, cotton, animals, railroads, and other economic resources of the South, especially during General William Tecumseh Sherman's indiscriminate shelling of Atlanta and ferocious march through Georgia and South Carolina. Sherman defended his actions as essential to victory, saying "if we must be enemies, let us be men, and fight it out as we propose to do, and not deal in such hypocritical appeals to God and humanity."[21] After the mayor of Atlanta begged Sherman to spare pregnant women, mothers, and small children "the woes, the horrors and the suffering," Sherman invoked military necessity: "My orders are not designed to meet the humanities of the case, but to prepare for the future struggles."[22] These actions all likely complied with the code, and some scholars have argued that only violence and destruction such as pillaging and private plunder by troops that extended beyond acts needed to accomplish the military objective were violations; and these, they argue, were unauthorized by Sherman.[23] Yet the boundlessness of Lieber's idea of acts in support of military necessity, which in Sherman's march included taking food and other supplies to live off the land, amounted to an invitation to indiscipline and brutality.

Lieber died in 1872, but his effort to condition humanity in war on the requirements of military necessity has had a long legacy. In 1868, the Declaration of St. Petersburg, an international treaty banning the use of small, inflammable projectiles was predicated on Lieber's thinking. Lieber's views on the treatment of prisoners, pillaging, and many other subjects influenced a convention adopted at a conference held in The Hague in 1899 designed to prevent war and restrict the means and methods of warfare.[24] In a peace conference in The Hague in 1907, governments adopted the so-called Martens Clause, an overarching rule holding that gaps in the rules of war must be governed by "usages established by civilized peoples, from the laws of humanity and the dictates of the public conscience."[25] The clause established that gaps in explicit prohibitions on conduct cannot imply that the conduct is permitted.[26] But it also allowed commanders to use weapons and tactics that they claimed balanced military necessity and humanity.[27] During the Philippine–American War of 1899–1902, Lieber's code was invoked by commanding officers to defend the use of concentration camps and torture of prisoners, including waterboarding. Channeling Lieber, General John Bell argued that a short and severe war was "better than a benevolent war indefinitely prolonged."[28]

Before World War I, the U.S. Army revised the Lieber Code as the Rules of Land Warfare, expanding it to contain 443 articles and maintaining Lieber's core idea of reconciling humanity and necessity. The current version of the Department of Defense's Law of War Manual still pays homage to Lieber's code, calling it a "canonical law of war document for the United States," though it acknowledges that "parts of it no longer reflect current law."[29] That is an understatement. Lieber's ideas of a "fragile equipoise" between humanity and military necessity, including regarding health services, though often hailed, is now severely constrained by the law of war.[30] The propriety of conduct involving the wounded and sick, their caregivers, or hospitals can no longer be judged by the justice of the war or the need to bring it to a swift and successful conclusion. That profound departure from Lieber's conceptualization is the legacy of Lieber's contemporary, Henri Dunant.

# HENRI DUNANT AND THE PRINCIPLE
# OF HUMANITY

Born in 1828, Dunant was the son of devout Calvinists in Geneva who engaged in work to help orphans, prisoners, and the poor. Dunant took after his parents, feeling a need to spread a gospel of love and humanity expressed through volunteer work, and founded a League of Alms.[31] When the bank he worked for sent him to North Africa, Dunant was fascinated by the region even as he was appalled by the exploitation of labor he witnessed. He sought business opportunities in Algeria and tried to start an agricultural company. After difficulties obtaining financing in Paris and being rebuffed in obtaining the land and water rights he needed, Dunant came up with the unlikely notion of going directly to the French emperor, Napoleon III, for help. Dunant was undeterred by the fact that the emperor was in the midst of a military campaign in which he commanded tens of thousands of troops in a war against Austria.

In June 1859, Dunant brought two memos he sought to give the emperor to the town of Castiglione, Italy, about one hundred miles from Milan. One of them extolled the virtues of Napoleon III and the other described his proposed project.[32] As Dunant arrived, the French army and its Sardinian allies were mobilizing against the Austrians in what would become the battle of Solferino. Dunant never got to speak with Napoleon III, but he was a witness to the largest battle in Europe since Waterloo, with three hundred thousand soldiers stretched over more than twelve miles, often fighting hand-to-hand. At least five thousand soldiers were killed and more than twenty-three thousand were wounded. As he later wrote in his evocative and passionate memoir of the battle, *A Memory of Solferino*, "the fighting rages on all sides and grows more and more furious. Compact columns of men throw themselves upon each other with the impetuosity of a destructive torrent that carries everything before it."[33] The close combat became "sheer butchery," followed by cavalry charges that trampled men and severed their heads and limbs.[34] After an entire day of ferocious fighting, a storm erupted, its cold rain and hail adding to the misery of the soldiers, especially those wounded on the field. With the French prevailing on the battlefield, the Austrians finally withdrew, but "though the Army, in its retreat, picked up all the wounded men it could carry in military wagons and requisitioned carts, how many unfortunate men were left behind, lying helpless on the naked ground in their own blood."[35] As night fell, the dead were everywhere. The wounded soldiers begged for water, comfort, and death to end their misery. There was no one to attend to them, as at the time anyone entering the battlefield was considered a belligerent and subject to attack, no matter what their purpose.[36]

The next morning Dunant surveyed the scene: "When the sun came up on the 25th, it disclosed the most dreadful sights imaginable. Bodies of men and horses covered the battlefield; corpses were strewn over the roads, ditches, ravines, thickets and fields; the approaches to Solferino were literally thick with dead."[37] The modern cylindrical bullets used in the battle had caused "agonizingly painful fractures" and "frightful" internal injuries.[38] Wounded survivors remained in agony: "The poor wounded men that were being picked up all day long were ghastly pale and exhausted. Some, who had been the most badly hurt, had a studied look as though they could not grasp what was said to them; they stared at one out of haggard eyes, but their apparent prostration did not prevent them from feeling their pain."[39] The torment of the wounded continued, and despite the efforts of the quartermaster corps and local volunteers to collect them and take them to field hospitals or into local villages, many of the soldiers lay abandoned. The wounds of many of them became infected by dirt, dust, and the absence of water to clean them.

The wounded rescued from the field did little better. Surgeons worked through the night to amputate limbs, but there were too few of them and little water and food. The lack of medical attention for wounded soldiers was not uncommon in mid-nineteenth century European wars. In France, conscription of new recruits was seen as a way to replace wounded soldiers, rendering medical care a lower priority for the army. A long period of peace after the first Napoleonic wars also reduced the medical corps.[40] In England, in the years following the battle of Waterloo in 1815, the British army had become ill-funded and lacked administrative coherence. The medical staff was poorly trained and lacked commitment to their function. As one historian noted, medical officers' "knowledge was limited and their interest in the men was less."[41]

With medical services inadequate and the needs overwhelming, Dunant jumped in. He organized local citizens to find bandages, enlisted boys to carry water, and drafted tourists, journalists, and businessmen to come to the aid of the wounded soldiers. Local and military doctors contributed to the effort to save lives, performing hundreds of amputations in gruesome conditions. Writing of French doctors treating the wounded, Dunant was in awe. They "not only did everything that was humanly possible without distinction of nationality; they grumbled and complained at their inability to do more."[42] He saw them as heroic: "Surely, if those who make the slaughter can claim a place on the roll of honor, those who cure, and cure often at the risk of their lives, are entitled to their due of esteem and gratitude."[43]

Witnessing the carnage and participating in the response to it profoundly changed Dunant. He saw nothing heroic or energizing about war. His book is empty of consideration of whose cause was just and whose was not. His instincts were pacifist, though he believed avoidance of war unlikely or even hopeless. What, then, to do? His answer was to try to ameliorate the suffering of the wounded: "In an age when we hear so much of progress and civilization, is it not a matter of urgency since unhappily we cannot always avoid wars, to press forward in a human and truly civilized spirit to attempt to prevent, or at least alleviate, the horrors of war?"[44] He saw all the wounded as sharing a common humanity, and so all were equally deserving of care. As Dunant put it, his view was based on "the moral sense of the importance of human life; the humane desire to lighten a little the torments of all these poor wretches, or restore their shattered courage; the furious and relentless activities which a man summons up at such moments: all these combine to create a kind of energy which gives one a positive craving to help as many as one can."[45] This imperative to reduce the suffering of the wounded transcended any judgment about their allegiances or of the justice of the cause or country for which they fought.

The principle of humanity embraced by Dunant arises out of a belief that life itself is intrinsically valuable so that each person is and should be treated as an end, not a means. In contrast to Lieber's consequentialist approach to morality in war, the principle of humanity is an approach to conduct based on that independent moral belief.[46] Jean Pictet, author of encyclopedic commentaries on the four modern Geneva Conventions of 1949, described the principle of humanity in circumstances of war: "Assisting human beings plunged into suffering by a common destiny—human beings among whom all distinctions have been wiped out by suffering."[47] Dunant's cry for humanity profoundly influenced the law of war because of its "prophetic power to restrict the excesses of war," as humanitarian and scholar Hugo Slim has written.[48] It gives no weight to the purposes of the war, whether it is just, nor to the need to quickly prevail and bring the war to an end.

The principle of humanity has not only undergirded the Geneva Conventions for more than 150 years, but has also become enshrined as a foundation of modern humanitarian practice, adopted by aid organizations, the UN, and donors who respond to disasters. The UN's humanitarian agency expresses the principle as, "Human suffering must be addressed wherever it is found. The purpose of humanitarian action is to protect life and health and ensure respect for human beings."[49] As applied to humanitarian aid, invoking the principle of humanity may mask issues such as the priorities among recipients and the power relations between those offering aid and those receiving it.[50] But these questions don't arise with respect to attending to and protecting the wounded and sick in war.

Perhaps paradoxically, though, in invoking humanity in *A Memory of Solferino*, Dunant said nothing about the rules of war, particularly how the wounded and sick should be protected from harm, the obligations of combatants to offer care, or the role of civilians in their treatment. Instead, he concluded his book with a call to create voluntary societies to provide care for the wounded and sick and for the establishment of a new international organization to lead the effort. He suggested that nations agree to the creation of such societies through a "convention inviolate in character" that "might constitute the basis for societies for the relief of wounded in different European countries."[51] Dunant's book had enormous influence in Europe, an impact sometimes compared to the reception of *Uncle Tom's Cabin* (a book Dunant deeply admired) in the United States and Victor Hugo's *Les Misérables* in France.[52] Although *A Memory of Solferino* was first privately printed, Charles Dickens published excerpts and its growing popularity led to translation into five languages. It stimulated a movement across Europe to put his idea of voluntary societies into practice. A year after its publication and two months before President Lincoln issued the Lieber Code, Dunant, with the help of Gustave Moynier, who chaired a Geneva aid society, and four other men, founded a new organization, the International Committee for the Relief to the Wounded. It was to be dedicated to mobilizing volunteers to attend to wounded combatants. The name was later changed to the International Committee of the Red Cross.

Even as the movement for an international convention gathered momentum, Dunant did not consider how it should affect the rules of war. Yet if volunteers were going to be authorized to go on the battlefield, they had to be immune from attack or arrest. During Napoleon III's Italian campaign, of which the battle of Solferino was a part, doctors were locked up in Milan's fortress.[53] At Solferino, some volunteers were shot. J. H. C. Basting, the chief medical officer of the Dutch Army, who had been impressed with *A Memory of Solferino* and translated it into Dutch, came up with a solution: the convention should guarantee the protection of the volunteers and declare that medical personnel be considered neutral in the conflict, as they play an exclusively humanitarian role.[54] The two men agreed, too, that volunteers could be identified by wearing a distinctive uniform or emblem to signify their role.

Dunant and four founding colleagues convened an international meeting in October 1863 to discuss these ideas, calling it the Geneva International Conference to Study Ways of Overcoming the Inadequacy of Army Medical Services in the Field. It took place in the then-elegant, recently completed Palais de l'Athénée, built to house the Geneva Arts Society. Fourteen governments, mostly European, as well as relief societies, attended. Dunant's proposal for voluntary societies proved controversial. The French argued that no civilian volunteers should be present in the battlefield. One delegate suggested that the solution was more mules to transport wounded soldiers off the battlefield. The British, having been inspired by the work of Florence Nightingale, had established a well-functioning medical corps and saw no need for voluntary societies, but rather wholesale reform of military medicine.

Nightingale came from a very different background than Dunant, a privileged and rich British family, but like Dunant's, one committed to good works. On a trip to Germany in 1850, she visited a Lutheran home for sick and deprived people and felt inspired by divine purpose to become a nurse despite Victorian conventions against nursing as a proper career for an upper-class woman. Her talents both in nursing and management were so considerable that, within a few years, she was running a hospital for ailing governesses in London, all the while receiving financial support from her father to live in a manner consistent with upper-class expectations. During a cholera outbreak at another London hospital, she mobilized to improve the hygiene practices of hospital staff.

When England sent troops to Crimea in 1853, almost no provision had been made for their medical care.[55] Nightingale prevailed upon the Secretary of War, Sir Sidney Herbert, to send her to the front. In a report for a commission on the sanitary condition of the army, she described what she found on arrival at the hospital in Scutari (Üsküdar), a district in Istanbul. She wrote, "I have been well acquainted with the dwellings of the worst parts of most of the great cities of Europe but have never seen any atmosphere which I could compare with it." Ventilation and heating were nonexistent. Privies "poured their poisons into the corridors and wards; the sewers being loaded with filth, untrapped and without ventilated openings,. . . the sewer gases blew into the wards and corridors." Walls were saturated with organic matter, rats ran under the divans where men were placed, blankets were few, and those available covered with filth and vermin. Water was unfit to drink. The conditions all contributed to outbreaks of dysentery, typhus, typhoid, cholera, and other diseases. The mortality rate among the troops was 60 percent from disease alone, a rate higher than that in London during the great plague.[56] More than 1,400 soldiers died in the hospital in the month after she arrived. She went to work to improve sanitation, correct ventilation and sewer problems, provide clean linens and clothing, and obtain clean water. She kept meticulous, voluminous records of her approach and collected epidemiological data on sickness and death rates. The results were remarkable. Within a few months, the number of deaths per month in the hospital declined to under two hundred, and then to under ten. She reported that mortality had declined to a level lower than among British soldiers at home.[57] After the war, her work stimulated wholesale reform of military medicine in the British army.

Dunant admired Nightingale's work in Crimea and sent her a copy of his book. For her part, Nightingale was unimpressed with his approach to care for the wounded on the battlefield as they relied on voluntary action. She wrote, "A society of this kind would take upon itself the duties that are in fact incumbent on the government of every country" and would likely result in relieving "these governments of a responsibility that is really theirs and which they alone are in a position to assume."[58] Dunant disagreed, believing that voluntary societies were essential because reform of military medical services was impossible.[59] The delegates were not convinced by her experience or argument. Misogyny very likely played a role. A French delegate dismissed the notion that nurses could withstand the rigors of a military campaign. Despite his knowledge of Nightingale's work, and the heroic work of women in Solferino, Dunant wrote:

> It must not be thought that the lovely girls and kind women of [the region of] Castiglione, devoted as they were, saved from death many of the wounded and disfigured, but still curable, soldiers to whom they gave their help. . . . What was needed was not only weak and ignorant women, but, with them and beside them, kindly and experienced men, capable, firm, already organized, and in sufficient numbers to get to work at once in an orderly fashion.[60]

Even as Dunant wrote, the American nurse Clara Barton had already overcome opposition by the U.S. War Department and military surgeons to begin voluntary action to collect and distribute medical supplies for wounded soldiers. After much cajoling, she gained permission to work on the front lines of the Civil War, where she became known as the American Nightingale and the Angel of the Battlefield.

Although Dunant and his colleagues prevailed at the conference in authorizing the development of voluntary societies to provide care in war, Nightingale's prescription proved just as influential. Both left a legacy. Militaries have a responsibility and must have the capacity to ensure the health of their soldiers as well as others who are wounded during fighting. Humanitarian organizations nevertheless play a critical role in offering care to the wounded and the sick. Even as humanitarianism grew, military medicine continued to improve along with the scientific understanding of treatment of disease. At the time, though, the tension between the two approaches was reflected in the American Civil War, as the Union Army opposed the establishment of the U.S. Sanitary Commission, a private group that reported on health conditions in army camps but ultimately, mostly through the work of women, offered supplies, food, clothing, and succor for wounded Union soldiers.[61]

Dunant's and Basting's proposal to protect hospitals, ambulances, and military medical corps, however, did not stimulate the opposition some of Dunant's allies expected. The conference passed a broad resolution calling for the protection of the wounded, ambulances, military hospitals, and everyone offering medical care, be they volunteers, military medical officers and staff, or inhabitants of the country providing care to the sick and wounded. It called for the identification of voluntary societies through a distinctive sign to offer its members protection. To move the recommendations forward, in 1864, Switzerland convened another conference, to draft an international convention. In addition to European states, Brazil, Mexico, and the United States attended. Francis Lieber wanted to go but Lincoln and Secretary of State William Seward declined to send him as the Civil War still raged.[62]

As at the 1863 conference, the proposal for the immunity of health care from attack generated little pushback, as it posed no threat to the military tactics of the major powers. Some, including Prussia, believed it could protect its own health workers, whether their own military surgeons, or volunteers.[63] No one seems to have taken a position similar to Lieber's, whose code had been promulgated the year before, that qualified the immunity of hospitals and caregivers on the basis of military necessity. The conference adopted a Convention for the Amelioration of the Condition of the Wounded in Armies in the Field, the first international treaty on the treatment of the wounded and sick in war.[64] For the first time, it imposed a legal obligation on militaries to collect and care for wounded and sick combatants, "to whatever nation they may belong" (Article 6). It authorized "any inhabitants of the country . . . to bring help to the wounded," and, through their presence in a home, "ensure its protection" (Article 5). It prohibited belligerents from attacking these caregivers or military medical personnel, military hospitals, and ambulances, as long as they accommodate the wounded and the sick (Article 1). It authorized a special emblem on an armband to identify health workers—the now-familiar red cross.

All the major European powers ratified the Convention. Dunant and his colleagues, believing that the Convention was founded on the values of Christian civilization, did not envision signatories beyond Europe, but Japan and the Ottoman Empire joined as well, with an accommodation to Islam by authorizing the use of a red crescent as an emblem.[65] The Europeans' surprise was almost certainly a product of the ignorance of a predominant branch of the Islamic tradition that embraced principles of protection of noncombatants in war, principles such as proportionality, humanity, compassion, nondiscrimination, equality, and fraternity.[66] After the American Civil War, Clara Barton, traveling in Europe, learned of Dunant's book and the creation of the establishment of the International Committee. Returning home, she campaigned for the U.S. ratification of the Geneva Convention. She was at first rebuffed by President Rutherford B. Hayes, who told her that ratification wasn't a necessity because the United States would never again experience a conflict like the Civil War. Undeterred, she founded the American Red Cross, and continued campaigning for ratification, finally succeeding in 1881.

Lieber's and Dunant's ideas developed independently, one written in the midst of war, the other in its wake; one composed by a warrior, the other by a humanitarian; one by a person for whom judgments about the justice of war were central; the other by one who cared little for a war's legitimacy; one a code for militaries, the other an international treaty. Yet some of the similarities between the medical dimensions of the Lieber Code and the Geneva Convention remain striking. They agreed that inflicting harm on wounded or sick soldiers no longer in combat was an abomination and, on the contrary, that combatants had affirmative obligations to care for them. They also agreed that medical personnel, hospitals, and ambulances should not be attacked. Yet, one profound difference separated them. Dunant and the Convention took an absolutist protective stance, opposing any military action that would harm wounded combatants and the facilities and medical personnel who treated them. By contrast, Lieber held that compassion for the wounded and sick and their caregivers must be tempered by the need to win a just war, and quickly—that is, military necessity. Over time, Lieber prevailed to the extent that his concept of military necessity influenced the views of armies ever since. But Dunant won the day in allowing military necessity as a justification for noncombatant harm only as specifically and narrowly permitted in later versions of the Geneva Conventions, thus deeply contracting the scope of allowable noncombatant harm, and in expanding protections of health care beyond what either Lieber or Dunant envisioned.

In the early twentieth century, the Geneva Convention was revised and expanded. One revision, a seemingly technical change, has become momentous for the protection of health workers in war. The 1864 Convention deemed military medical personnel and inhabitants of a war zone who provide medical care to be neutral, a legal status that meant that they supported no side in the conflict, comparable to Switzerland's traditional posture in war. That designation was problematic for health workers, though, as both military and civilian health workers have allegiances to one side that render them nonneutral but should not disentitle them to protection for their health-care work. Indeed, Dunant lauded the citizens of the Milanese town of Castiglione for offering succor to wounded German and Austrian soldiers despite the "profound hatred" the Milanese had for "their race, for their leaders, and for their Sovereign." He wrote, too, that the women of Castiglione showed "the same kindness to all these men whose origins were so different, and all of whom were foreigners to them. 'Tutti fratelli' [all are brothers] they repeated feelingly."[67]

Recognizing the problem, Louis Renault, in 1906 a distinguished French diplomat, international law scholar, and soon Nobel Prize winner, proposed an amendment to the Convention. He explained that doctors could not shed their nationality or military allegiance when treating the wounded and sick. Indeed, he said, "they are, in actual fact, enemies, albeit enemies with a special task, and protection and special immunities must be accorded to them precisely to enable them to perform that task."[68] Renault proposed eliminating the word "neutrality" in the context of medical care and replacing it with the phrase "respect and protect" toward the wounded and sick and health workers, facilities, and transports. "Respect" is meant to convey that medical caregivers are immune from attack or interference, and "protect" conveys an affirmative obligation by combatants to keep them from harm. His argument carried the day and the language he proposed has endured. References to neutrality in the context of health care disappeared from the Geneva Conventions. As later chapters will describe, though, the idea persists that political, religious, ethnic, or national allegiance of health workers, all breaches of neutrality, may result in the forfeit of their protection.[69] Instead, current law holds that they lose protection only if they commit acts outside their humanitarian function harmful to the enemy, for example, by participating in the fighting or hiding weapons in health facilities. For that reason, I do not use the commonly employed phrase "medical neutrality" in this book.

Dunant lived for another four decades after the Geneva Convention was adopted, but by the late 1860s, his life had collapsed. His investments soured, leading him to declare bankruptcy; then a court found that he had made false statements in the bankruptcy proceedings. Dunant was forced out of what was renamed the International Committee of the Red Cross and eventually left Geneva for Paris, where he lived in poverty for decades, sometimes reduced to sleeping on park benches. Long ignored by the growing Red Cross movement, in the 1890s, a series of newspaper and magazine articles restored his reputation. He became a leading advocate for disarmament and mediation to avoid war, and received the Nobel Peace Prize in 1901. Until the end, he remained worried about war and the fate of humankind. As he was dying in 1910, his last words were reported to be, "Where has humanity gone?" It would be worse than he imagined.

## TWENTIETH-CENTURY CATACLYSMS AND THE STRENGTHENING OF PROTECTION

In the decades that followed the adoption of the original Geneva Convention, new conventions were added. In 1899, conventions signed in The Hague extended protections to the wounded and sick at sea (which later evolved into the Second Geneva Convention) and called for bombardments to spare, as much as possible, hospitals and places where the sick and wounded are collected. In 1929, a third Geneva Convention addressed prisoners of war. Contempt for, not compliance with, the new rules, though, became evident from the start. Less than ten years after the adoption of the Geneva Convention in 1864, the Franco–Prussian War of 1870–71 and the siege of Paris revealed both the need for the Convention and the challenges to adherence. Hospitals on Paris's south bank were shelled, some doctors and nurses were executed, and patients were killed in their beds.[70] During World War I, Germany employed the new technology of airplanes to bomb London with incendiary devices and Britain responded with its own bombings of Germany.[71] Germany repeatedly sank hospital ships.[72] During the war years and their immediate aftermath, the International Committee of the Red Cross published complaints alleging 80 breaches of the Geneva Convention, including artillery attacks on medical installations and the execution of military and Red Cross medical personnel.[73]

In the 1930s, Benito Mussolini's campaign against Ethiopia employed newly sophisticated air power to target Red Cross field hospitals and ambulances at least 17 times.[74] In December 1935, the Italian Air Force launched two waves of air assaults, with 18 planes in all, against the city of

Dessie. One bomb went through the roof of a field hospital that had a prominent red cross painted on it; another hit a well-marked health facility operated by the Ethiopian Red Cross. Three weeks later, after days of reconnaissance by Italian planes, four of them attacked a Swedish Red Cross field hospital in Melk Dida. Six bombs hit the hospital, killing eighteen people instantly and wounding fifty, many of whom did not survive. Witnesses reported bomb craters and fire everywhere. Italian documents revealed it was a deliberate attack in retaliation for the killing of a downed Italian pilot by local Somalis.[75]

Marcel Junot, a delegate of the International Committee of the Red Cross in Ethiopia, wrote that, by February 1936, "everywhere our ambulances fled from the Italian bombing, fell into the hands of the enemy, or escaped only in the nick of time."[76] In one incident, he wrote, an Italian plane dropped ten large bombs, twenty smaller bombs, and a number of incendiaries on a hospital tent compound marked with a large Red Cross flag spread on the ground. The second bomb hit a tent where an operation was taking place, killing the patient on the table.[77] An Austrian doctor told Junot that the Red Cross emblem offered no protection, so he removed it from his hospital tents and worked under cover. The ICRC was seen as falling into "sad irrelevance" as the attacks continued.[78] While denying responsibility, Italy sought to shift the blame on Ethiopians as an inferior race who could not grasp the meaning of the laws of war. Italy also falsely claimed that Ethiopians used medical facilities for military purposes. Popular magazines in Italy featured covers depicting Ethiopians soldiers hiding in hospitals.[79] Though extensive international press coverage highlighted Italy's deliberate attacks and generated outrage around the world, during and after the war the politics of the League of Nations led to investigations but no action against Italy. Ethiopia again tried to bring cases to the post–World War II UN War Crimes Commission, but politics again interfered, as opposition by the British and the postwar Italian government squelched those efforts as well.[80]

The Italian airstrikes were deliberate, but as air power developed in the first half of the twentieth century, an enormous gap in the protection of health care in the Geneva Convention emerged: military attacks that did not distinguish between legitimate military targets and hospitals or civilian structures. These assaults did not target hospitals, but these were nevertheless hit because of the indiscriminate bombing. In the 1920s, a proposed international treaty would have outlawed bombing of infrastructure other than munitions factories and communications and transportation facilities used for military purposes. It was never adopted. The horror of the indiscriminate bombing of cities during the Spanish Civil War depicted in Pablo Picasso's painting, *Guernica*, proved a prelude of what was to come. At the beginning of World War II, the British Royal Air Force abided by the stillborn treaty to protect infrastructure, but incrementally retreated from its restrictions. Prime Minister Winston Churchill quickly came to embrace indiscriminate bombing of cities even before the German bombing of London, Coventry, and other cities. Hospitals, churches, and homes were all victims of the strategy of total destruction, designed to wreck Germany's economy and sap its population's morale. In 1940, Churchill said that nothing would defeat Hitler other than "an absolutely devastating, exterminating attack by heavy bombers from this country upon the Nazi homeland."[81] His rationale channeled Lieber in asserting that a war to save democracies against totalitarian forces was just, leaving leeway for the imposition of untold suffering to make victory possible.

Although Churchill occasionally expressed qualms about the deaths bombing caused, once saying, "Are we beasts? Are we taking this too far?"[82]—he never relented from the strategy. When the United States entered the war, it followed suit. Both countries employed strategic, indiscriminate bombing of German cities throughout the war, reaching its apex in the first months of 1945. The infamous firebombing of Dresden in February killed 25,000 people and destroyed 75,000 homes in just a few hours, but it is far from an isolated case. More than 17,000 people were killed in the bombing of the town of Pforzheim, almost 3,000 in Berlin, and at least 4,000 in Würzburg. The list could go on. In all, about 350,000 people were killed in the bombing of German cities, almost all of them not involved in the military industry.[83] The same strategy was used in the war against Japan. In March 1945, the United States dropped napalm-filled bombs on

Tokyo, killing an estimated 100,000 people in a single night. It followed with the incendiary bombing of 66 more cities, killing hundreds of thousands more civilians. The intense heat, fire, and destruction from the burning napalm were so cataclysmic that historian Tami Davis Biddle of the U.S. Army War College wrote that, in the atomic bombing of Hiroshima and Nagasaki a few months later, "no moral threshold was crossed that had not been crossed much earlier in the year."[84]

The stunning level of death and the horror of melting eyes and flesh from the incendiary and atomic bombing of these cities has overshadowed the medical crisis that followed. In his classic book, *Hiroshima*, John Hersey describes the gruesome burn and crush injuries the hundred thousand immediate survivors of the atomic bomb suffered, and the efforts of the single uninjured doctor, Dr. Terufumi Sasaki, in the city's largest hospital, to cope. Ten thousand severely injured survivors sought relief at a hospital with only six hundred beds and a decimated staff. Hersey wrote, "bewildered by the numbers, staggered by so much raw flesh, Dr. Sasaki lost all sense of profession and stopped working as a skillful surgeon and sympathetic man, and he became an automaton, mechanically wiping, daubing, winding, wiping, daubing, winding."[85] In the aftermath of the war, far from recoiling at the morality and consequences of the use of these weapons, British and American military planners argued that the strategic bombing of cities remained a needed option in a potential future war against the Soviet Union. In a speech to the Naval War College in 1947, General Albert Wedemeyer, Chief of Army Plans and Operations, said that a future conflict would likely become a "war of extermination."[86]

Though not as apocalyptic, another concern for health care arose at ground level during the war in Europe. Civilian health workers who either cared for wounded combatants, especially resistance fighters in occupied territory, or failed to report them to authorities, were punished, even executed. After the war, some health workers who provided care under the auspices of an occupying authority were prosecuted for treason as medical care to enemies was equated with taking up arms against one's country.[87]

The atrocities of World War II brought pressure to strengthen the protection of civilians in the Geneva Conventions. The tensions of the Cold

War, along with demands for the inclusion of fighters challenging colonial empires in the conventions, made for difficult negotiations in 1949. Additionally, unlike in 1864, many proposals for revision would seriously constrain military tactics. The governments nevertheless found a way to agree to update and expand the conventions. One provision addressed the arrests and punishment of health workers for care to enemies. It permitted inhabitants and relief societies to "collect and care for the wounded or sick of whatever nationality" and prohibited anyone from being "molested or convicted for having nursed the wounded or sick."[88]

The centerpiece of the revisions, though, was a new, fourth convention dedicated to protection of civilians in armed conflict. For the first time, wounded and sick civilians, along with pregnant women, became immune from attack unless they took direct part in hostilities. Civilian hospitals and medical staff members were equally protected so long as they did not "commit, outside their humanitarian duties, acts harmful to the enemy."[89] These harmful acts are limited to practices such as using hospitals to store munitions, billet soldiers, fire weapons, or employing ambulances to transport weapons or fighters. Even when misused, a warning was required before attack. As in 1864, the revised and new conventions left no room for Lieber's view that hospitals should be protected only "as much as the contingencies and necessities of the fight will permit" (Article 116). The only deference to military considerations in the fourth convention regarding wounded and sick civilians concerned the capacity to search and care for them and security needs during evacuation and care. As one scholar put it, "Codification has resulted in a progressive trend toward emphasis on the humanity prong of the military necessity–humanity balance."[90]

Even with these advances in protection, the United States and its allies successfully defeated proposals to adopt the principle of distinction between military and civilian objects in attacks, which would have prohibited indiscriminate bombing. The opponents sought both to avoid a retrospective judgment of their bombing of German cities in the war, and to retain latitude to detonate nuclear weapons in the future.[91] Nor did the negotiators adopt the principle of proportionality, which prohibits attacks that, while having a legitimate military objective, may be expected to cause death or injury to civilians or damage to civilian objects that are excessive in relation to the concrete and direct military advantage antici- pated. The principle of proportionality takes Lieber's concept of military necessity as a justification for harm and turns it inside out: even if a tactic is deemed militarily necessary, it may still be prohibited because of the disproportionate civilian harm it will likely bring. The principle of propor- tionality similarly rejects the idea that collateral damage to civilians is always acceptable as long as the target is a military one.

Reformers also failed in their efforts to apply the expansive provisions of the revised Geneva Conventions to civil war, as the Lieber Code had done. From their inception in 1864, only wars between states were covered by the Geneva Conventions. The ICRC pressed the conferees to extend the conventions to internal conflicts. Though the idea had other- wise wide backing, colonial powers objected that extending the conven- tions could legitimize rebel groups, and the U.S. did not want to apply the conventions to Communist insurgencies. The contentious issue resulted in a compromise: a single article, identical in each of the four 1949 conven- tions, applying to noninternational wars. One clause of the article provided that "The wounded, sick and shipwrecked shall be collected and cared for" and that individuals not in combat "shall be treated humanely." This general statement, though an advance in protection, lacked the specific obligations the conventions imposed on combatants in interstate wars, thus leaving enormous room for interpretation and, with it, harm.

Almost two hundred states ratified the 1949 conventions. They became so well accepted that their key provisions, including all those related to health care, have become what is called customary international law, which means that even entities that haven't agreed to them are bound by their provisions. Those bound include organized armed groups in civil wars. But the omission of the principles of distinction and proportionality had a cataclysmic impact, giving continued license to indiscriminate bombing. Over the next three decades, indiscriminate airstrikes killed well over a million people and destroyed innumerable hospitals. When the Korean war started less than a year after the adoption of the revised con- ventions, President Harry Truman initially ordered General Douglas

MacArthur, commander of U.S. and UN forces in Korea, to avoid indiscriminate bombing. MacArthur refused requests from his generals to incinerate North Korean cities and forbade attacks in urban areas. As the allied military campaign in Korea struggled, though, the command adopted a policy of purposeful destruction of North Korean cities through firebombing with napalm, as well as dropping nonincendiary bombs.[92]

On November 5, 1950, MacArthur ordered General George Stratemeyer, his air commander, to firebomb the North Korean city of Sinuiju. Three days later, seventy-nine U.S. bombers dropped more than five hundred tons of napalm-filled bombs on more than a square mile in the center of the city of sixty thousand people. The commander of the assault reported afterward that "the town was gone."[93] General Stratemeyer said that all the targets were "military ones," which was true to the extent that hospitals were not specifically targeted. The Air Force, though, said the strikes constituted a "maximum attack," that destroyed 90 percent of the city, thus placing severe doubts upon Stratemeyer's claim to the media that bomb runs had stayed away from the city's hospital areas.[94] What followed was a campaign of firebombing that, according to the Air Force, partially destroyed eighteen of North Korea's twenty-two cities.[95] The U.S. and its allied forces dropped more bombing tonnage in Korea than in the entire Pacific theater in World War II. Five times as much napalm was inflicted upon Korea as in the whole of World War II.[96] Historian Charles Armstrong wrote that U.S. planes ran out of targets as every city, town, and industrial target of possible interest had been destroyed.[97] By the war's end, well over one million North Korean civilians had been killed, representing between 12 and 15 percent of its entire population, a higher per capita civilian death rate than in any other war in modern history. North Korea's estimate of one thousand hospitals destroyed is considered realistic.[98]

Throughout the bombing campaign, the Pentagon and the UN command were subjected to withering criticism by the Soviet Union, which proposed a condemnatory resolution at the Security Council. General MacArthur and Secretary of State Dean Acheson argued that only military targets were bombed, and that the campaign sought to avoid harm to civilians. Eighteen months and stunning levels of destruction later, the *New York Times* reported that the Pentagon insisted that napalm is "an extraordinarily effective weapon that should be used discriminately," and that the "overriding consideration for a field commander is the security of his troops and the selection of the best weapon in his arsenal for a given tactical situation."[99] This flexibility in its use, combined with a highly elastic concept of military target, meant that vast portions of civilian society were obliterated.[100] Military officials vigorously resisted entreaties from the ICRC, American critics, and others to stop the campaign, or at least offer civilians safety zones. Again, the Pentagon argued that the law of war only prohibited intentionally targeting civilians, which it denied.

After the war, the ICRC continued to push to outlaw indiscriminate and disproportionate attacks and, failing that, its 1958 commentaries on the Geneva Conventions urged belligerents to spare hospitals in aerial attacks.[101] Its admonition was largely ignored. In the Vietnam War, the U.S. flew more than 126,000 B-52 bombing sorties, dropping the equivalent of 640 atomic bombs and 400,000 tons of napalm on North and South Vietnam. Thirty-seven million pineapple bombs, cluster munitions loaded with 250,000 lethal ball bearings, rained down as well. A single B-52 could deploy more than 25,000 Guava munitions, each of which contained 300 steel balls, and which can still be found in Vietnam, Laos, and Cambodia today.[102] Credible estimates of civilian deaths that resulted from the bombing are in the hundreds of thousands of people. Many hundreds of thousands more civilians were also killed in bombing runs in Laos and Cambodia that lasted for years. Because the bombing objectives were largely military, or deemed so, and civilians were not specifically targeted, the American position, as in Korea, was that they did not violate the Geneva Conventions.

Unlike in the largely unknown and unopposed war in Korea, however, the Vietnam war was politically charged, with the indiscriminate bombing a central element of disgust and opposition. Norms on indiscriminate bombing were also starting to change toward greater protection of civilians.[103] "Hey, hey LBJ," demonstrators chanted, "how many kids did you kill today?" President Lyndon Johnson, exquisitely attuned to the opposition to the war, often ordered restrictions on bombing tactics in order to reduce civilian casualties. In Operation Rolling Thunder, a forty-three-month bombing campaign against North Vietnam from 1965 to 1968 designed to disrupt supply routes into South Vietnam and force Ho Chi Minh to negotiate peace, Johnson required White House approval of bombing targets. Even with Johnson's restrictions, the CIA estimated that through the end of 1966, two-thirds of all casualties in the campaign were civilians, amounting to around twenty-five thousand people.[104] The number would double before the campaign ended.

Pentagon planners and lawyers deeply opposed the limitations as a self-imposed straitjacket on military effectiveness that, echoing Lieber, they claimed compromised the prospect of victory. W. Hays Parks, who served twenty-four years as the Pentagon's leading expert on the law of war, and whose views were widely shared in the U.S. military, cited military necessity to justify the bombing runs. He defined it even more broadly than Lieber, as based on the "overall campaign or war" rather than the particular military circumstances in battle. Parks also argued that the duty to avoid excessive civilian casualties was limited to those "blatant" acts that "shock the conscience of the world because of their number," and that are "tantamount to total disregard for the safety of the civilian population."[105] Today those views sound both cavalier and legally absurd, but at the time even prominent legal experts critical of the Vietnam War did not entirely disagree with the Pentagon's view of the law. In 1970, Telford Taylor, a law professor at Columbia University who served as counselor to the prosecution during the Nuremberg war crimes trials, wrote a widely read book, *Nuremberg and Vietnam: An American Tragedy*. It was a painful reflection on the atrocities committed by his own country's military forces in Vietnam, including the My Lai massacre, retaliatory killings, and the U.S. "body count" strategy that encouraged the killing of enemy soldiers who could have been taken prisoner. He castigated the lack of accountability of senior military and political officials for these war crimes. Yet on the question of bombing, he commented sardonically, "After the experience of the Second World War one might have supposed it to be common knowledge that heavy bombing near populated areas—even if strictly military objectives are targeted—inevitably kills people and destroys their buildings." But, he added, "I can see no sufficient basis for the war crimes charges based on the bombing of North Vietnam."[106]

In 1972, President Richard Nixon launched a new bombing campaign, dubbed Linebacker, designed to repel North Vietnamese troops entering South Vietnam, and to attempt to force peace negotiations. His restrictions on bombing were looser than Johnson's, and the continuing use of napalm, cluster bombs, and white phosphorus, and the willingness to bomb in poor weather led to at least thirteeen thousand deaths.[107] Later that year, Nixon launched Linebacker II, also known as the Christmas bombings, in an effort to destroy infrastructure and supply lines in the cities of Hanoi and Haiphong. The bombing restrictions now were tighter, including the use of laser-guided weapons and target maps that identified hospitals and schools. Even so, in just eleven days, more than 1,500 civilians were killed.[108] Telford Taylor was accompanying peace activists in Hanoi at the time, and was present when the 940-bed Bach Mai hospital in Hanoi was bombed. After returning, Taylor wrote an op-ed for the *New York Times*, reporting that even though most of the hospital's patients had been moved before the bombing, he was told that about 25 members of the hospital staff were killed. But, he added, "Despite the concentration of the attack, it is impossible for me to believe that the hospital was the target of the raid, which was probably directed at the airfield and nearby barracks and oil storage units."[109] He essentially agreed with Hays Parks's view that no violation had been committed.[110]

Sustained and vocal opposition to the Vietnam War, the high number of Vietnamese civilians killed, and the changing norms on civilian deaths in war, all helped stimulate support for the ICRC's long campaign to bring the principles of distinction and proportionality into the Geneva Conventions and expand coverage to civil wars.[111] Geopolitical stars also began to align, with the proliferation of nuclear-armed states and interest expressed by the Soviet Union and newly independent states in strengthening protections to fighters in colonial wars.[112] After three years of preparatory work and four years of negotiations, in 1977, two sets of amendments, known as Additional Protocols to the Geneva Conventions, brought additional legal protections for health care and civilians in war.

At last, the principles of distinction and proportionality became enshrined in law. The first Protocol, applying to interstate wars, required that only military objects may be attacked, and it prohibited attacks that purposefully or by their nature do not distinguish between military and civilian objects. Article 57 elaborated the rules, requiring that combatants take precautions in attacks, "doing everything feasible to verify that the objectives to be attacked are neither civilians nor civilian objects subject to special protection but are military objectives." It also obligated combatants to adopt means and methods of attack with the goal of avoiding, "and in any event, minimizing incidental loss of civilian life, injury to civilians and damage to civilian objects." Embracing the principle of proportionality, it stated that combatants must "refrain from deciding to launch any attack which may be expected to cause incidental loss of civilian life, injury to civilians, damage to civilian objects, or a combination thereof, which would be excessive in relation to the concrete and direct military advantage anticipated." Even when all these restrictions are met, it provided that, if during an operation the attacker determines that the conditions cannot be met, it must be suspended.[113] Although ambiguities remained in determining what constitutes a military advantage and how proportionality is measured, these provisions of Protocol 1 represented a sea change in the law of war, finally enabling the law's protection of health care, and civilians generally, to catch up with the long-established means of warfare.

Protocol 1 did more than that, devoting twenty-four articles to the protection of medical care. It expanded the definition of individuals protected, now including all civilians in need of medical assistance or care, such as newborns and those suffering from a mental disorder. All must be respected, protected, and treated without distinction, regardless of affiliation, ethnicity, religion, or other factors, unless they take direct part in hostilities. The same applied to health facilities, now defined to include all facilities organized for medical purposes including the prevention of disease. Civilian ambulances and other medical transports became protected as well. It vastly expanded protections for health workers, too. Building on the 1864 and 1949 conventions, it authorized local aid groups, such as the Red Cross and Red Crescent societies, to collect and care for the wounded and sick and admonished that "no one shall be harmed, prosecuted, convicted or punished for such humanitarian acts" (Article 17).

In an even more remarkable innovation, Protocol 1 prohibited punishment of anyone for having engaged in any medical activities compatible with medical ethics or to compel the person to engage in acts that violate medical ethics (Article 16). That means that a belligerent may not punish any health worker, in whatever setting of practice, who provides ethically mandated, impartial, and professionally appropriate care to someone it deems an enemy, spy, terrorist, or subversive.[114] Protocol 1 also contained additional and very broad provisions relating to public health. It did not allow military forces to attack objects indispensable to the survival of the civilian population including food, crops, livestock, and agricultural supplies, and waterworks, no matter what the motive. Nor were they permitted to use methods of warfare that could be expected to harm the natural environment in a way that would undermine the health or survival of the population.

By the time these changes were discussed, changing norms about conduct in war meant that they were relatively uncontroversial. By contrast, the proposals to expand the protections of the Geneva Conventions to civil wars caused furious and acrimonious debate, as they were characterized on one side as protecting freedom fighters in wars of national liberation, and on the other side as encouraging and coddling terrorists. In a reprise of the vexing questions General Halleck brought to Francis Lieber, there were debates over whether insurgents should be given prisoner of war status rather than treated as criminals, what uniforms and command structures were prerequisites for protection, and whether conflicts short of war should be included. These disputes threatened to derail the negotiations. In the end, the governments reached a compromise, adopting a second, more abbreviated Protocol for what the treaty called noninternational armed conflicts. Protocol 2 omitted the principles of distinction and proportionality, but the norms of conduct in war have changed so dramatically that today the two principles are accepted as customary law, thus applying to civil wars. Protocol 2 also excluded application to civil disturbances and violence short of war and was far less expansive on the protection of the wounded and the sick, and health services than Protocol 1. Still, Protocol 2's medical provisions included the most critical protections: that the wounded and the sick must be protected and respected, treated humanely, and receive medical care, "to the fullest extent practicable and with least possible delay" and without distinction on any but medical grounds.[115] It permitted the civilian population to offer to collect and care for the wounded and sick and contained a requirement like that of Protocol 1 prohibiting punishment of a health worker for acting in conformity with medical ethics.

The Protocols had limits. They contained no accountability or enforcement mechanisms, only a procedure that permitted governments to agree to reviews of their conduct by an independent commission, whose findings would not be public. No reports by combatants were required, nor any mechanisms for review of conduct in war. Protocol 1 was ratified by 174 countries and Protocol 2 by 160. A number of countries with sizable militaries, including the United States, India, Iran, Iraq, Israel, Pakistan, and Turkey did not, mostly because of the constraints it imposed on fighting an insurgency (the U.S. also declined to ratify Protocol 1, on other grounds). Despite these dissenters, many of the Protocols' provisions, including principles of distinction and proportionality, were soon recognized globally as customary law binding to all parties in internal conflicts. Organized armed groups under a command that is responsible for the conduct of subordinates are also bound under customary international law. In the U.S., the two principles, along with many other provisions of the Protocols, were incorporated in the Pentagon's Law of War Manual, jettisoning Hays Parks's expansive view of allowable harm to civilians. Disagreement exists whether both Protocols' prohibition on punishment of health workers for acting in accord with their ethical obligations constitutes customary law. The International Committee of the Red Cross takes the position that they are.[116] Some scholars argue otherwise.[117] The Pentagon's *Law of War Manual* makes no reference to any such duty, though it does not explicitly reject it. Notably, though, in 2016, the U.S. cosponsored a UN Security Council resolution that affirmed a norm against punishing health workers for engaging in ethically required medical duties.[118]

The two Protocols expanded protection for the wounded and sick, addressing more questions than Dunant considered or even imagined. They resolved the law on three of the major vulnerabilities health workers and facilities face in contemporary war: indiscriminate and disproportionate attacks that destroy hospitals, violence inflicted on health care in civil wars, and punishment for treating enemies in accordance with their ethical obligations. Some gaps remain, though these are minor compared to vastly strengthened protections for health care in the most fraught circumstances of modern war. Humanity gained a stronger foothold in the laws of war protecting the wounded and sick.

## DIGNITY AND RIGHTS: THE TRIUMPH OF DUNANT?

The elegant Palais de Nations sits on a hill in Geneva with a stunning view of Lake Geneva. Built in the 1930s as the home to the League of Nations, at the time it was the largest building in Europe besides the Versailles Palace. Every May, in the gorgeous spring weather, almost 200 Ministers of Health and other officials gather there as the World Health Assembly, the governing body of the World Health Organization. In May 2011, I went there to lobby the leadership on behalf of sixteen medical, human rights, and humanitarian groups, urging the WHO to become more actively engaged in ending violence against hospitals and health workers in conflicts throughout the world. The timing of launching the initiative turned out to be fortuitous. The Arab Spring prodemocracy protests that had begun in Tunisia in December 2010 had just reached the tiny Persian Gulf kingdom of Bahrain. Protesters there called for a new constitution to protect political freedoms and end discrimination against the majority Shi'a population.

At first the government made a few concessions to the demonstrators. But as protests continued, it imposed a state of emergency, brought in troops from Saudi Arabia and Gulf States to enforce it, and used lethal force, including high-velocity weapons and shotguns, killing some protestors and injuring hundreds of others. The authorities arrested thousands of people, some held in incommunicado detention, and tortured many of them. Security forces denied passage of ambulances seeking to reach people who had been shot and physically assaulted doctors, nurses, and emergency responders seeking to attend to the wounded. The country's main hospital, the Salmaniya medical complex, became both a security zone and a site of protests as wounded demonstrators arrived. Security forces arrested and tortured patients inside the hospital.[119] As in protests in Egypt and Syria, doctors participated in the protests while also providing medical care for the injured. Security forces responded by interrogating and arresting dozens of doctors and nurses, including the head of the Bahrain Medical Society. The charges against them ranged from refusing to come to the aid of a person in need to unauthorized possession of weapons to seeking to overthrow the government.[120] While in detention, many of the doctors and nurses were tortured and forced to sign false confessions. The government suspended more than one hundred health workers from their jobs.

International condemnation of the crackdown led the government of Bahrain to transfer the prosecution of doctors and nurses arrested from military to civil courts. The Bahrain Medical Society spoke out against the government's suppression of peaceful protests and violent interference in medical workers' duties to provide emergency care. The group called for the removal of the Health Minister.[121] To no avail: most of those who were tried were convicted, and sentences were harsh. One of the doctors, Dr. Ali al-Ekri, a pediatric orthopedic surgeon, was arrested at the Salmaniya Medical Complex on March 17, 2011, while in the operating room after treating wounded protestors. He was tortured into signing a false confession and the court disallowed the evidence of coercion used to obtain it. He was convicted of weapons possession and sentenced to 15 years in prison. In 2013, twenty-one of the convictions of the doctors and nurses were reversed on appeal.[122] But Dr. al-Ekri served five years in prison.[123]

Even before the convictions on trumped-up charges, the upheaval disconcerted WHO's director general, Dr. Margaret Chan. In her opening speech to the World Health Assembly, she directly alluded to and condemned the assaults.[124] Under pressure, Bahrain's acting Minister of Health, Dr. Fatima Al Balooshi, held a press conference during the Assembly to defend the government's conduct, but her remarks reflected the obtuseness as well as the brutality of the government as she accused the doctors and nurses of criminal acts.[125] Neither Dr. Chan nor the delegates to the Assembly particularly cared that the Geneva Conventions did not apply to the political violence in Bahrain, as it was not at war. The distinction between political and armed conflict was irrelevant to the underlying wrongs, that injured people were denied care because they were political adversaries, and that providers of care were punished for offering it.

If the Geneva Conventions did not apply, international human rights law did. Human rights treaties impose obligations on governments toward all people in their territory, prohibiting the arbitrary arrests, denial of the rights to due process, free speech, and assembly, and torture in detention inflicted by Bahrain. But for those engaged in efforts to protect human rights, some questions arose: Did international human rights law prevent Bahrain from denying medical care to people it claimed were trying to overthrow the government? Did it forbid arresting doctors and nurses for providing treatment to them? If so, did the Bahrain doctors and nurses who engaged in political activities forfeit their rights? The same questions arose in Arab Spring protests elsewhere. In Cairo, police and military forces assaulted doctors who had set up field hospitals in Tahrir Square, the epicenter of the protests. Military personnel destroyed some of the field hospitals and took supplies from others. Some doctors were arrested.[126] As in Bahrain, many of the doctors active in the emergency medical response were themselves committed to revolution.[127]

The answers to these questions derive from the history, values, and concerns of international human rights law. The 1949 Geneva Conventions were but one of a flurry of responses to World War II atrocities and their aftermath. The year before, the newly formed United Nations adopted a Convention on the Prevention and Punishment of the Crime of Genocide. To address the needs of millions of displaced people in Europe, in 1951 it agreed to a Convention on the Status of Refugees. And in a development that was to shape values, policy, and international law for decades to come, the United Nations established a Human Rights Commission, chaired by Eleanor Roosevelt. It was tasked with drafting a declaration of universal human rights. Latin Americans and others from less developed countries provided much of the intellectual heft in conceptualizing human rights.[128] Roosevelt drove it through politically. She had championed civil rights in the United States for decades and possessed the moral stature and political skills necessary for guiding a contentious process forward—one further complicated by escalating Cold War tensions.[129] After a tortuous drafting process, the statement ultimately became the Universal Declaration of Human Rights, which envisioned a world where everyone's human dignity is respected as "the foundation of freedom, justice and peace in the world."[130]

Coming just after a war in which respect for human life was largely extinguished and the notion of rights might have seemed a cruel joke, the declaration was at once a statement of values, an aspiration to realize them, and a thinly disguised political manifesto. Its values went far beyond the relief of human suffering in war on which the Geneva Conventions were founded. Its ambition was to promote, as it stated in the preamble, "the inherent dignity and equal and inalienable rights of all members of the human family." It was an act of defiance as well. The rights it asserted were adopted in the face of the worst wrongs security forces could commit, a time when cynicism about respect for human dignity would have been understandable. Instead, it not only stood as a stirring rejection of the thinking that brought the atrocities, but asserted values that were inimical to the deeply entrenched practices of some of its own leading signatories. The declaration demanded no discrimination based on race at a time when the United States was racially segregated by law. It called for democracy and self-determination when European powers would not consider autonomy or independence for their colonies in Africa and Asia. It urged political freedom when the Soviet Union was a vicious totalitarian regime. In retrospect, it seems miraculous that the declaration was adopted at all.

The declaration proceeded from the belief that advancing human dignity requires both protection of political freedom and affirmative steps to achieve economic and social security. It recognized both traditional political and civil rights, but also social and economic rights, such as to health, food, work, and housing, which the declaration called "indispensable" to human dignity. The declaration was not binding on anyone, but over time, the rights it recognized were incorporated into international human rights treaties that established legal obligations on governments to respect rights, to protect rights from interference by third parties, and to fulfill rights by positive, concerted action. The rights to health and life established by these treaties filled gaps left open by revisions to the Geneva Conventions by applying them to political violence short of war, and by setting out governments' obligations to ensure availability of access to health care in all circumstances.

The right to life contained in the declaration and, later, the International Covenant on Civil and Political Rights, includes a responsibility on governments not to arbitrarily or discriminatorily deny or obstruct life-saving care for injuries people suffer. Governments are obligated not only to refrain from taking away life, but to ensure access to and protect health care, while also taking steps to establish conditions necessary to sustain them.[131] The right to health—more formally, the right to the highest attainable standard of physical and mental health—is contained in the International Covenant on Economic, Social, and Cultural Rights. We tend to think of the right to health as a right to health care that imposes affirmative obligations on governments to provide services, such as vaccinating children, establishing primary health care systems, conducting disease surveillance, and ensuring access to health care. But it also requires governments to *respect* health care, that is, not to interfere with or obstruct the enjoyment of the right, such as through policies or practices of discrimination or by denying or interfering with care for the wounded and sick.

Both rights apply during times of internal upheaval arising out of political crises and violent insurgencies.[132] Governments may not deny health care as a punitive or discriminatory measure. Government security forces and law enforcement agencies may not attack the wounded and sick, nor health workers. They must respect medical ethics and refrain from punishing health workers for providing care no matter who the recipient of care is.[133] National security cannot be invoked to limit the right to health unless the government meets a very heavy burden to show that the restriction is consistent with law (including international human rights standards), serves legitimate aims, is necessary for the promotion of general welfare in a democratic society, and is the least restrictive means of achieving its objective.[134] In a report to the UN General Assembly, Agnès Callamard, UN Special Rapporteur on Extrajudicial, Summary, or Arbitrary Executions, pithily explained the implications of the right to life for violence against health: "Saving lives is not a crime."[135] A group of other UN experts wrote that the right to health demands that "doctors must not be arrested, charged or sentenced for acting within their professional duty of ensuring medical impartiality."[136]

These developments all provided the legal scaffolding for the powerful anger stemming from the prosecution of doctors and nurses in Bahrain for doing their medical duties. Under severe international pressure, Bahrain's government created an Independent Commission of Inquiry to examine human rights violations during the protests. It devoted considerable energy to reviewing the medical dimensions of government conduct. It found some cases where doctors discriminated against Sunni patients, or permitted their political activities to interfere with their medical duties, either of which might warrant professional discipline.[137] But these were minor concerns compared to the commission's finding that security services violated human rights law by arresting patients because they had been injured in demonstrations, attacking medical staff members attending to the wounded, and mistreating patients and health workers at the hospital.[138]

The emergence of human rights concepts and law also profoundly influenced the law of war. The relationship between human rights law and the Geneva Conventions can be complicated, as some of the obligations in the two bodies of law conflict with one another. An obvious example is that under the law of war, a soldier is entitled to kill an enemy soldier in battle, an act that in peacetime would be considered a violation against the prohibition against extrajudicial execution. In cases like that, the Geneva Conventions govern because it more specifically addresses the conduct. In most cases, though, both sources of law apply and complement one another.[139] Each branch of law adds dimensions to the protections and rights of civilians in armed conflict. For example, the right to health requires governments engaged in armed conflict to expend resources and take measures to safeguard health institutions, ensuring that health care remains available and accessible to the population.[140] Governments' duties also include efforts to reach vulnerable people.[141] They must also address the frequent indirect consequences of war on health, such as increases in infectious diseases and rising child mortality.[142] Special measures may be needed to address obstacles to access to care because of insecurity.[143] In internal conflicts, human rights law rather than the Geneva Conventions is often relied upon in accountability proceedings against governments. For example, the European Court of Human Rights issued judgments on Russian responsibility for harming civilians in Chechnya exclusively on the basis of human rights law, including the right to life.[144] Similarly, a concurring judge in the Inter-American Court of Human Rights explained that prosecuting a doctor for providing medical care to alleged terrorists would violate the right to life.[145]

Even more profoundly, human rights law has infused the very foundations of the Geneva Conventions. The principle of humanity that undergirds the conventions is focused on preventing and ameliorating human suffering. Human rights law is premised on a more expansive vision, the promotion of human dignity in all its forms and in all aspects of life. Its ambition is to enable all people to have opportunities and protections that enable them to develop their capacities and pursue their aspirations in an environment of personal, economic, and social security. In the past few generations, promoting human dignity has been incorporated into the conceptualization of the purposes of the Geneva Conventions.[146] This objective, expanding beyond Dunant's thinking, renders Lieber's approach to civilian protection, which paid no heed to the dignity and worth of human beings, even more problematic.[147]

Dunant would surely have been thrilled by this evolution. But he might well have been made despondent by the events following the adoption of the Additional Protocols and the incorporation of human rights ideas into the Geneva Conventions. The flouting of their requirements continued in their wake in the last quarter of the twentieth century, most notably in internal wars. For example, after ratifying both protocols in 1978, El Salvador became embroiled in a civil war marked by massacres, persistent cruelty, and the killing of between thirty and seventy thousand civilians, the vast majority of them by government security forces.[148] The Reagan administration, seeking to stop what it saw as a Communist insurgency, supplied the government with more than $4 billion in aid, trained elite military units, and provided helicopters and other weapons.[149] It turned its back on massive human rights violations its client government committed, which brought the term "death squads" into the vocabulary of violence.

In one respect, though, El Salvador signaled a turning point. It was one of the first times independent medical human rights investigators doggedly documented and disseminated findings about atrocities against the wounded and the sick and health providers in war. Two of the participants in early investigations, Dr. Carola Eisenberg and Dr. Robert Lawrence, went on to become founders of Physicians for Human Rights, and later became my mentors. In 1983, Dr. Lawrence's team published a paper in the *New England Journal of Medicine* that departed from the dispassionate language of medical journals to recount "the systematic use of terror in ways that are hideous and frightful."[150] Doctors who protested the killing and kidnapping of patients and doctors in hospitals were themselves killed or disappeared. The risks health workers faced was brought home to the team in the worst possible way. In one hospital the team visited, they were hosted by Dr. Roberto Rivera Martelli, an obstetrician devoted to caring for the poor. Less than a month after the team left, Dr. Martelli was abducted from his clinic by armed men and was never again seen.[151] The government especially obstructed health care to rural areas where rebels were active. The need for medical help was so compelling that Dr. Charlie Clements, who later became president of Physicians for Human Rights, went to El Salvador, not to investigate but to offer care. He experienced firsthand and later wrote compellingly about the consequences of the violence to indigenous communities and his frustrating efforts to offer them health care.[152]

By 1989, a million people had fled El Salvador and hundreds of thousands of others had been displaced. Another team of medical investigators traveled to the country that year, this time affiliated with Physicians for Human Rights, which had been founded three years before. Another of PHR's founders, Dr. Jack Geiger, along with Dr. Eisenberg and other investigators worked to write one of the organization's earliest reports. The investigators found that the government of El Salvador continued, year after year, to obstruct passage of medical supplies and provision of care in rural areas, justifying their actions on the grounds that the supplies might reach rebel groups. The government impeded vaccination campaigns and, in one case, its troops attacked health clinics serving an insurgent group, killing five medical personnel and five patients.[153]

Violence against health care characterized other conflicts, too. In the last decades of the twentieth century, large scale assaults on health care took place in Bosnia, Burundi, Chechnya, Colombia, Croatia, East Timor, Kosovo, Mozambique, Nepal, Nicaragua, the occupied Palestinian territory, the Philippines, Rwanda, and Sierra Leone.[154] In Nicaragua, the Ministry of Health estimated $25 million of damage to health facilities that were destroyed or looted of equipment and supplies; at least forty-two health workers were killed.[155] The attackers clearly found military advantage in doing so, a trend that continued into the twenty-first century. Despite its rejection in the law, Lieber's idea of military necessity survived in practice, influencing and rationalizing the conduct of combatants toward health care. The concept was and remains a psychologically powerful justification for violence against health care. While unlikely to cite Lieber, they often act on his premises, that "the exigencies of war" and the "contingencies and the necessities of the fight" permit the infliction of harm on patients, health institutions, and personnel. The idea of military necessity, moreover, easily morphs into military convenience. The case studies that follow depict how Lieber's logic remains in competition with Dunant's demand for humanity, and challenges us still.

# 2

## DENYING CARE TO ENEMIES

A CENTERPIECE OF the Geneva Conventions from its inception, and reaffirmed since, is the obligation of impartiality, to provide care to the wounded and sick irrespective of their affiliation or allegiance. The obligation parallels a responsibility of health care providers that is both grounded in their ethics and deeply felt by them. Combatants, however, breach it with regularity. They find advantage in denying care to enemies or killing them in their hospital beds. This chapter looks at how the resistance to the requirement of impartial care played out in the war in Chechnya in 1999–2000, in violent incursions of government security forces into hospitals in Afghanistan, and in the denial of care to whole populations in the ethnic states of eastern Myanmar, where itinerant health workers were targeted for seeking to serve displaced and suffering people.

### THE BANDIT DOCTOR: CHECHNYA

At the end of January 2000, four thousand Chechen rebels and civilians evacuated the province's capital of Grozny after a long assault by Russian forces that left the city in rubbles. Hundreds of them were killed or wounded in the retreat, mostly from antipersonnel landmines. Three hundred survivors, many with gruesome injuries from landmines, managed to make it through deep snow to a hospital, though it had been partially destroyed by Russian rocket attacks in the town of Alkhan-Kala, outside Grozny. There, a Chechen surgeon, Dr. Khassan Baiev, whose own house in the town had been blown up in prior attacks, worked in the basement to try to save as many people as he could. Dr. Baiev operated around the clock for three days. Exhausted, he fainted twice. By the end of the third day, his hands wounded by the work, he had performed sixty-seven amputations and seven brain surgeries. In a memoir of his experience, he wrote, "I had cut through so much bone that the teeth at the center of my hacksaw blade became dull."[1]

One of Dr. Baiev's patients was Shamil Basayev, a notorious Chechen rebel commander, whose leg had been shredded by a landmine in the retreat. Dr. Baiev had known Basayev as a boy, but now the Russians had a million-dollar bounty on Basayev's head because of his long history of attacks on Russian forces. Western journalists had gotten word of Basayev's presence, and as Dr. Baiev amputated his leg, Reuters photographed the scene and a video of it appeared on Russian TV. Dr. Baiev and his colleagues knew that Russian soldiers, in search of Basayev and other Chechen fighters, would soon arrive as part of their *zachiska*, house-to-house "clean-up operations," that included roundups and often executions of young men. The wounded fighters and civilians in the hospital would be vulnerable, so Dr. Baiev and his colleagues decided that they had to remove them from the hospital.

With the permission of Bislan Gantimirov, an ethnic Chechen working as a local administrator for Russia, Dr. Baiev put some of the wounded on three buses, aiming to transfer them to a hospital in another city, Urus-Martan. Dr. Baiev traveled on one of the buses with the wounded. At a bridge, Gantimirov's men turned back the buses, refusing passage until the wounded rebels retrieved their guns from Alkhan-Kala and turned them over to the Russian troops. The buses returned to Alkhan-Kala. The *zachiska* had already started, but the men managed to retrieve the guns and Dr. Baiev brought them back to the bridge. He then realized he had been double-crossed: Russian forces had blocked the bridge with tanks to prevent people from leaving Alkhan-Kala during the *zachiska*. He still tried to secure passage across the bridge for the wounded, but was refused. While trying to negotiate for his patients, he overheard a Russian officer say, "Have you found that fucking bandit doctor yet."[2] Later that afternoon, Russian soldiers forced the buses, still carrying the wounded, to go to a "filtration camp," ostensibly to separate fighters from civilians, but known to be a detention facility where men were beaten and tortured. Meanwhile, the soldiers locked Dr. Baiev in a shipping container, where he spent a freezing night. The next morning, village women remonstrated, demanding his release. The Russians soldiers on guard, apparently unaware that he was a wanted man, let Dr. Baiev go.

Dr. Baiev returned to Alkhan-Kala, where he learned that Russians had ransacked and booby-trapped the hospital and executed seven of the patients who had remained there. He was disconsolate, telling my then-PHR colleague Doug Ford, who was investigating human rights violations, "These were my patients. I knew them; I knew their life stories, I had operated on them; this was a terrible blow to me."[3] A few days later, a Chechen who worked for the FSB, the successor to the Soviet KGB, warned Dr. Baiev to leave Chechnya immediately as the Russians were planning to arrest him. With the help of the FSB officer, he began a harrowing escape through six Russian checkpoints and made it to the city of Nazran, in the neighboring province of Ingushetia. There he met a Reuters journalist, who introduced him to Doug as well as to Peter Bouckaert from Human Rights Watch. After consulting with them, Dr. Baiev decided to hold a press conference to tell the world what was happening in Chechnya. Concerned for his safety, they also encouraged him to get out of Russia, and helped him quietly fly to Moscow. Human Rights Watch arranged a secret meeting at the U.S. embassy, which issued him a visa to come to the United States.

When I met him in Washington, Dr. Baiev still had the bearing of the gifted martial arts athlete he had been, but remained traumatized by his experience. Additionally, he had left his country and family, spoke almost no English, and was depressed that he couldn't practice medicine in the

United States. Yet he had no regrets about doing what he believed was his medical duty, to treat all in need (after he was granted asylum, his family joined him in the U.S.). There was irony, too in the Russians' targeting him. Dr. Baiev had also saved the lives of wounded Russian soldiers. Doing so almost cost him his life. Just a month before the Russians sought him out during the fighting in Alkhan-Kala, a Chechen commander, Arbi Barayev, and his men came to Dr. Baiev's hospital. They accused him of opening a hospital for Russian soldiers. Barayev's men tied up Dr. Baiev. Barayev said, "He deserves to die. He has opened a hospital for Russian soldiers," and shot his rifle at the ceiling, continuing, "he is treating our enemies."[4] The men held a mock Sharia court and Barayev's men called for his execution. In his defense, Dr. Baiev protested that his hospital served the community and treated many Chechen fighters as well as Russian soldiers and had even evacuated a large group of Chechens to save them from Russian forces. He said he lived by the Koran, was dedicated to helping the needy, and that he had even treated Barayev himself when he had been injured early in the war.

In the midst of this confrontation, an explosive went off, wounding two Russians and four of Barayev's men. The latter ordered Dr. Baiev to attend to the injured rebels first, but he insisted on treating the Russians, who needed more urgent care. "Don't touch those pigs," one of Barayev's men shouted, and fired again at the ceiling. "I'll shoot you." Dr. Baiev wrote that he responded, "In this hospital I give the orders."[5] The men backed off. Dr. Baiev toiled to save the victims' lives for thirty-six straight hours, during which an intense Russian artillery barrage blew out the door frame and a window of the hospital. When Dr. Baiev finally left the hospital, he saw much of the town on fire. As he walked home, Russian contract soldiers, known for their indiscipline and brutality, stopped him, accusing him of treating Chechen rebels. They kicked and punched him, then threatened to shoot him. They ultimately decided to use him as a human shield as they walked through the town, but after women in the town furiously screamed at the soldiers, they let him go.

The enmity between Chechens and Russia has a long and tragic history. Chechnya is more than a thousand miles south and a world away from

Moscow in the North Caucasus region. Ethnic Chechens are largely Muslim and for centuries have been considered hostile by the Russian government. During the Second World War, suspicious of Chechens' loyalty, Stalin deported a half million of them deep into the Soviet Union. More than a hundred thousand Chechens died during the forced removal, or shortly thereafter. Many of the survivors were sent to labor camps. Not until the late 1950s were they and their descendants permitted to return to their province, where many found their farms ruined and their homes occupied by strangers. After the fall of the Soviet Union, a violent Chechen separatist movement grew, leading to two wars with Russia in the 1990s. The second war, launched by President Vladimir Putin in 1999, pitted Chechen rebel forces against ill-trained and indifferently commanded recruits and contract soldiers in the Russian army. The conflict was bitter and ruthless, characterized by torture, disappearances, and attacks on medical facilities and the wounded and the sick.[6] It was too dangerous for humanitarian workers to offer aid in Chechnya, as they risked murder and kidnapping for ransom. Respect for the obligations not to interfere with health care for wounded enemies and not to punish health workers was entirely absent.

At the end of 2000, Dr. Baiev's application for asylum in the United States was granted. Around the same time, I traveled with a Czech physician and humanitarian, Ondrej Mach, to the region to continue PHR's investigations of ongoing human rights violations in Chechnya. The danger of kidnapping made it highly risky to go into Chechnya, so we interviewed displaced persons in camps in the neighboring Russian province of Ingushetia, where as a safeguard against abduction we were accompanied by a guard carrying an AK-47. Gas pipes crisscrossed the pathways in the camp to keep the endless rows of tents warm. It seemed like an explosion waiting to happen, but the residents had more pressing issues on their minds: disappeared sons, brothers, and fathers. Interviews with young men apparently arrested for the "crime" of being of military age revealed that many were forced down into large open pits, living on floors that were alternatively frozen or full of sludge. Families sometimes went back into Chechnya to search for their sons and look for the right Russian soldier to bribe to obtain their release.

We also heard stories about the widespread destruction of health facilities and received photos of hospitals that had been severely damaged or destroyed by Russian bombing. Physicians told us about the pressure not to treat wounded Chechen fighters and described the arrest of two doctors interrogated and later arrested while working in a hospital. But we also heard that despite the dangers, these doctors, like Dr. Baiev, were committed to treat all patients. Standing up in the face of demands not to treat fighters' enemies was dangerous, but as I have heard from health workers in conflicts all over the world, not that unusual. They embraced the idea of medical impartiality—treating patients based on need, without consideration of nationality, religion, or political or military allegiance. That commitment has become deeply engrained both in the ethos and ethical codes of the medical professions and in law.

The Geneva Conventions have long imposed a duty on combatant forces to provide care for the wounded and sick impartially, but the medical duty of impartiality in accepting individuals as patients is of more recent vintage. In the United States, for example, the organized medical community long resisted any requirement of impartiality in decisions on who to treat to avoid having to take on African American patients. The American Medical Association instead elevated the idea of physician autonomy in its ethical principles, including being "free to choose whom to serve."[7] During the civil rights upheavals of the 1960s, it lobbied heavily against federal enforcement of antidiscrimination law in the context of patient selection.[8] Eventually, the AMA bowed to social and legal pressure. Its ethical principles still assert that "physicians are not ethically bound to accept all prospective patients," but say they may not discriminate on the basis of factors "that are not clinically relevant to the individual's care."[9] International organizations of physicians and nurses have adopted even more express prohibitions on discrimination in patient selection, including those based on political or military affiliation in armed conflicts and situations of political violence. The World Medical Association, founded after World War II to set global ethical standards in the aftermath of Nazi perversion of medicine, and of which the AMA is a member, declared that medical ethics in war, including the duty of impartiality, are the same as medical ethics in peacetime. It required that physicians accept patients without consideration of sex, race, nationality, religion, political affiliation, or any other similar criterion. It later was explicit in stating that an enemy is entitled to equal care.[10] The International Council of Nurses similarly required nurses "to respect human rights," and not to restrict their services based on consideration of factors such as race, gender, sexual orientation, or politics.[11]

This view is now broadly accepted in the health professions, illustrated in a symposium conducted by the American Journal of Bioethics. The editors asked Israeli, American, and British bioethicists to consider two cases concerning physicians' duties to treat the most unsympathetic of all patients in Israel, Palestinian terrorists. The first case involved a twenty-five-year-old Palestinian leader of Hamas who directed suicide bombings that had killed forty-six Israelis and injured more than a hundred. In a battle with Israeli soldiers, they shot him in the abdomen. He received emergency care in a Palestinian hospital, but in critical condition, he was transferred to Hadassah Hospital in Israel. He remained in the intensive care unit for twenty days, and was then discharged and put on trial. He was sentenced to life imprisonment. The second case involved another Palestinian, wounded during the siege of a church in which his group took hostages. His comrades initially prevented him from leaving the church, but after twelve days, and in septic shock, he was also brought to Hadassah Hospital. He remained for a year while undergoing numerous operations to deal with complications (some a result of delays by Palestinians in getting him to treatment), at a cost of more than $350,000. During his hospital stay, he sometimes was housed in the same ward as Israelis injured in terrorist attacks and often received priority in treatment because of his severe medical condition. All but one of the commentaries argued that the physicians have an ethical duty to treat the wounded Palestinians, including during the second man's year-long hospital stay.

As Chiara Lepora and colleagues explained, "medical role morality" includes impartiality as well as the duty to maintain health and prevent diseases, disability, or death for all patients.[12] The principles of humanity and justice are also germane, as Benjamin Gesundheit and colleagues, who posed the questions to other scholars, noted that many Israeli doctors are children or grandchildren of survivors of the Holocaust. They wrote, "We make a point of valuing every human life, and, above all, of not discriminating in any manner—treating everyone who comes through our doors."[13] All but one scholar rejected the claim that the moral worth of individuals could be taken into account in determining entitlement to care, as justice does not permit them to make such judgments. Michael Davis explained, "The question [of moral worth] assumes that the right to medical care can be forfeited by acts done before coming under a physician's care. The assumption seems wholly foreign to how the principle of justice operates in a medical context." He warned that "dehumanizing one's enemy is, of course, a long first step toward committing atrocities."[14] The only partial dissenter in the group, Ari Zivotofsky, cited the Jewish sage Maimonides for the view that "compassion to the wicked is cruelty to all human beings."[15] His view, however, only extended to defending a government's decision to decline its resources to pay for a year of hospitalization when its own citizens needed services, not to deny the doctors' responsibility to treat the terrorist.

Take another case. A scene of cheering spectators celebrating runners nearing the end of the Boston Marathon in 2013 turned to violence and panic as bombs contained in the backpacks of two terrorists suddenly exploded. When the police tracked down the two brothers responsible for the attacks, the police killed the elder one and wounded the younger one, Dzhokhar Tsarnaev. He was brought to Beth Israel Deaconess Medical Center in Boston and put in the care of Doctor Stephen Odom, the surgeon on call. Journalists asked Dr. Odom how he felt about saving the life of a man who had committed such a horrific act. "What would the alternative be?" he replied. "Even people who are incarcerated for terrible stuff still get care. It's just what we do."[16]

The papers in the bioethics journal and the Tsarnaev example differ in one respect from Khassan Baiev's surgery on Shamil Basayev. In Israel and Boston, the alleged perpetrators of the crimes were in custody, and indeed were eventually tried and sentenced for their crimes. Notwithstanding the recognized duty of impartiality in patient selection, treating them may have triggered strong emotions or even personal moral qualms. The doctors and nurses did not, however, have to consider the possibility that, after treatment, a person who committed horrific acts would be back on the street, with a new opportunity to kill or maim Israelis or Americans. By contrast, after lifesaving treatment, Basayev might, and indeed later did, resume his command and orchestrate attacks on Russia. The original Geneva Conventions of 1864 partially addressed this concern by requiring that enemies who have been treated and released be sent home with a commitment not to fight again. That idea proved unworkable, though.[17] As a result, in 1906, revisions to the convention provided three options: to imprison the soldier, ask a neutral third state to do so, or return the soldier home. Aside from the awkwardness of trying to implement these rules, they did not address circumstances where wounded soldiers were treated by civilians—as permitted by the convention—and outside of the control of military forces. From the beginning, moreover, two rules remained constant: first, care to a wounded fighter may only be denied if the individual engages in an "act of hostility," such as continuing to shoot; second, the civilian providing care, like Dr. Baiev, cannot be punished for providing ethically mandated treatment, no matter what the prospects for future violence by the wounded soldier once recovered.[18] They are treaters and healers, not judges and prognosticators.

The rules forbidding interference in care or punishment of caregivers for treating a fighter not in custody often seem counterintuitive, militarily troubling, and psychologically difficult for some commanders and soldiers. The possibility of the enemy patient getting back into the fight is one of the reasons soldiers, whether part of state armed forces or armed groups, find it rational and justifiable to kill enemies in hospitals and to punish health workers whose work might have the effect of facilitating an enemy's return. In their view, allowing treatment of wounded enemies could put their own forces at greater risk. When the Russians confronted Dr. Baiev about treating Basayev, they may have had reason for concern that if and when Basayev recovered from his injury, he would resume command and launch attacks on their forces and installations. Why, then, should they permit him to be treated? And why should they allow a doctor to be the means by which he could return to the fight? The logic resembles Lieber's notion of military necessity that takes into account war's "exigencies" and "contingencies," not Dunant's concept of humanity. Bioethicist Michael Gross adds a gloss to this logic, arguing that health workers have two distinct moral duties, one to people in need of care and another to their own nation, especially when treating an individual who might commit acts of violence once recovered. When they conflict, he writes, a responsibility to nation—military necessity—can prevail.[19]

While his argument has surface appeal, it turns out to be very problematic. It puts the health professional in the untenable position of making judgments about the person's acts, culpability, and future conduct. From a practical standpoint, the doctor lacks competence to judge the military situation, and in any event would have to make decisions without full knowledge of the facts.[20] Moreover, it would mean a fundamental departure from the health professional's role. As one MSF doctor said about judgments about the acts and likely future conduct of a wounded person: "That is for police, not doctors." Gross's position is also boundless, permitting the principle of humanity and the duty of impartiality in care to be suspended whenever a wounded or sick soldier is not in custody, thus allowing men and women deemed enemies to die based on mere speculation about their possible future hostile acts.

That position is, finally, contrary to both the rules of war and traditions persisting for over a century and a half. The many iterations of the Geneva Conventions recognized Gross's concern but accepted the primacy of humanity over worries about future actions of a recovered fighter. The 1864 convention extended immunity of civilian doctors from attack and punishment, regardless of who they treated. The commentaries to the first 1949 convention emphasize that the absence of exceptions to the principle of humanity is based on a conscious choice by governments. They state: "It should be made clear to everyone that, in adhering to the Geneva Convention, the States have agreed to sacrifice national interests to the dictates of conscience, and that the Convention, by the predominance of which it gives to humanitarian sentiments, is a breach in the barrier of hostilities between nations and their enemies."[21] As noted in chapter 1, the choice of "predominance of humanitarian sentiments" regarding medical care in conflict has strengthened over time, particularly expressed in the protocols' prohibiting punishment for acts consistent with medical ethics. So, it remains that civilians providing the care, like Dr. Baiev, cannot be punished for offering treatment, no matter what the likely actions of the wounded soldier once recovered.

The conventions, however, offer government security forces the means to learn if an enemy is receiving care from a civilian health worker. The 1977 protocols allow governments to enact laws to require health workers to breach medical confidentiality and report the identity of patients suffering injuries from violence, such as gunshot wounds. Such laws are common in civilian life around the world.[22] In wartime, these provisions can compromise the purposes of the Geneva Conventions in discouraging the wounded and the sick, especially combatants from armed groups, from seeking care for injuries because of the risk of being reported to authorities and arrested.[23] The laws also raise the stakes for civilian health workers forced to disgorge the names of their patients to security forces, which poses both ethical quandaries and risks of retaliation. As a result, the commentaries to the protocols urge states not to use their authority to compromise fundamental principles of medical ethics.[24] Others have proposed invoking human rights law, which requires governments to respect medical ethics without exception, to avoid caregivers having to share information on their patients.[25] Both approaches seem unlikely to be adopted. With the legal authority to pursue their enemies in health facilities, the practice has become common in conflicts throughout the world, leading not only to compelled reporting of names of patients, but to violence inside hospitals, as discussed in the next section. To avoid the harms stemming from sharing patient information, military commanders and political leaders must commit to respecting medical ethics and patient privacy during hospital search operations.[26] They should issue operational instructions, provide training, and inflict discipline to ensure that health care can be offered safely to the patient and without risk to the provider.

Russia had long affirmed commitment to the Geneva Conventions, but it invented reasons why they didn't apply to that conflict, and its conduct demonstrated contempt for them.[27] Without the inculcation of the values and law in training and expectations of accountability of leaders and troops, external pressure must be brought to bear. There were attempts, particularly through cases brought to the European Court of Human Rights. Because Russia was a party to the European Convention on Human Rights, Chechens brought hundreds of cases concerning disappearances and other atrocities before the court, and it issued more than a hundred judgments against Russia. The government, however, ignored them and showed not the slightest interest in holding its soldiers to account for crimes they committed. It prosecuted no one. There was little domestic pressure on the government to refrain from brutality, as President Vladimir Putin manipulated media coverage of the atrocities and marginalized NGOs reporting on Chechnya.[28] Russia refused to abide by the court's judgments to provide compensation to victims, make policy changes, and ensure accountability for perpetrators.[29]

Diplomatic pressure on Russia was tepid. The Clinton Administration's priority in engaging with Russia was to promote market-based democracy and reduce its stockpile of nuclear weapons. This led it to pull punches about Russia's conduct. The then-secretary of state, Madeleine Albright, was quoted at the time as saying, "the last thing we should be doing is trying to turn Russia into an enemy."[30] In a hearing before Congress in April 2000, Senator Patrick Leahy asked Deputy Secretary of State Strobe Talbott whether Russia's atrocities amounted to war crimes.[31] Talbott declined to answer.[32]

While living in the United States, Khassan Baiev received a scholarship with Operation Smile, an organization that sends surgeons around the world to repair cleft palates. He traveled to Colombia, Vietnam, Japan, and Russia. In 2010, he returned to live in his own house in Alkhan-Kala, and I spoke to him again as I was writing this book. He still felt an obligation to provide surgical care to the many Chechens suffering from traumatic injuries as well as to children with birth defects. In the twenty years since the war, 90 percent of the hospitals that had been destroyed in the war were rebuilt. The bigger problem was that doctors had left for Europe and hadn't returned. "People don't talk about the war," Dr. Baiev also told me. "They say that time heals all wounds but there is still a scar. I keep busy in medicine, leaving no time to think."

## THE PERILS OF IMPARTIAL
## HOSPITALS: AFGHANISTAN

When I visited Afghanistan in 2016, the blast walls that hid embassies and government buildings, the military vehicles on the streets, and the armed checkpoints were a constant reminder of the terrorist threat. They contrasted starkly with Kabul's noisy, crowded, and chaotic street life. I was there to attend a two-day meeting on improving protection of health programs from violence and disruption. In an earlier trip there, I stayed in a hotel that was barricaded from the street, but this time my hosts thought I would be safer in an NGO compound. Rather than hiding behind fortifications, the NGO's strategy was the opposite. The compound blended into a local street, with only sleepy guards out front. Upon arrival, though, I was given not-very-reassuring instructions on what to do in case of an armed attack. It consisted of getting to a safe room in a dark basement as quickly as possible, barricading myself in, and coming out when the shooting stopped.

For health-care providers, the dangers were far greater. They had to contend not just with demands of armed groups but with violent incursions by Afghan security forces. Their vulnerability was in some ways paradoxical, as Afghanistan's Ministry of Public Health, with support from international donors, had vastly expanded access to primary care for rural Afghans, who suffer some of the highest rates of disease and premature death in the world. Though not without setbacks, the government was justly proud of reducing death of women in childbirth and young children.[33] Too often, though, security forces' violent intrusions into and forced closures of hospitals and clinics imperiled care. Yet another paradox: as in many countries in conflict, the ministry's policy was to care for all, civilians and combatants alike, in areas controlled by the government

or by the Taliban.[34] The policy was not just based on public health principles but security strategy. The executive director of a health services organization (who asked that neither he nor his organization be named for
security reasons) told me that impartiality in patient care was the organization's only means to remain in business and keep patients and staff safe.
Patients were never asked about their affiliations or beliefs. However, this
very commitment to impartiality sometimes puts the facilities, staff, and
patients at risk from government military forces.

At dinner one night in Kabul during my 2016 visit, the country director
of the Swedish Committee for Afghanistan told me about an attack earlier
that year at its clinic in Wardak province, not far from Kabul, but an area
largely controlled by the Taliban. As helicopters hovered over the facility,
elite Afghan security personnel accompanied by international forces
stormed into one of the committee's clinics in the middle of the night.
They removed two injured patients and a young boy accompanying one of
the patients. During the attack the soldiers kicked in doors and beat and
handcuffed the entire staff, including a midwife and an ambulance driver.
The hospital director later said, "They were yelling at us, 'You are serving
the Taliban.'" The security forces killed the three people removed from the
hospital, including the boy. In defending the action, a spokesman for Wardak province's police chief was unapologetic, saying "Those killed in the
hospital were all terrorists."[35] Not surprisingly, after the raid, the number
of patients who came to the clinic declined. The Swedish Committee
demanded an investigation and accountability.

Three years later, in July 2019, I called Khalid Fahim, the program
director for the Swedish Committee of Afghanistan in Kabul, to find out
if there had been any government investigation of the incident or any further violence. He explained that the government had never furnished his
organization with an investigative report of the Wardak attack, but that
no further attacks by Afghan military forces had taken place in the province. Just a few days after our call, though, special forces of the Afghan
National Directorate of Security, part of the government's intelligence
apparatus, again attacked a Swedish Committee for Afghanistan hospital
in Wardak. Commando units arrived in helicopters at night, apparently in

search of a Taliban official. Before they entered, they shot and killed a man accompanying a patient. The commandos conducted a room-by-room search looking for the Taliban official. They removed a guard and a lab technician and fatally shot both.[36] The same month, again in the middle of the night, special forces arriving in helicopters invaded an NGO clinic in a part of Helmand province controlled by the Taliban. They physically attacked patients and abducted the doctor in charge of the clinic.[37] The imperiousness of security forces in Afghanistan was demonstrated, too, in another 2019 incident in the Taliban stronghold of Zabul province in southern Afghanistan. After hospital guards didn't open a gate fast enough to satisfy the Afghanistan National Police, they shot one guard and beat another. Once inside, they used small arms fire and arrested a patient on suspicion of being a Taliban member.[38]

Search of a hospital by security forces to make an arrest is lawful under the Geneva Conventions. Hospitals are not sanctuaries where individuals who make war on their governments are immune to capture. But the obligations to respect and protect the wounded and sick and health workers apply. Thus, violence, disruption of medical activities, and detention of staff are off limits.[39] Yet violence in hospital searches by Afghanistan's security forces has been a prominent feature of the war. Medical staff have been assaulted, kidnapped, arrested, or killed. Patients in medical distress may be removed, costing them their lives. Sometimes a facility has had to close for days or weeks. As word gets out about the raid, patients, fearing harassing interrogations or arrest, stop coming for the health care they need. When antigovernment armed groups learn that their comrades have been removed from the hospital, they may no longer view the hospital as impartial and attack or loot it and kidnap staff to treat their wounded elsewhere.[40] In the 2019 Wardak attack, the Taliban retaliated for the government's intrusion and killings by forcing a week-long closure of forty-four of the seventy-seven health facilities in the province. It claimed that Sweden had not done enough to prevent such attacks. More than five thousand patients a day were affected by the closures.[41]

Violent intrusions into health facilities by security forces in conflicts is common. A 2014 report by the ICRC found that armed entry to health facilities by state security forces is one of the most frequent sources of violence affecting health care in conflicts. Police or soldiers typically enter with massive force, wielding automatic weapons and engaging in a military-type action to secure the facility. Force protection doctrines, designed to minimize the vulnerability of or loss of soldiers in military operations, can also have a deleterious impact on health facility searches. One program director in Afghanistan told me the attitude of commanders on the ground is, "our lives are in danger, not yours." The soldiers intimidate and demand information from staff about patients deemed enemies and threaten the staff with violence or arrest if they do not cooperate. In some intrusions, the medical staff may itself be viewed as a threat to the security and the success of the operation. The report also found that during searches, access to portions of hospitals or the entire facility may be sealed off, preventing doctors and other medical staff from accessing patients.[42] At other times, military forces enter the health facility to kill or abuse enemies treated there.[43] Moreover, while only government forces are permitted entry, because only they have authority to search and arrest, armed groups follow their lead.

In these circumstances, medical impartiality in care becomes not an element of security but a risk to it. During the 1999 war in Kosovo, for example, Serbian police forced expulsions of some ethnic Albanian patients from hospitals, sometimes causing their deaths, jabbed their batons into the wounds of patients, and extinguished cigarettes on the backs of their hands or broke their ribs. Women in labor were denied entry to state-run obstetrical clinics.[44] In South Sudan, government soldiers entered hospitals suspicious of anyone with gunshot wounds and killed enemy fighters.[45] A health worker there told an investigator from the NGO Watchlist on Children in Armed Conflict that, during a clash, a government official demanded that hospital staff "come and treat the soldiers in the barracks." One of the rebel troops present thereupon threatened the staff that if they agreed "it would be the end of it all."[46]

Militaries generally lack operational rules to prevent harm in hospital searches, and hostile, dehumanizing attitudes toward the patients sought can come into play. Comments made by officials during and after the first Wardak attack made it clear that they believed that the hospital should not be treating enemy combatants at all. The executive director of a health program in another insecure province in Afghanistan told me that both government police and military forces say, "you are providing care for our enemies." He explained, "Anyone in power doesn't like that you serve their enemies." In 2017, he said, government armed forces closed one of his organization's health facilities for more than a year, objecting that opposition forces were being treated there.

There is an alternative approach. The ICRC has issued extensive recommendations on how to avoid harm to patients and staff in hospital searches.[47] In U.S. combat operations in Iraq and Afghanistan, in the early years of the U.S. wars there, commanders conducting searches had the option of employing aggressive "shock and speed" techniques rather than "kinder, gentler approaches."[48] Criticism of violent entries into health facilities in Afghanistan led the headquarters of the U.S. and coalition forces to issue an order in 2011 prohibiting searches of health facilities except in exceptional circumstances and even then only with approval by a two-star general. The search also had to be coordinated with the director of the facility. The order also required that, in these searches, troops refrain from use of force except in self-defense.[49] The order remains a rare exception in military practice. For example, the U.S. Army *Law of War Manual* states that it is "not prohibited to capture the wounded and sick, even if they are in the care of military medical units or facilities, or civilian hospitals," without any mention of restrictions or constraints on conduct during armed entry and search except that needed medical care must continue to be provided.[50] Even the order in Afghanistan seems not to have been applied to Afghan special forces the U.S. has trained, equipped, and supported. More broadly, militaries don't adjust search and arrest tactics to ensure compliance with obligations to patients and staff in a health facility. Military commanders need to commit to the norms of the Geneva Conventions, offer clear guidance to frontline troops on appropriately conducting searches of hospitals, and discipline the troops and commanders when there are breaches.

Outside pressure can help. In recent years, Afghan security and political leaders have been under considerable pressure to reduce civilian casualties. The UN Mission in Afghanistan publishes a detailed quarterly report on civilian casualties, which has considerable influence in Afghanistan and in international forums. The mission also engages with Afghan security officials to discuss incidents and demand competent and thorough investigations. The United States, which provides three quarters of the funding for the Afghan security forces, often uses its leverage to seek to reduce civilian casualties. NGOs have also provided advice and assistance. In 2017, President Ashraf Ghani removed hundreds of weak military leaders, replacing them with more capable and professional generals and colonels, and committed to rooting out corruption in the military.[51] The same year the government established a National Policy for Prevention and Mitigation of Civilian Casualties, which focused on thorough investigations of incidents, sharing of information, and victim compensation. NATO trained more than four hundred security officials in civilian casualty reduction. The efforts brought some progress, especially in incident investigation.

Even so, two years later, civilian casualties increased, leading the Afghan government to establish new guidance.[52] It also convened a high-level board to identify areas of improvement for civilian casualty mitigation. In response to the Wardak attack in 2019, the Swedish Committee for Afghanistan met with high-level officials of the Afghan government, including the national security advisor. Promised investigations and new guidelines and protocols for entering health facilities, however, were not forthcoming, at least publicly. At the same time, special forces from the intelligence agency, the National Directorate of Security, were operating independently of the Afghan army and largely escaped both reforms and outside pressures to abide by the law. Violent hospital searches were part of a pattern of lethal search operations by these security forces, often in conjunction with CIA paramilitaries, that began in 2015 to seek out Taliban fighters in homes and elsewhere. The program was expanded in 2017 and characterized by Secretary of State Mike Pompeo as "unforgiving, relentless."[53] In 2018, 64 search operations by Afghan security, mostly special forces, and often accompanied by CIA paramilitaries, resulted in the deaths of more than 220 people, up from 63 deaths in 26 search operations in 2017, which in turn represented an increase from 2016.[54] The trend continued in 2019, when the number killed rose to 278.[55] In the first quarter of the year, progovernment forces, 80 percent of which were Afghan security forces, were responsible for killing 72 civilians in search operations,[56] more civilian casualties than antigovernment forces.[57] For the first half of 2019, the UN found civilian casualties "shocking and unacceptable." It also determined that efforts to reduce them had been insufficient.[58]

Late in 2019 I asked a health program director in an insecure province whether the Ministry of Defense or Ministry of Public Health addressed his concerns about the conduct of Afghan troops in hospital searches. He responded, "Unfortunately the Ministry of Public Health did not help." The director explained that the ministry is "with us in principle and they raised the issue in Cabinet meetings with the Ministry of Defense and Ministry of Interior, but on the ground nothing happened." The governor of the province also supported the health program, saying "We are with you." But the commanders on the ground paid little heed, and interference with health care continued with impunity. After an attack by special forces that killed four brothers in the same family in September 2019, President Ghani accepted the resignation of the head of the country's main intelligence agency, ordered an investigation, and restricted their search operations, but the results were not released to the public.[59] The CIA and Department of Defense also declined to take any responsibility or even acknowledge the misconduct of Afghan special forces in connection with the assaults, part of a pattern of lack of accountability for CIA and Afghan special forces.[60]

The abdication of responsibility by the Ministry of Public Health and government, as well as the CIA and Pentagon, have left it to health agencies and the local community to seek to improve security in their facilities. Joanne Liu, former international president of MSF, insisted bluntly, "War stops at the door to our hospital."[61] Similarly, Markus Geisser, who ran the ICRC operation in Kandahar, Afghanistan from 2009 to 2011, told me that health providers "make all possible efforts that health facilities they supported one way or the other remain absolutely free of guns and avoid arresting people inside the facilities." He added, "I think in an ideal world a hospital is one of the best examples of humanitarian space." Many health facilities have signs on entrances that arms may not be brought inside, though there is no requirement in the Geneva Conventions that military forces abide by the rule. When MSF returned to Afghanistan in 2009 after a long hiatus, it insisted on a written memorandum of understanding with the Afghan government prohibiting weapons in health facilities.[62] The government also agreed not to conduct interrogations on patients unless they were medically fit to respond. In later agreements with MSF, the Afghan government agreed to further restrictions. For example, no military or security activities were allowed inside MSF facilities, and security forces entering must be unarmed. The agreement also required a judicial warrant under law and prior notification to the facility. Most NGOs, especially local ones, running health clinics and hospitals, though, lack the clout and influence of MSF or ICRC to demand such rules.

The burden of protecting health facilities from violent entry should not be on health providers. Until political and military leaders demand that hospitalized combatants and civilians not be dehumanized or deemed unworthy of care, and hold their troops accountable for respecting the wounded and the sick, the abuses will likely continue.


## ENEMY COMMUNITIES: MYANMAR

In June 2012, in the town of Mae Sot, Thailand, a community health worker serving remote, vulnerable ethnic communities in northern and eastern Myanmar—formerly known as Burma—told my then-Johns Hopkins colleague Katherine Footer and me, "Because we are health workers for our people, if they [the soldiers] know this they will kill us."[63] The health workers were targeted by the national army, called the Tatmadaw, in a fifty-year-long war, largely unknown in the West, in which ethnic groups in a large swath of the country sought autonomy from an oppressive central government. For the Tatmadaw, the enemy was not an individual health worker who treated a wounded adversary, but entire ethnic communities. We were there because health organizations serving these communities approached us to help improve their documentation of assaults against and threats to their health workers. As a first step, we listened to the stories of more than two dozen community health workers and learned more from organizational managers in Mae Sot and in rural mountainous areas to its south.

Mae Sot, home to sixty thousand people, sits on the Thai side of the Thai-Myanmar Friendship Bridge. Burmese influence is everywhere, most noticeably on faces painted with *thanakha*, a yellow paste on a person's cheeks and nose, often in elaborate geometric shapes, and common in Burmese culture. The outskirts of Mae Sot contain refugee camps for tens of thousands of people displaced in the armed conflict in five states on Myanmar's eastern and northern borders with Thailand and China. Right across the bridge from Mae Sot lies Myanmar's Karen state, where the Karen National Union, dating from 1948, has claimed to be a legitimate government representing three million people. Mae Sot became a hub for NGOs documenting human rights violations, providing support for prodemocracy activists, and Karen groups offering health care for refugees and conflict-affected villages in eastern Myanmar. But unlike a typical war-based international organization company town, Mae Sot lacked ubiquitous white Land Cruisers and large expatriate staffs. Since the early 2000s, Myanmar has imposed heavy restrictions on international humanitarian organizations to operate in the rebellious regions of eastern Myanmar.[64] Local organizations, including the social service arms of entities like the Karen National Union, provided primary care to ethnic populations who had been subjected to state repression and displacement. In areas controlled by opposition forces, they set up clinics.

The armed conflict dates to the origins of the modern Burmese state after World War II. The new government thwarted ethnic minorities' demands for autonomy, leading to armed conflict. In the Karen state, the Karen National Union combined a military wing, the Karen National

Liberation Army (KNLA), with a social service apparatus, the Karen Department of Health and Welfare, begun in 1956. The war has been relentless and cruel, even more so after a military coup in 1962 that ended any prospect of autonomy for the ethnic states. In 1968, the Tatmadaw began a counterinsurgency strategy called Four Cuts, designed to deny rebel groups access to food, resources, information, and recruits, in part by forcing civilian populations to leave areas where opposition armed groups might support and protect them. Civilians became the enemy. The Tatmadaw signed cease-fire agreements with some groups in the mid-1990s and launched new counterinsurgency campaigns against others, including the Karen National Union.[65]

The Karen Human Rights Group documented the dynamics of the assaults on villages. They included Tatmadaw shelling of villages from surrounding hills, entering a village and burning schools, clinics, or houses, and/or summarily executing residents who had not successfully fled. They often laid landmines or destroyed livestock as they left. At times, during night patrols, soldiers shot or detained civilians. Tatmadaw soldiers responded to fire from the KNLA by indiscriminately shelling villages, or conducting retaliatory attacks.[66] The army took people's land and subjected the local population to extortion, arbitrary arrest, forced labor, torture, sexual violence, and indiscriminate killing.[67] In so-called black zones, where there was active conflict, the Tatmadaw soldiers were permitted to shoot people on sight. Between 1996 and 2011, the year before our arrival, the Tatmadaw destroyed or forced abandonment of more than three thousand five hundred villages in the ethnic states.[68] By 2012, it had internally displaced more than four hundred thousand people in the region and more than one hundred thousand others had fled as refugees.[69] The use of population displacement as a military strategy has become all too common in war over the past half century, bringing the terrible euphemism "ethnic cleansing" into the global vocabulary, especially during the war in Bosnia in the 1990s. The International Crisis Group, which focuses on the political dimensions of conflicts, noted in 2017 that in South Sudan, "Warring parties tend to view civilians as integral elements of their enemy's economic, political and social support system." During incidents of "revenge violence," it concluded that "civilians are likely to be treated not as distinct and protected but as part of an armed group."[70]

War, human rights violations, and displacement had dire health consequences in Myanmar, which exacerbated the abdication of government responsibility for population health across the country. During the long period of military rule, wealthy members of Burmese society purchased expensive private care, while the vast majority of the population, mostly poor, was largely abandoned. Over the decade before we arrived, Myanmar allocated only between half a percent and 3 percent of its national budget to health care.[71] The military, by contrast, received a third of the budget. Myanmar ranked 190 of 191 countries in health at the turn of the twenty-first century. The government's response to lymphatic filariasis, a treatable infectious disease that causes disfigurement and disability, is illustrative. Transmission of the disease can be controlled by a drug that costs only one dollar per person per year. Myanmar's neighbor Thailand has virtually eliminated the disease, but an estimated two million people suffered from it in Myanmar in the early 2000s. Later, the government actually cut funding for preventing and treating it.[72]

Myanmar devoted even fewer resources to the contested areas in the rebellious ethnic states. Clinics in urban areas under government control were inadequately staffed and of poor quality. Midwives who traveled from village to village were only compensated for their work by fees, largely unaffordable to an impoverished population.[73] The vicious combination of poor nutrition, inadequate vaccination coverage, and scant access to health care resulted in the death of one in five children before the age of five. Human rights violations, too, took a huge toll. Forcibly displaced women in the eastern states had a far higher likelihood of anemia, lack of access to health care, and unmet needs for contraception.[74] Physical abuse by soldiers, forced labor relocation, and food destruction exacerbated the likelihood of early death, especially among women and children.

Local organizations stepped in to meet many of the people's health needs. The Karen Department of Health and Welfare operated sixty-one clinics serving almost two hundred thousand people in 2012.[75] The Mae Tao clinic, in Mae Sot, was founded by Cynthia Maung, a politically active physician, after the military government crushed a prodemocracy movement that she supported. It provided care to refugees in Thailand and soon expanded its work to provide care in eastern Myanmar.[76] She also cofounded the Burma Medical Association to support health-care services in the region. By 2012, it supported thirty-nine clinics.[77] The Four Cuts strategy, however, left many thousands of displaced people without access to these and other clinics. Dr. Cynthia, as she is known, joined with prodemocracy activists from the ethnic communities, along with medics from the Karen, Mon, and Karenni states, to start the Back Pack Health Worker Team. Its mission was to serve displaced people in insecure areas where the Karen Department of Health and Social Welfare, the Burma Medical Association, and other groups could not safely operate freestanding clinics. It worked not just in areas that were contested, labeled "brown" in Four Cuts jargon, but also in "black" zones, areas where people were forcibly relocated and the Tatmadaw were instructed to shoot on sight. Back Pack's name comes from its mission and operational strategy. To provide community-based health care to vulnerable, displaced people, its four thousand health workers walked from village to village to offer care and public health advice. The health workers, who often came from the communities they served, were trained for about six to nine months in Mae Sot and returned to work in their own villages. The local supervisors, who were given the designation of "field-in-charge," as well as some others, came to Mae Sot twice a year for additional training, and we arranged to meet them there.

For hundreds of thousands of people living in the most contested and dangerous areas, Back Pack's three-to-five-member teams became the only health-care providers.[78] The organization aspired to create a sustainable system to meet the population's needs for primary medical care, including treatment of infectious disease, war trauma injuries, and maternal and child health. Its approach was highly sophisticated. Back Pack designed its programs by carrying out public health assessments. It adopted diagnosis and treatment protocols based on international guidelines and collected data on outcomes for evaluation and health planning. Working through village authorities, it trained traditional birth attendants and offered health education programs on hygiene, water, and sanitation, including diarrhea prevention, nutrition, landmine education, HIV prevention, and family planning. Each team served a number of villages. The medics also quietly cooperated with government-trained midwives and helped villagers get to clinics in more secure areas when a team's own capacity was insufficient to meet a medical need.

Earlier in 2012, the Karen National Union and the government agreed to a cease-fire in Karen state, but the precariousness of health care in the war remained fresh in the minds of the eighteen male and nine female health workers with whom we spoke from Back Pack and other organizations. The health workers were reserved, perhaps a product of the huge gulf in our national, cultural, economic, and educational backgrounds. Speaking with a Western academic into an audio recorder may have contributed to the sense of distance. Yet the health workers seemed far from intimidated. Instead, while modest, they conveyed pride in their professionalism and ethical seriousness, commitment to their health mission, and confidence in their skills. They had long accepted the security risks in the work they did.

Despite, or more likely, because of their mission, the Tatmadaw viewed the medics as targets, just like the civilians they served.[79] The risks they faced were in part a product of their ethnic identity, their close ties to communities and, for some, a past affiliation with an armed group. Dr. Mahn Mahn, a founder and director of Back Pack, said in a radio interview the year before we arrived, "Since our health workers are from the communities we serve, when the communities undergo hardship, our workers tend to suffer as well."[80] While impartial in their work, their allegiances and those of their organization were clear. But the Tatmadaw saw any support, expressed openly or by offering services, for a rebellious population, as an illegitimate political and military act. Additionally, as one health worker told us, because their medicines were not generally available in eastern Myanmar, the Tatmadaw assumed that the medics were affiliated with military groups. A twenty-six-year-old woman from another ethnic group, the Kachin people, told us, "From my perspective, if they know we are from [health organization name redacted] they will conclude that we are supporting rebels, without thinking that we are working for people. They just think we support armed groups." This attitude also helps explain why health services were often singled out for violence. One health worker told us, "The Tatmadaw came and burned the clinic. They didn't burn the whole village, they burned only the area of the clinic." A Karen woman described a time when soldiers shot at her team leader in the midst of a 2008 attack on a village. She said that soldiers "dismantled the doors [of the clinic] and took all the medical supplies. They left nothing. They even took the Christmas tree." Another female Karen medic told us that if they set up a clinic in a village, it had to be temporary: "The security isn't good, and we can't set up our clinic permanently at a place because the enemy can come at any time, so we don't dare keep medicines in our clinic."

Between 1998 and 2011, nine medics and one traditional birth attendant were killed by the Tatmadaw or from landmine injuries.[81] Health workers told us that the Tatmadaw often subjected them and their colleagues to physical violence, threats, or confiscation of medications.[82] Much of the violence was connected to attacks on villages. One health worker told us the story of a medic who was in the midst of providing care in a village. When the Tatmadaw arrived, they killed him. To increase their security, medics tried to figure out troop movements before they approached a village. "Sometimes the Tatmadaw set up at the village in daytime, and we dare not go at that time," a Karen health worker explained. "But if there was a patient in need of care we went into the village at night, when the forces [went] back to their base."[83]

Their work is itinerant, so the medics had to worry about encountering the Tatmadaw during their travel between villages, which were sometimes a three-day hike apart. They avoided roads but even furtive walks through the forests were risky. A Karen health worker recalled a 2010 incident during which "our team leader had to cross the road one time. He suddenly met the Tatmadaw and fled. . . . The Burmese Army shot at him, but he escaped."[84] A Karen male medic said that he "stopped traveling with medicines after I was asked for money at the checkpoints." Occasionally, health workers had to avoid certain villages altogether. A Karen man, who had long experience as a medic, told us, "The blood bank could not bring blood because the Tatmadaw had positions on the way. The patient died. If they had seen me with blood it would have been difficult for me, they would have arrested and killed me."[85] In other cases, they had to take circuitous routes, losing valuable time. A male Karen medic told us, "Sometimes we take longer than usual or are not allowed to go at all because we could be put at risk. Therefore, we avoid the usual route and spend at least double the amount of time going another way." Entire programs suffered from the insecurity. "We had a malaria program, a TB program, school health, reproductive health, traditional birth attendant training, Vitamin A, D, worming, and lastly our universal provision," one medic said. "Altogether, ten programs."[86] They had to discontinue all but two until security gradually improved area by area. They had little hope of restraint from the Tatmadaw, which was well protected from pressures to obey the law (as evident again in 2021 in its attacks on doctors during 2021 protests).

Back Pack medics were not entirely without security. Village leaders shared intelligence with them, and villagers and sometimes KNLA soldiers escorted them through the forest. In our study, we found that "the collective sense of purpose and commitment by the community to ensure safe access to health care was evident across interviews and well-illustrated by one health worker: 'We all cooperate together, not only health workers, but regional community leaders, village leaders, and regionally based health care organizations.'"[87] These initiatives were part of larger strategies communities undertook to protect themselves from Tatmadaw-initiated violence, food thievery, and forced displacement. They included negotiations with local Tatmadaw commanders, managing trade-offs in their relationships with soldiers, subterfuge in revealing food production, and intelligence gathering in determining when it was essential to flee.[88] In some cases, communities resorted to the use of landmines and local armed guards.[89]

These relationships to communities, moreover, were part of the Back Pack ethos and agenda. It had an explicitly prodemocracy agenda linked to its health work and was very public about expressing its views. In its 2012 report, which coincided with a time of hope that a political transition to democracy in Myanmar was possible, it emphasized that "meaningful political negotiations to address the underlying political and socioeconomic issues driving the conflict have not yet occurred," and that a sustainable peace depended on the establishment of democracy.[90] The people they served were seeking autonomy from the central government. From Francis Lieber's point of view, they were properly labeled as enemies, and could be made to suffer for it. As his code set out, "the inoffensive individual is as little disturbed in his private relations as the commander of the hostile troops *can afford to grant in the overruling demands of a vigorous war.*"[91] The latter phrase meant "the private individual of the hostile country is destined to suffer every privation of liberty and protection, and every disruption of family ties," other than being murdered, enslaved, or carried off.[92]

There is no doubt that the Tatmadaw commanders viewed Back Pack, as well as the communities it served, as their political and, indirectly, military enemies, a view reinforced by the security the KNLA sometimes provided and the intelligence Back Pack received from sympathetic troops. Perhaps more surprisingly, some of Back Pack's international donors expressed concern about Back Pack as being too political, and not sufficiently humanitarian. They were uncomfortable with its alignment with the Karen National Union's agenda and the KNLA. Whereas Back Pack believed democracy was essential to advance population health, the donors saw its relationships and commitments as inconsistent with the neutral stance they expected of a humanitarian organization.[93] Other donors had reservations about Back Pack because its health workers operated illegally in Myanmar, despite their having no other choice as the government would not allow them official authorization to practice.

These criticisms and concerns were an expression of a larger debate within the humanitarian and donor community about the role of neutrality in aid work. Neutrality, meaning not taking a position on one side or another in the conflict, is one of four principles—the others are humanity, impartiality, and independence—initially promulgated by the International Committee of the Red Cross and then adopted by the UN as the foundation of humanitarian practice. Most aid groups express fealty to the four principles as part of their organizational ethos. A commitment to neutrality is said to demonstrate that the group cares only about relief of human suffering and meeting people's needs, and thus leaves politics aside. Its strictly neutral stance is a major reason why the ICRC only rarely openly criticizes a belligerent for violations of human rights or humanitarian law, or releases information it has about those violations. In its view, doing so is a political act. Instead, the ICRC tends to condemn violations of international humanitarian law generally, without specifying the perpetrator, and to call on all parties to abide by their obligations. That stance is controversial because it demands public silence in the face of atrocities, but it remains a means to enable the organization to gain the trust of all belligerents and engage in confidential dialogue with them toward access to populations in need and increased compliance with the law.

For Back Pack and for indigenous health workers in conflicts throughout the world, the debate over whether they should embrace neutrality is beside the point. They are committed to impartiality in care and humanity toward all, but neither of these values is dependent on neutrality. In any event, they could not shed their identities as members of the very ethnic groups that have been under assault by oppressors for half a century. They could not be expected to feign indifference to the political aims of the Myanmar government to quash aspirations for democracy and self-governance, nor to the Tatmadaw's military objectives. It was also pointless to make such an effort, as the Tatmadaw acted as though the medics had allegiances to the communities from which they came. That is why neutrality is not an ethical obligation in health practice, nor should it be. Health workers can take a political position on the issues of the day, express those positions in public, and still adhere to their ethical obligations including impartiality. Similarly, military-affiliated health workers are not, and cannot be, neutral, but nevertheless have been, from the original Geneva Convention, protected. Unfortunately, neutrality is often conflated with the duty of impartiality. The latter requires treating everyone without regard to characteristics such as race, gender, political beliefs, ethnicity, or political affiliations. Impartiality does not require the health worker to be personally indifferent to politics.

The demand for neutrality is more than a mistake about morality and ethics in humanitarian practice. It has an insidious implication, that neutrality is a prerequisite for immunity from attack or arrest. According to this view, health workers are entitled to protection from attack only to the extent that they have no political position, or at least don't act to advance it. In an otherwise thorough and sound report, for example, the independent commission that examined human rights violations during Arab Spring demonstrations in Bahrain took doctors to task for participating in political demonstrations near the country's main hospital. It stated that "it is difficult to reconcile" these activities with the "full exercise of their medical responsibilities."[94] The commission drew this mistaken conclusion notwithstanding their entitlement to act politically so long as it did not compromise their compliance with ethical obligations. Its posture is not only wrong but dangerously puts health workers at risk of violence or arrest.

As explained in chapter 1, more than a century ago the Geneva Conventions abandoned the idea that health workers should be deemed neutral, as that characterization misrepresented health workers' duties, affiliations, and functions. Rather, the conventions were revised to entitle all health workers to protection and respect, including military medical workers who indubitably affiliate with one side in a conflict. Under Protocol 2, those protected include individuals assigned to medical duties by an armed group that is a party to a conflict. Health workers may also act politically to address social and political wrongs while also offering health care to individuals in need. Similarly, from a human rights perspective, health workers are not excluded from rights such as freedom of expression and assembly on account of their medical work. For the people living in ethnic communities in Myanmar, requiring neutrality of health workers would mean abandoning a population in desperate straits.

A second objection to Back Pack's work was that its work amounted to support that advanced the military objectives of the KNLA by better enabling displaced populations to resist the Tatmadaw. Though not addressing health workers, in his book *Killing Civilians: Method, Madness, and Morality in War*, humanitarian practitioner and scholar Hugo Slim provides a sound perspective on activities of civilians that may contribute to the objectives of one side of a conflict.[95] Slim frames his discussion around the concept of "innocent civilian." He recognizes that vast numbers of civilians are not "innocent" in the sense that children are innocent. They have political views and may have strong political commitments and agendas, as Back Pack certainly did. The activities of such groups may not be wholly beyond support for the war effort, for example, procuring food for an army. Back Pack's medics offered support for indigenous populations, and in that way countered Tatmadaw efforts to undermine the well-being of communities and to deny them democratic governance. As Louis Renault had pointed out in 1906, health workers are in some sense genuine enemies of the regime, but of a special, protected kind. And as Slim explains, combatants need to recognize the reality of people's lives and allegiances, and the goal must be to keep all noncombatants immune from harm, lest war become an environment where everyone affiliated in some way with, or who supports the enemy, becomes a target.

The Geneva Conventions and customary international humanitarian law embody, in a practical way, Slim's argument. They seek to draw a line between civilian activities that are protected and those that are not. Civilians must not be subject to attack or punishment unless they play a "direct part in hostilities." The ICRC devoted seven years of consultations with more than fifty experts to issue eighty-five pages of interpretive guidance on the meaning and application of this phrase. It concluded that "direct participation in hostilities" applied only to acts likely to affect military operations or inflict death or injury on enemies. Further, it argued that there must be a causal link between the act and the harm, and that the actor must specifically intend to cause the harm.[96] The guidance denied that sympathies, allegiances, participation in governance, or economic activities that are helpful to one side disentitles people to protection as civilians. The ICRC position has been hotly debated, but with respect to health care, its reasoning is reinforced by other provisions in the Geneva Conventions. They state that medical units are protected unless they commit, "outside their humanitarian function, acts harmful to the enemy."[97] Providing health care is not such an act.

If the law is on their side, health workers' affiliations, identification, or sympathy with one side of a conflict nevertheless puts them in jeopardy. The risk is great not only in war but in situations of political volatility, protest, or violence, when health workers provide care for people who join protests against governments and sometimes participate in protests themselves. Chapter 4 discusses the targeting of health workers during Arab Spring protests in Syria. Much the same was evident in other parts of the Middle East. At the start of the Arab spring demonstrations that led to the downfall of President Hosni Mubarak in Egypt, many physicians had dual motives: supporting the revolution and treating the wounded. They saw the two in harmony and some linked them more explicitly, that treatment of demonstrators also was a means to sustain the protests.[98] Many of them were harassed by police and some were arrested.[99] Later, as the protestors' unity frayed, some doctors retreated to an exclusively medical ethics mindset, feeling an obligation to treat all in need, including those whose political positions were anathema to them. Those values were especially challenged in a third phase, when doctors themselves faced a high risk of attack during the violence designed to bring down the Muslim Brotherhood.[100] Regardless of their motivations in these different phases—political, ethical, humanitarian, or some combination thereof—their entitlement to immunity from arrest or attack for engaging in medical work remained the same.

The antigovernment protests in Sudan in 2018–2019 were even more fraught for doctors. Physicians were recognized as leaders of a protest movement for democracy and reform. Security forces responded violently against the protesters and targeted physicians, including for providing medical care to wounded demonstrators. One of them, Dr. Babiker Abdul Hamid, was killed as he attended to an injured protester. By April 2019, more than 130 doctors had been arrested, 56 of them in a dormitory for physicians in training.[101] On June 3, Sudan security forces killed more than a hundred protesters engaged in a sit-in in Khartoum. In its aftermath, the security forces invaded hospitals to chase down the wounded, threaten patients, and destroy equipment. They beat people trying to enter hospitals and demanded that doctors discharge injured patients, in some cases threatening to shoot them if they did not. Eight hospitals had to close and security forces destroyed mobile clinics set up to treat injured protesters.[102] According to Dr. Ahmed Al-Mandhari, director of the WHO for the Eastern Mediterranean region, "health care workers appear to have been targeted for fulfilling their professional duties."[103] In protests in the United States after the killing of George Floyd by police in Minneapolis, street medics, including those with medical or Red Cross insignia, were assaulted by police in multiple cities.[104]

In these circumstances of armed conflict or political upheaval, health workers were responding to both a medical and political crisis. Whatever their views, allegiances, and political activities, they carried out their medical work with integrity and compassion. Whether they were motivated by political beliefs or professional obligations does not matter. For very different reasons, the motivations of the health workers likely didn't matter to the armies or regimes that oppressed them, contemptuous as they were of the obligation they owed to protect and respect health care and alleviate suffering. On the contrary, the forces wanted to increase the suffering of all the people under the health workers' care, whether members of an indigenous ethnic group or members of a political movement, and punish those who got in their way. This attitude would become even more pronounced in the global campaign against terrorism.

# 3

## COUNTERTERRORISM

The Devouring Monster

OUNTERING TERRORISM BECAME a global priority at the end of the twentieth century—and brought a vast extension of the logic of denying health care to enemies and punishing their caregivers. In the past thirty years, laws and enforcement policies proliferated that authorized arrest and imprisonment of health workers who provide care to people deemed terrorists, or who belonged to terrorist organizations. They restricted humanitarian aid to populations in need if living in areas controlled by groups designated as terrorist. In the 1990s, harbingers of the new laws emerged in prosecutions of physicians in Turkey and Kosovo for offering care to alleged terrorists. At the time, the U.S. and other Western countries labeled the charges as violations of human rights. Now, though, they and governments throughout the world have created legal regimes that similarly criminalize health care in the name of counterterrorism, thereby undercutting the principle of humanity, the ethical and humanitarian law obligations of impartiality, and the human rights to life and health. They deny care wholesale to populations in need and put health workers at risk of incarceration for doing their duty.

## ENEMY OF THE STATE: TURKEY

Dr. Şebnem Korur Fincancı never set out to be controversial, much less someone who Turkey's governor of Istanbul called an enemy of the state. Growing up, her family encouraged her to follow her uncle's career as an academic physician. She chose forensic medicine only after learning that her competition for a residency spot in pathology was the daughter-in-law of a professor. Still, she was intrigued by the specialty, as it combined medical skills with what she told me at dinner in Istanbul in 2018 is the ability to see "all aspects of society, where the violence starts, and how to protect people from violence." She didn't know at the time that, even as she progressed through a distinguished academic career, her scientific and medical skill and integrity in making and reporting forensic findings would get her into trouble.

The circumstances in which she had to work were clear the first time I met her. Partly but not exclusively as a result of an armed insurgency by the Kurdistan Workers' Party (known as the PKK) that began in 1984, Turkey exemplified a national security state. In 2000, my wife Margaret and I had dinner with Dr. Fincancı and a few others from the Human Rights Foundation of Turkey at a restaurant near Taksim Square, the lively area of central Istanbul with upscale hotels, trendy and touristy restaurants, and live music into the wee hours. A live band was playing as we conversed and ate. Suddenly the music stopped. Three or four police officers had entered the restaurant and demanded identity cards from every diner. Margaret and I handed over our American passports with some concern. The police took everyone else's documents as well and left. "What happens now?" I asked. Dr. Fincancı said they would likely come back later, return the identification cards except, perhaps, one belonging to a person they decided to take into custody without explanation. If that happened, she said, they might release the person later that night, the next morning, or not at all. An hour or so later, the police did come back, identification documents in hand, and no one from our group was apprehended.

Over the years, I saw Dr. Fincancı at human rights meetings, where she represented human rights organizations in Turkey. But it wasn't until 2018, at another dinner in Taksim Square—this time at a rooftop restaurant down a side street no tourist would ever find—that I learned of the contradictions of her professional life. On the faculty of Istanbul University, she was one of the most respected forensic physicians in Turkey. At the same time, the government repeatedly claimed that she was associated with terrorists. The saga began a few years before she started her residency in the late 1980s, when a military coup overthrew Turkey's civilian government. More than half a million people were arrested, many of them tortured. In trials that lacked due process, almost half of those arrested were convicted of crimes related to subversion, membership in a leftist organization, or similar political offenses. Many journalists were sent to prison, and more than a million-and-a-half people were blacklisted. The Turkish Medical Association's activities were suspended for three years. The Forensic Medicine Institute of Turkey, associated with Istanbul University, came under the jurisdiction of the Ministry of Justice.

What got her into trouble was torture. During the 1980s, the PKK bombed government buildings, kidnapped and assassinated officials, and attacked Turkish diplomatic and commercial activities in Europe. The government designated the PKK as a terrorist organization. Suspected PKK militants were arrested in the thousands, as were people having nothing to do with the PKK. Almost all were tortured, even those arrested after civilian rule was restored. Some of them died. Under Turkish law and practice, forensic practitioners examined individuals who died in detention. The government pressured the examiners not to suggest in an autopsy report that injuries found on someone who died in custody were likely attributable to torture. In the very first week of Dr. Fincancı's residency in 1985, a judge asked the Forensic Medicine Institute to conduct a review of an autopsy conducted two years previously on a prisoner. The report revealed serious injuries to the man, but the examiner hadn't made any findings whether the detainee's injuries were likely to be the product of torture. When Dr. Fincancı reviewed the report, she saw that it revealed injuries to the man's feet consistent with the practice of falanga, the severe beating of the feet. She also found musculoskeletal injuries that probably resulted from the man's suspension by his arms and being forced into a contorted position. No alternative explanation could account for the injuries. At a training and case discussion at the institute, she reported what she found, but received pushback. "A professor argued that foot injuries could have been caused by jumping, and injuries under the armpits from hitting himself against a wall," she recalled, and explained to me that the alternative theories were "medically ridiculous." The lesson was disturbing: "I witnessed how they covered up all these findings." That day, she vowed to work on these cases and tell the truth when she found torture of prisoners.

As she saw other cases of prisoners who had died of torture in detention, she started to read more about the problem, both globally and in Turkish detention facilities. Between 1989 and 1995, at least eighty health professionals were detained for reporting torture or treating its victims.[1] Dr. Vincent Iacopino, later my colleague at Physicians for Human Rights, surveyed doctors at a medical conference and found that a third of respondents who responded to a question about whether police influenced their report answered affirmatively. The fact that half of those surveyed did not answer that question may well have signaled their fear. Follow-up interviews revealed that police in southeastern Turkey threatened doctors who reported torture and sometimes demanded that doctors sign medical reports to attest that there were no signs of torture.[2]

In 1989 Dr. Fincancı joined the newly established human rights committee of the Turkish Medical Association. By the early 1990s, Amnesty International and other local and international human rights organizations had begun to report beatings, suspension by arms and legs, use of electrical shocks to genitals, and blunt trauma in Turkish prisons. In 1990, thirty-two prominent intellectuals and human rights groups founded the Human Rights Foundation of Turkey, dedicated to the rehabilitation of torture survivors. It became part of a global network of rehabilitation centers for survivors of torture funded by the United Nations and other donors. The need for such an organization was reinforced the following year, when Turkey enacted a tough anti-terror law that criminalized many nonviolent political activities and extended criminal liability to members of organizations that aided terrorist groups.[3] The new law allowed prosecutions in special state security courts, which had less transparency and due process than regular courts, and no independent judges. Individuals arrested could be held for fifteen days incommunicado or thirty days in southeastern provinces operating under a state of emergency because of the conflict with the PKK.

As the number of detainees subjected to torture grew throughout the 1990s, so did the government's pressure on doctors not to report torture and to falsify medical examinations of detainees in custody to avoid findings of torture. In 1999, the government arrested Dr. Cumhur Akpinar, charging that his findings that detainees had been tortured amounted to aiding an illegal organization (he was subsequently acquitted).[4] The government also looked askance at medical treatment for members of the PKK and their families. It alleged that Dr. Zeki Uzun, a gynecologist fluent in the Kurdish language, provided treatment to members of the PKK by taking Kurdish women as patients. Dr. Uzun was arrested in his office by anti-terror police, who blindfolded him and demanded that he sign a confession that he was a doctor for a terrorist organization. He was held in detention for a week, during which time security agents repeatedly beat him on his head and chest and subjected him to near suffocation with a plastic bag.[5] At his trial, a convicted PKK member testified that Dr. Uzun had provided medical care to women associated by marriage to a member of the PKK or otherwise affiliated with the organization.[6] Dr. Uzun was ultimately acquitted, but the message was clear: doctors were not to treat anyone remotely affiliated with the PKK. In preparation for Dr. Uzun's trial, a physician instructed to determine whether he had been tortured in detention was so terrified that the doctor conducted his "examination" from ten meters away from Dr. Uzun. He wrote a medical report that Dr. Uzun was not tortured, a finding refuted after his release by a thorough and independent medical examination.[7]

Meanwhile, Dr. Fincancı's academic career took off. In 1990, after completing her residency, she was appointed to prestigious faculty positions at Istanbul University. But in her reviews of medical reports required when a prisoner died, she repeatedly found and reported evidence of torture. The pressures on her built. "One day," she told me, "the Minister of Justice called and told me that I am [a] member of a leftist organization." His reasoning for that belief was that "I had provided a medical legal report for someone who belonged to a leftist organization. And because of that I was a member of a leftist organization." She laughed off the call, but the Minister was serious. A few months later, an inspector came to the Institute of Forensic Medicine to review her work. After the review, in 1996, the same year doctors affiliated with the Human Rights Foundation of Turkey began to face arrest, she was discharged from the Institute on a flimsy pretext.

Despite her firing, Dr. Fincancı's work continued to be respected by her peers, so she retained her academic position at Istanbul University. She also contested her discharge from the Forensic Institute and was eventually vindicated. Harassment continued. In 2000 she was accused by the Governor of Istanbul of being an "enemy of the state," and he urged that she be forbidden to work at the Forensic Institute. When recounting so many such incidents to me, she laughed, at ease with her decision and untroubled by the risks she took. That year, apart from the unsettling police appearance at the restaurant, I witnessed two aspects of the government's intimidation of physicians who documented torture or treated its victims. During my visit to Istanbul, one of Dr. Fincancı's colleagues who joined us at dinner, Dr. Önder Özkalıpcı, a physician with the Human Rights Foundation of Turkey who conducted medical examinations of victims of torture, took me to a state security court to witness proceedings there. A Turkish doctor was on trial for reporting evidence of torture he found when he examined its victims. As was common in these cases, the proceedings often stretched out for months and even years. A few days later, I traveled to the city of Izmir for a meeting of international health and human rights organizations that had spoken out in defense of Turkish doctors who had been arrested and imprisoned for medical care to alleged terrorists. As the meeting was about to start, police barged in and informed the group that the meeting was forbidden. We left the building and hung out on the street. After an hour or so the police departed. Our Turkish colleagues explained that their coming was just routine intimidation and encouraged us to continue with the meeting. We went back inside to hold the meeting; the police didn't return.

The following year Dr. Fincancı was fired again from the Forensic Institute. Even so, she continued to advance in her academic career, but professional respect only went so far. During the academic year 2004–05, she was accused on a university listserv of being a member of the PKK. "I found [the accusations] ridiculous. I was sure of myself," she told me. "I was a professional and always tried to do my job in the best way I could manage. . . . I try to find the truth. It is my obsession," Dr. Fincancı said. She went on, "Fellow faculty members recognize that. . . . It's an issue of medicine. I try to do my best with my medical knowledge not my political affiliations and they all know that." In 2009, still fearless, she managed to keep navigating government demands while maintaining her professional position and integrity, made ever more difficult as the government expanded criminalization of health care to alleged terrorists as the conflict with the PKK remained unresolved. Dr. Fincancı became president of the Human Rights Foundation of Turkey.

In 2012, Turkey broadened its terrorism offenses to deem a person who aided a terrorist organization to be a member of the organization.[8] In 2013, nationwide protests against the government brought a violent response by the police, who injured eight thousand demonstrators. The government offered no first aid to the wounded protestors, so the Turkish Medical Association and other groups created makeshift emergency aid stations in mosques, shopping malls, and elsewhere, some of which the police assaulted. In the aftermath of the protests the government enacted a new law rendering it a criminal offense to provide emergency medical care without permission from the Ministry of Health.

The Secretary-General of the Turkish Medical Association, Ilhan Bayazıt, responded, "The government sees the helping of injured protesters as a political act, and they want to stop it."[9] Two doctors were charged under the law with "protecting perpetrators by extending them first aid" and were sentenced to ten months imprisonment.[10] The government also brought a lawsuit against the Turkish Medical Association and the Ankara

Medical Chamber, a local medical association, charging them with having established health-care units illicitly and without control and supervision.[11] The case was ultimately dismissed. Soon thereafter, the conflict in southeastern Turkey flared up. In 2015, youth militias from the PKK barricaded parts of cities there. In July, Turkish security forces responded with a campaign against the PKK in the region, including 24-hour curfews in twenty-two cities and towns, some of which lasted weeks. Turkish security forces shelled towns, including civilian apartment buildings, and leveled neighborhoods. Arbitrary arrests and torture followed.[12] The curfews prevented almost all access to emergency medical care, including passage of ambulances and private vehicles carrying the wounded and sick, and cut off access to food, water, and electricity.

In the city of Cizre, with a population of a hundred thousand people, eight health centers were closed for almost three months and three of them were destroyed during the shelling. Security forces took over hospitals to use as dormitories for their troops and to control access to medical care. Wounded people were often denied access to medical care in facilities that were available.[13] In five other cities, primary health centers providing care for an estimated half a million people were shut down.[14] During a second curfew in Cizre, lasting almost three months, between one and two hundred civilians were trapped in basements in an area of heavy fighting, many of them injured. All of them eventually died of their injuries or from lack of food or water.[15] Turkish security forces swept through the region, arresting or administratively punishing doctors who provided aid to fighters and civilians wounded in the violence.

In early 2016, the Human Rights Foundation of Turkey and other medical and legal groups launched an investigation into human rights violations during the fighting in Cizre. One day after the curfew was lifted in March, Dr. Fincancı participated as the team's forensic specialist. She visited ruined buildings including basements where more than 170 bodies had been retrieved. There she found the lower jawbone of a child, which contradicted the government's claim that all those in the basement were terrorists. Dr. Fincancı also examined the autopsy of a man who had been dragged along the street by a military vehicle. According to the government, the man was killed in clashes with the police and, as they suspected him of carrying bombs, soldiers dragged his body behind a vehicle so that, if bombs exploded, no one would be hurt. Dr. Fincancı's review of the autopsy, however, revealed the lie. She determined that he was alive when tied to the vehicle, and that all his injuries, including gunshot wounds, were inflicted while being dragged along the street. The Human Rights Foundation sent the report, along with photographs, to the European Court of Human Rights.

Two months later Dr. Fincancı was arrested. The pretext was that she had participated, along with fifty-six journalists, academics, and others, in guest editing a newspaper sympathetic to Kurdish claims for self-determination after its regular editors had been arrested. Of the fifty-six signatories, however, only three were arrested: Dr. Fincancı and two journalists who had also written human rights reports on the violence in Cizre. She was charged with making terrorist propaganda. After being jailed she was conditionally released after ten days, pending trial. One of her colleagues in the Cizre investigation, Dr. Serdar Küni, was also arrested for terrorism. He was charged with providing medical care to Kurdish rebels under a law that states that a person who offers aid to an illegal organization can be punished as though a member of it. Christine Mehta, a human rights investigator observing the trial, listened to the prosecutor argue, "He has treated people injured in illegal incidents." She reported that in response to the charges, Dr. Suni told the court, "I have been a practicing physician in Cizre for twelve years." He continued, "I have no connection with armed groups. I have always simply practiced my profession and given medical help to those who needed it."[16] He was convicted and sentenced to four years in prison. As of early 2020, his appeal was pending. Meanwhile, a second criminal case was brought against Dr. Fincancı for campaigning for peace. She was sentenced to two and a half years imprisonment, though released pending her appeal.

In the summer of 2016, there was an attempted military coup against President Recep Tayyip Erdogan. Within a week of the coup, 2,700 judges (a third of the entire judiciary), 15,000 teachers, and tens of thousands of civil servants and members of the military were suspended or dismissed.

Many were detained. Every university dean in the country was suspended. About fifty hospitals and health clinics, including leading facilities in Ankara and Istanbul, were shuttered because of alleged ties to Fethullah Gülen, who President Erdogan claimed was behind the coup attempt. Tough counterterrorism laws were invoked against members of the medical community. Prosecutors alleged that Ali İlker Baştan, a Turkish dentist, had treated Gülen while visiting the United States, which the prosecution equated with "membership in a terror organization," and "involvement in activities on behalf of a terror organization." Baştan denied knowing or treating Gülen, explaining that his travel to the U.S. was for conferences and educational programs.[17] In April 2018, the court convicted Dr. Baştan and sentenced him to seven years and six months detention, to be served under house arrest.[18]

At our dinner in 2018, Dr. Fincancı told me she expected to be convicted at her trial for allegedly making terrorist propaganda. She was as matter of fact about the prospect as in describing her career, concerned only that her incarceration would be painful for her family. Medical and journalism groups from within Turkey and around the world denounced and campaigned against the prosecution, and the pressure apparently brought results: in July 2019, she was acquitted. In July 2020 her conviction for campaigning for peace was also reversed. She said, "I think it is an appropriate decision. We are the only country where demanding peace is criminalized."[19] Still president of the Turkish Human Rights Foundation, her work continued.

## FROM PERSECUTION TO PROSECUTION: KOSOVO

Dr. Luan Jaha entered medical school in Pristina, capital of the then-Serbian province of Kosovo, in 1988, on the cusp of what was to become Serbia's severe repression of the province's ethnic Albanian majority. A year later, Slobodan Milošević, who demagogically promoted Serb

nationalism within Yugoslavia, became president of Serbia. He successfully maneuvered passage of constitutional amendments that revoked
Kosovo's semiautonomous status within Serbia. Soon thereafter, the government expelled thousands of ethnic Albanians from the civil service,
universities, and secondary education, and curbed their employment in the
state-dominated medical system. By 1998, only 10 percent of the physicians
in the state system were ethnic Albanians. Clinical training for medical
students in hospitals was off-limits.

Though a much quieter personality than Dr. Financı, Dr. Jaha had
firm convictions. As a student journalist in the late 1980s, Dr. Jaha was
arrested for stories he wrote and detained for a few days before the Supreme
Court ordered his release. With the onset of repression, he decided it
would be safer to transfer to a medical school in Croatia, then still part of
Yugoslavia. After graduating in 1992, he remained in Croatia, where he
completed additional training. Upon gaining his license as a physician in
1994, he returned to his hometown of Rehovec in Kosovo. Because, as an
ethnic Albanian, he was not permitted to work in a public clinic, he, like
so many other Albanian physicians with few options, set up his own
practice.

Milošević's brand of Serb nationalism led to the breakup of the state of
Yugoslavia and a brutal war with Croatia and then Bosnia from 1991 to
1995. It was characterized by genocide, mass rape, and ethnic cleansing.
One hundred thousand people were killed. Kosovo escaped that war, but
during the 1990s, under the leadership of Ibrahim Rugova, Kosovar Albanians engaged in nonviolent resistance to the draconian restrictions on
their personal, professional, and political lives. A shadow Kosovar Albanian legislature voted for independence, which the Serbian government
refused to recognize. Kosovar Albanians conducted elections and established parallel systems of social services, health care, and medical
education. An internationally supported NGO, the Mother Theresa
Society, opened more than one hundred clinics to serve more than three
hundred and fifty thousand people discriminated against in state health
services. The resilience of the ethnic Albanian population through the
1990s, though, was tested by the escalation of severe human rights

violations by Serbia against it. In 1994, the UN General Assembly condemned Serbia for police brutality, discrimination against ethnic Albanians, harassment and imprisonment of Albanian political figures, intimidation of Albanian journalists, dismissal of doctors from clinics and hospitals, and the elimination of the Albanian language from official use.[20] By 1996, an organization calling itself the Kosovo Liberation Army (KLA) called for armed resistance.

At the start, the KLA neither gained traction among the population, nor had military impact on Serbia. Soon, though, the KLA obtained vast amounts of arms after Albania's weapons stocks were looted during a period of anarchy. At the same time, it gained popular support as nonviolent resistance had done nothing to ameliorate the repression. In July 1998, Rehovec, where Dr. Jaha practiced, happened to be the site of the KLA's first attack on Serb security forces in a city. Although the KLA offensive initially succeeded, Serb and Yugoslav federal forces pushed the KLA back. Dr. Jaha responded to the crisis by treating wounded civilians and KLA fighters. The following month, in a bus station in the nearby city of Prizren, a police officer from Rehovec recognized Dr. Jaha and arrested him. The officer told Dr. Jaha that the police had been looking for him, characterizing him as a doctor for the KLA. Dr. Jaha said he responded, "I am not a soldier, just a civilian doctor."

The officer brought him to prison. An investigating judge informed Dr. Jaha that he was accused of violating articles 125 and 136 of the Federal Republic of Yugoslavia penal code for organizing medical services for the KLA. Section 125 of the code outlawed acts of violence and "some other generally dangerous action out of hostile motives against the [Socialist Federal Republic of Yugoslavia]." Article 136 prohibited membership in or assistance to organizations engaging in hostile acts against the state.[21] Prosecutors took no heed of another part of the criminal code regarding a physician's responsibility to treat those in need. Remanded to a detention facility, he was interrogated and tortured. Dr. Jaha's captors beat him with rubber sticks on his legs, arms, and hands, subjected him to electric shocks, and suffocated him with a bag placed over his head. At one point Dr. Jaha lost consciousness. The beatings continued almost every day for six weeks.

At night, he heard others being tortured. Ultimately, he succumbed. He said, "I signed a paper that I was in charge of the KLA medical service. It was the only way to stop the beatings."

Fortuitously, in October 1998, while Dr. Jaha was in detention, an attempt to avoid war and to address the fate of the now more than two hundred thousand refugees and displaced people from the escalating conflict was underway. U.S. special envoy Richard Holbrooke reached an agreement with Milošević. It required the regime to withdraw some security forces from Kosovo and participate in peace talks, and authorized two thousand unarmed civilian human rights monitors from the Organization for Security and Cooperation in Europe to patrol in the province. The deal also put pressure on judges to release doctors who were arrested for providing medical care to the KLA. The wheels to secure his release were greased as well by bribes paid by Dr. Jaha's family to the prosecutor and judges. Charges against him were dropped. Once released, Dr. Jaha thought it too dangerous for him to remain in Rehovec, so he traveled to Pristina, where he sought work with an international organization. He met investigators from Physicians for Human Rights who were seeking information about the fate of doctors who had been arrested for charges similar to those brought against Dr. Jaha. With his excellent English and his knowledge of the medical community, Dr. Jaha was hired.

The PHR investigators found cases of other Kosovar doctors arrested in the summer and fall of 1998. Another doctor from Rehovec, Dr. Shani Bajraktari, an ophthalmologist, was also arrested in the wake of the KLA attack in July 1998. Government forces learned that he, like Dr. Jaha, had provided medical aid to wounded KLA soldiers. A Serb neighbor sheltered Dr. Bajraktari, but the police eventually discovered and detained him. He was released after a brief interrogation, but in September he was detained again when in Prizren. This time, Dr. Bajraktari was beaten until he signed a confession that he worked in a KLA clinic. The indictment brought against him equated medical treatment for members of the KLA with membership in a terrorist organization:

In the time from April to the end of September 1998 in the areas of Orahovac [Serbian for Rehovec], as a member of terrorist organization called KLA, he took part in the acts of violence to create insecurity among the citizens, by working in [state hospital] in Orahovac. He took part in a meeting of medical workers in the elementary school and accepted the role of organizing health care and treatment for the members of KLA after they committed terrorist attacks.

Working under the advice of supervisors in the so-called 'KLA,' he left his work place in the Orahovac clinic several times and went into the village of Drenoc led by a person named Mensur to the illegal KLA ambulanta [clinic] where he delivered medical care to so-called "KLA" members wounded in armed conflicts. He also went to the village of Gajrak where he examined and treated so-called "KLA" members by undertaking surgical interventions. He took part in the supply of dressings and medicines and transport of the same to illegal clinics. In an effort to hide these activities, he explained his absence from work as taking vacations. By doing this he has committed—the act of terrorism from Article 125 of the Penal Code of Yugoslavia.[22]

When he appeared before a judge, Dr. Bajraktari denied the charges and was beaten again in the courtroom. After months in jail, Dr. Bajraktari's case came to trial, and he received the support of Serbian neighbors. He nevertheless was convicted and sentenced to three-and-a-half-years' imprisonment. With the help of a bribe, he was released on bail pending appeal, and ultimately fled to Albania, where he remained until the war ended.

PHR's investigators found fourteen doctors charged with these and similar crimes and incarcerated. Twelve of them were tortured.[23] Another of them was Dr. Zaim Gashi. Before the war he served patients from all ethnic groups in the small town of Sferke and collaborated with his Serb medical colleagues. In 1998, he completed training in emergency medicine and went to the village of Kpuz, northeast of Rehovec. Soon a frightening odyssey began. Serb troops shot artillery into Kpuz, setting it on fire and forcing its inhabitants, including Dr. Gashi, to flee. He eventually made it back to Sferke, where he provided care for twenty-five thousand internally displaced persons, local citizens, and members of the KLA, which controlled the village. In September, Serb forces retook the town. Dr. Gashi fled again, this time to the town of Panore, taking whatever medical equipment he had left with him in his car. Soon thereafter, Serb paramilitary forces entered Panore, burned and looted it, and captured him along with other Kosovar Albanians. When Serb forces learned he was a doctor, they asked him to treat a wounded Serb soldier, which he did; then he was moved, along with other Kosovar Albanian men, to a detention facility. During six months in detention, he was beaten repeatedly as he was interrogated. When Dr. Gashi was brought to trial in February 1999, he cited the Hippocratic oath as obliging him to provide care for all in need. The police demurred, telling him he had no responsibility to provide medical care to the KLA. He was convicted and sentenced to six months imprisonment and released for time served. When I spoke to Dr. Gashi in Pristina ten years after these events, he told me that he still experienced pain in his back and shoulders from the beatings.

Serb forces supplemented the arrests with a terrifying, sustained campaign of intimidation, violence and threats against doctors. During late 1998, three physicians were targeted and murdered.[24] Other physicians were summoned for "talks" with the police, who demanded information about their activities, affiliations, patients, and the names of other doctors. Many doctors feared offering care to wounded civilians, much less to KLA soldiers, and stayed away from areas where civilians might be attacked. Even house calls were risky. One doctor told a PHR investigator, "Every time we go into the field to see a patient, we run a big risk from the police."[25] Others' clinics were burned by Serb forces. Many Kosovar Albanian physicians abandoned medical practice, moved to the countryside, fled to the mountains along the Albanian border, or left the country. The Albanian population, already under enormous stress, was left with far fewer resources for their medical needs. Meanwhile, Serbian military forces commandeered hospitals and clinics for use as military bases and weapons storage facilities, and placed antiaircraft artillery on their roofs.[26] PHR investigators learned of more than seventy instances where patients, some of them critically ill, decided it was too risky to seek care.[27]

Having sat by for more than two years in the face of atrocities in Bosnia, President Bill Clinton felt pressure to act to stop Milošević's depredations in Kosovo. In March 1999, after peace talks broke down, and with support from NATO, he ordered the bombing of the Serbian military and some civilian installations in Serbia. In response, Milošević forcibly expelled almost a million ethnic Albanians from Kosovo, most fleeing to neighboring Macedonia and Albania. His forces increased attacks on members of the medical community who remained. On the first day of the bombing campaign, Serbian police came to the home of the chief of surgery of Djakovica Hospital and slit his throat. Another doctor was killed the following day, and within a few weeks, nine had been murdered.[28] Others were hunted down as they moved from place to place to avoid detection. Serb forces destroyed more than one hundred health facilities, mostly local clinics, took over almost sixty others for military purposes, and expelled dozens of patients and health workers from hospitals, often beating them in the process.[29] The few nurses and doctors who had managed to hold onto their jobs in state-run clinics or hospitals were expelled. In April, one renowned doctor, Flora Brovina, who also was a writer, poet, and human rights activist, was abducted by Serb paramilitaries and brought to Serbia. She was interrogated for weeks, then accused of providing medicine and treatment to wounded combatants. She was sentenced to twelve years' imprisonment.[30]

A cease-fire in June 1999 ended the conflict. Refugees began to return to Kosovo as fifty thousand troops from NATO members and other countries were sent to keep the peace. Kosovo soon declared its independence. Milošević and four others were eventually indicted for crimes against humanity by the International Criminal Tribunal for the former Yugoslavia (he died before a verdict), though the indictment contained no charges relating to the arrests and prosecution of the doctors or abuses of patients. In the immediate aftermath of the war, despite the NATO presence, vicious reprisals against ethnic Serbs in Kosovo began. Within weeks, all Serbian physicians either retreated to Serbian enclaves within the country or left Kosovo.

Most of the ethnic Albanian doctors who had fled Kosovo or were expelled returned. Dr. Jaha and Dr. Bajraktari resumed their practices. Dr. Gashi completed a residency in internal medicine with a subspecialty in gastroenterology. The doctors could once again obtain privileges to practice in hospitals and the community's leaders took control of Kosovo's medical school. Yet the decade-long experience of discrimination and exclusion, followed by arrests, torture, and flight, could not be shaken off. After conversations with Kosovo Albanian physicians soon after the war ended, my colleague Jennifer Leaning and I wrote that "many expressed a profound sense of moral confusion and weariness." We learned that "they felt 'unprepared—both psychologically and in terms of their training—to come to terms with what they had experienced and the implications that experience might have for future medical practice, in terms of focus, commitment, priorities.'"[31] They also felt ethically at sea. From a professional standpoint, they wanted to create a culture of human rights in health care amidst the ongoing postwar tensions and uncertainty. They sought to be a part of the global medical community, sharing its values and ethical commitments. Most of them accepted the idea of impartiality and equal access to health care for all people. Yet they remained conflicted about their duties. One said:

> I was among those who were arrested and sent to prison in Serbia. I could never describe my feelings about this. I thought they would kill me or burn me or cut me into small pieces. There were many times I thought of ending my own life to end this situation. Now you ask me to treat one of them. I would say that I would do the best I could but my hand would be shaking the entire time. . . . All of your personal feelings must be put under the table because of your commitment to the Hippocratic Oath as doctors . . . but these feelings are very raw and new.[32]

Others felt that that their own losses and the suffering of their families made it "too soon" to talk about human rights. One told us: "It is very difficult to put aside the feelings of the last ten years . . . I worry that I will have trouble treating a Serb patient without having a feeling of hate inside. I don't think I can forgive them for teaching me how to hate."[33] The conversations yielded proposals to the Organization for Security and Cooperation in Europe and the ICRC to build human rights into medical education and to create a new medical society to promote human rights in health. But almost uniformly, the doctors were not ready to work with Serb physicians. They wanted Serb doctors to apologize for excluding them from the health system and for complicity in or toleration of the violence, arrest, and imprisonment of Kosovar Albanian physicians. Even had the Serb doctors apologized (they did not), the Kosovar Albanian physicians were not willing to allow those doctors to hold positions of authority in hospitals or the medical school.

Ten years later, I returned to Kosovo, with Dr. Jaha as my guide. After the war, the WHO engaged in a misguided effort to create a new health care system without any input from the doctors. Dr. Jaha and many other doctors maintained their private medical practices outside the new system. Serb doctors remained in Serb enclaves, entirely segregated from Kosovar Albanians.[34] The Kosovar Albanian physicians remained grateful that throughout the ordeal, they felt support and solidarity from human rights organizations, the United States, and NATO. Even a decade later, though, many of the doctors we had spoken to earlier were still suffering from the trauma of exclusion and war. They also felt vulnerable to episodes of intermittent violence. The postwar interest in creating a new medical society and medical education programs premised on human rights and ethics had waned.

After the war, sustained international pressure led to the release of Dr. Brovina in November 2000. It wouldn't be long, though, before the United States, undercutting norms of humanity and human dignity, adopted the very posture that Serbia and Turkey did in bringing charges and threatening doctors for providing care to alleged terrorists.

# COUNTERTERRORISM LAW AND
# THE DENIAL OF HUMANITY

During the 1990s, the U.S. State Department's annual global reports on human rights condemned Turkey for the arrests and prosecutions of doctors for honest forensic evaluations of torture and rehabilitation of its victims, and Serbia's arrests and prosecutions of doctors in Kosovo for providing medical care to members of the KLA.[35] Dr. Khassan Baiev, the Chechen doctor, personally benefited from U.S. commitments to the immunity of health workers from punishment for engaging in medical activities. The American embassy in Moscow helped him flee Russia in 2000 and he was granted asylum in the United States because of his well-founded fear of persecution at home. Had he applied a few years later, however, his application might well have been denied for having treated a terrorist, Shamil Basayev. A Nepalese medic who sought to obtain asylum in the United States ran into this very stumbling block. During a Maoist insurgency in Nepal that lasted from 2001 to 2005, the government issued a directive that health workers had to get government permission before treating rebels.[36] The medic, initials BT, was kidnapped by Maoist rebels at gunpoint and forced to treat their compatriots suffering from gunshot wounds and burns. BT was eventually able to escape from the Maoists, but soldiers of the Royal Nepalese Army arrested him for violating the government's directive. They beat him with the butt of a gun and sticks, stuck pins in his fingertips, cut his fingers and hands, and threatened to kill him. BT managed to flee the country and make his way to the United States, where he applied for asylum. The parallels to Dr. Baiev's case are apparent, except that BT provided care to the rebels only under duress.

An immigration judge granted BT's claim for asylum. The government appealed, arguing that BT had provided support to the Maoists in the form of medical care, and as a result was not eligible for asylum under its view of the law. According to its interpretation of new U.S. immigration laws, companions to draconian criminal laws, medical care for a designated terrorist organization amounted to "material support" for terrorism.

In a friend-of-the-court brief, colleagues and I argued that the Geneva Conventions precluded punishment or other adverse action against BT for adhering to his ethical obligations during the conflict. The Board of Immigration Appeals sided with the government and reversed the grant of asylum to BT. It stated that medical care was like any other form of material support for terrorism, such as arms or money. It wrote that BT's actions in providing care "that may have saved the lives of Maoist rebels clearly furthered the ability of the Maoists to continue in pursuit of their terrorist activities."[37] Happily for BT, four years after his initial application, the Department of Homeland Security granted him asylum, but only because his actions were coerced. It did not change its position that medical care could amount to material support for terrorism.

BT's case was a product of the transformation of global and domestic counterterrorism law and policy that began in the 1990s. Over the course of a decade, the tentacles of new laws reached into medical practice and humanitarian aid. In that decade, terrorist acts directed against the United States became a major national security, foreign policy, and political issue. In 1992, al-Qaeda carried out its first terrorist attack, on a hotel in Aden, Yemen. The following year, Ramzi Yousef orchestrated the first bombing of the World Trade Center, killing six people and injuring more than a thousand. The same year, eighteen U.S. servicemen were killed in Somalia after their Black Hawk helicopter was shot down. Congress responded in 1994 by enacting a tough counterterrorism law to criminalize "material support" for terrorist acts, such as arms, funding, housing, services, or transport. In 1996, it created a companion law prohibiting material support for foreign terrorist organizations and amended immigration law to preclude entry of individuals who provided such support. The amendments also removed an exception for humanitarian assistance to persons not directly involved in terrorist acts. In its place it enacted a limited exception for medicine.[38]

During the 1990s, though, the new laws were not applied to health workers, which is likely why Dr. Baiev's asylum application sailed through with relative ease. Others, too, including some who fought with military forces opposed to governments, were granted asylum.[39] Then came the attacks on the World Trade Center and Pentagon in September 2001. President George W. Bush called for a "war on terror." In that war, his administration considered the entire world to be a battlefield. New legislation gave the government vast new powers to seek out and punish alleged terrorists. Less than three weeks after the attacks of 9/11, Bush had little difficulty persuading the UN Security Council to adopt a broad counterterrorism resolution. It required member states to take decisive action to deter and punish terrorist acts and organizations. Among other provisions, the resolution demanded that governments criminalize a wide variety of forms of association with or support for terrorists and terrorist organizations. It required that refugee and asylum procedures be adjusted to ensure exclusion of members of terrorist organizations.[40] Because governments could not agree on definitions of terrorism or terrorist organizations, it was left to countries to decide for themselves. In addition, using its authority under the UN charter, the Security Council expanded tough, legally binding sanctions against specific terrorist organizations and countries. It set up elaborate machinery within the UN system to track whether governments were complying with the sanctions.[41] In two instances, the UN sanctions' committee cited medical activities as an element to justify the imposition of sanctions.[42] In 2004, the U.S. Congress again expanded its already tough counterterrorism laws and immigration restrictions.[43]

Before the enactment of the UN resolution, only 31 countries had terrorism-specific legislation; soon afterward, 109 countries adopted one or more new counterterrorism laws.[44] Counterterrorism provisions were also incorporated into immigration laws. Many of the new laws allowed punishment despite an absence of intent to help a group commit acts of terror. Some did not even require knowledge that the organization is designated as a terrorist group. The discretion to decide what acts could be deemed terrorist led to stunningly broad definitions. Egypt, for example, defined terrorist organizations to include any group that disrupts public order or threatens the safety, security, or interests of society; or harms or frightens individuals or threatens their lives, freedoms, rights, or security; or harms national unity.[45] The laws generally were not specific about designating medical treatment or humanitarian aid for terrorists as an offense, but like the counterterrorism laws of Serbia and Turkey, were so broad as to easily apply to it. The United Kingdom's law outlawed giving property to terrorists. Experts believe it could be applied to medical supplies used in treatment.[46] Australia's vastly expanded counterterrorism laws effectively proscribed sending funds for humanitarian assistance to some conflict areas or providing medical supplies to a hospital or funds to employ a doctor.[47]

The fervor often turned many good-faith actions, political protests, medical care, and humanitarian assistance, into crimes. The breadth of the law led prosecutors to apply them even in cases that could reduce terrorist threats. In 2010, one of these cases reached the U.S. Supreme Court. The case, *Holder v. Humanitarian Law Project*, involved a nonprofit group that sought to provide training and assistance in negotiating peace agreements, petitioning the UN, and advocating in a nonviolent manner, to the Liberation Tigers of Tamil Eelam in Sri Lanka and the Kurdistan Workers Party in Turkey, both of which were designated as foreign terrorist organizations.[48] The court acknowledged that the nonprofit group's intent was to promote lawful conduct by these groups and end vicious conflict. It nevertheless upheld the constitutionality of the government's broad interpretation of material support laws and the authority of the government to pursue the organization under counterterrorism law. Its reasoning well illustrates the new thinking about terrorism and the power granted governments by the new laws. In ruling for the government, the court endorsed the government's view that the proposed training might well provide legitimacy to the recipient groups and also free up resources they could use to commit terrorist acts. It demanded no evidence that there be a basis for this belief and opined that there was no need for the government to show how the particular form of support offered actually supported terrorism. Its mere possibility sufficed to outlaw the assistance.

It took little time for the new laws to be applied to medical care and for security forces to abuse health-care workers who offered care. In Ethiopia, doctors who refused orders to refrain from treating injured protesters were arrested. Five of them went missing and then disappeared. Pakistan's Counter Terrorism Department raided a medical center, where it arrested two alleged terrorists and three doctors who were treating them. The doctors were released only because the authorities finally acknowledged that they did not know that their patients were militants. In 2012, the Nigerian army and police personnel arrested Dr. Muhammad Mari Abba, after he met with officials from a World Health Organization program in Yobe state. He was suspected of providing treatment to members of the insurgent group Boko Haram. In Australia, a nurse was indicted for violations of counterterrorism laws for, among other things, providing medical services to the Islamic State.[49] In Iraq, doctors and nurses who were forced by ISIS to treat its fighters had terrorism charges brought against them.[50] Human Rights Watch reported that a nurse was sent to a displaced persons camp because she worked in an ISIS hospital during the occupation.[51]

In the United States, a New York physician named Rafiq Sabir, who also worked in Saudi Arabia, told an undercover FBI agent of his interest in providing medical assistance to wounded *mujahideen* in Saudi Arabia who sought to expel "infidels" from the Arabian peninsula. Sabir swore allegiance to al-Qaeda and gave his phone number in Riyadh to the undercover agent so that *mujahideen* needing medical assistance could reach him. A few days later, on May 28, 2005, Sabir was arrested and charged with using his medical skills under the direction and control of a foreign terrorist organization to further its illegal objectives. Sabir claimed medical care should not be punished because of the exception for "medicine" contained in the law. The court rejected that interpretation, holding that providing or administering medicine was not covered. It also held that criminal acts include "a range of conduct that may not be harmful in itself but that may assist, even indirectly," a terrorist group, "such as being a doctor on-call to treat wounded jihadists in Saudi Arabia."[52] He was convicted. Under U.S. counterterrorism law, moreover, an aid group medic could be charged with offering expert advice, which does not require proof that the medic worked under the direction and control of a terrorist organization.[53] Sabir is hardly a sympathetic figure in his zeal to serve al-Qaeda, but we should also recognize that he was never accused or convicted of participating in a terrorist act, aiding or abetting one, planning one, or having the intent to commit any of these acts. His only offense was offering medical services to the wounded, as the Geneva Conventions and human rights law permit. The conviction chilled the ability of doctors and nurses to work in any war zone where they might treat wounded civilians in an area, such as Gaza, which is controlled by a designated foreign terrorist organization, Hamas.

Colombia represents perhaps the most distressing case of the power of counterterrorism law to undermine the Geneva Conventions and 1977 Protocols. During the government's long war with the Revolutionary Armed Forces of Colombia (FARC), dozens of health workers were killed and many more were threatened. Some were kidnapped or disappeared.[54] In 2007, Colombia's Constitutional Court agreed to abide by the protocols, including the immunity they provide for health activities consistent with medical ethics. Nevertheless, after the decision, prosecutors continued to obtain convictions and imprisonment of physicians for the crime of rebellion for providing care for members of the FARC. In these cases, the courts so narrowly interpreted the requirements for medical immunity as to render them null. In one case, the Colombian Supreme Court of Justice upheld the conviction of a physician who referred FARC members for specialized care, reasoning that though the doctor's medical activities did not support the FARC, they could have strengthened the group, enabling it to fight against government forces.[55] In another case, the failure of Dr. Moreno García to report his offer of treatment to the FARC was considered evidence of criminal intent.[56] Colombia's Ministry of Health and Social Protection has sought to support and protect health workers by writing a manual on medical duties in armed conflict and situations of violence that asserts the right of health-care personnel not to be punished or prosecuted for medical activities. It is not clear, though, whether prosecutors will adhere to the manual.[57]

The foundations of these new laws starkly and profoundly conflict with the letter of the Geneva Conventions, including the obligations to treat all combatants without distinction based on affiliation and to refrain from punishment of health workers for offering care impartially. Additional Protocol 2 of the Geneva Conventions also recognized that armed groups may have their own medical units and personnel. More profoundly, the application of the new laws to health services implicitly repudiates the principle of humanity that underlies the conventions and the concept of human dignity that is the bedrock of human rights law. As Naz Modirzadeh, director of the Harvard Law School Program on International Law and Armed Conflict explained, international humanitarian law and counterterrorism law are based on contrasting paradigms. Under the former, care for the wounded and sick is not only legitimate, but mandatory, because it is based on respect for every human being and the corresponding obligation to prevent unnecessary suffering.[58] The new counterterrorism laws are based instead on the belief that national security is such an overriding priority that it legitimates disallowing any resources or succor, including the provision of medical care, to terrorists or people under their control.[59] The laws are a contemporary expression of Lieber's elevation of military necessity in a just war over the avoidance of harm to people not in combat.

At a deeper level, the counterterrorism paradigm endorses the dehumanization of people designated as terrorists: their suffering becomes irrelevant as the paradigm casts aside their status as human beings in favor of national security goals. At a conference in Geneva in 2019, this view was forthrightly expressed by a senior military official fighting an insurgency in Africa. He asserted that his military abided by the law, but that "to treat wounded terrorists is to support terrorism." His view is no different from those expressed by militaries and police in Turkey, Kosovo, Chechnya, and Afghanistan. Agnès Callamard, the UN Special Rapporteur on Arbitrary and Extrajudicial Executions, captured the impact of the new paradigm, writing that counterterrorism law was fast becoming "a monster that is devouring international law."[60] She might have added that it is devouring the foundations of that law as well.

The dehumanization inherent in the counterterrorism paradigm became apparent in a different context almost immediately after 9/11, when American military forces detained suspected terrorists in Afghanistan, Guantanamo Bay, and secret CIA detention facilities. In January 2002, the White House counsel, Alberto Gonzales, questioned the applicability of the

Geneva Conventions to detainees the United States labeled as terrorists. In a now-infamous memo, Gonzales wrote that the new paradigm of counterterrorism requires the "ability to quickly obtain information from a captured terrorist" to prevent future attacks, and "renders obsolete Geneva's strict limitations on questioning of enemy prisoners."[61] The idea that terrorists—actually, suspected terrorists—deserved the same respect as any other human being evaporated. The explicit goal of interrogation methods adopted by the Bush administration, moreover, was to strip the detainees of their humanity. The objective of CIA interrogations was to "psychologically 'dislocate' the detainee, maximize his feelings of vulnerability and helplessness, and reduce or eliminate his will to resist our efforts to obtain crucial intelligence."[62]

To further dehumanization, the CIA employed methods long recognized as torture, including sleep deprivation, isolation (often with the detainee naked), bombardment with constant loud noise, suspension by cables, and waterboarding. Medical personnel were expected to, and did, participate in these efforts to strip the detainees of their humanity. Physician and psychologist consultants advised interrogators how to exploit detainee physical and mental vulnerabilities as part of the interrogation process and inflict grievous pain and suffering on them, limited only by ensuring that the detainees did not die or be left with permanent physical injury.[63] The CIA also ordered that medical care to prisoners not be provided in a manner that could undermine the anxiety and dislocation interrogation techniques were designed to foster.[64]

The breadth as well as the conceptual foundations of the new counterterrorism laws have extended to denial of medical care and humanitarian aid to people who have nothing to do with terrorists and may even be its victims. The ICRC estimates that more than 60 million people live in areas controlled by armed groups, many of them designated as terrorist organizations.[65] The new laws severely restrict furnishing aid in areas controlled by designated terrorist organizations, on the theory that doing so would either provide them legitimacy or enhance their power. The laws also inhibit the ability of aid organizations to act impartially by restricting to whom and where they offer services. Forcing aid groups to depart from impartiality can jeopardize their security, as armed groups may become suspicious that they are spies or in league with their enemies.[66] Sometimes the very process of negotiating deals with insurgent groups to gain access to populations risks running afoul of laws or economic sanctions that prohibit interactions with terrorist groups. The resulting limitations and, from a recipient standpoint, arbitrariness of aid, can also lead people living in these areas to lose trust that the aid group is committed to meeting community needs. Yves Daccord, former director general of the International Committee of the Red Cross, noted that the trust of the population, "which is absolutely critical to demonstrate impartiality . . . is becoming a rarer commodity."[67] In addition to outright prohibitions on aid, both donor and host governments impose complex and burdensome bureaucratic rules to guarantee that aid does not reach alleged terrorist organizations. Aid groups must vet local staff and provide assurances that the individuals have no connections to terrorism. Their banks, also subject to laws imposing economic sanctions and prohibiting the financing of terrorism, are often even more cautious than the rules require, making it difficult for aid groups to transfer funds to pay local staff and suppliers. And all the rules have a chilling effect on humanitarian operations as aid groups seek to avoid reputational, financial, and legal risk if accused of breaching counterterrorism laws and regulations.

The result of these laws and policies became evident in Somalia, which in the first decade of the twenty-first century was experiencing severe drought and famine. In 2008, the United States designated the group al-Shabaab, which controlled a large swath of territory, as a terrorist organization. The designation stopped all new grants for humanitarian aid in areas al-Shabaab controlled and restricted the work of organizations then working in those areas. In 2009, the U.S. suspended $50 million in previously programmed humanitarian aid funds.[68] In 2010, the UN Security Council adopted its first and only resolution creating an exception to counterterrorism funding restrictions for humanitarian activities for work in Somalia, but it only applied to UN agencies and their implementing partners. The United States, moreover, did not recognize the exemption and imposed new funding constraints.[69] The following year a new drought hit East Africa and led ultimately to an even more severe famine. Although some of the counterterrorism restrictions in aid groups' funding were relaxed for a time, the humanitarian response was nevertheless severely hampered by the operational limitations, confusing restrictions, and funding shortfalls.[70] These restrictions, in turn, contributed to the already frayed relationships between humanitarian groups and al-Shabaab, which increasingly saw the aid groups as extensions of Western power and policy.[71] It also accused them of collecting data and lacking "political detachment and neutrality" and threw them out of areas it controlled.[72] More than a quarter of a million people died in the famine. It is impossible to know how many died as a result of the restrictions on humanitarian access based on counterterrorism measures, but the number is likely high.[73]

Since the Somalia famine, the restrictions continued and sometimes took bizarre forms. Nigeria made it exceedingly difficult for humanitarian organizations to reach four million people who live in regions under the control of Boko Haram. In 2017, Nigerian officials charged that MSF's medical activities were a threat to national security.[74] In 2018, the U.S. Agency for International Development's office in Nigeria imposed a new rule that any aid group it funds must obtain written agency approval for assistance to individuals associated with Boko Haram—including "individuals who may have been kidnaped by Boko Haram or ISIS-West Africa but held for periods of greater than six months." The rule denied or at least delayed help to those who may need it the most, such as the more than 1,000 children kidnapped since 2013, including 276 girls taken from a school in the town of Chibok in 2014.[75] Around the same time, the British government froze cash assistance to tens of thousands of people living in camps or informal settlements in northeast Syria, many of whom had fled their homes to escape ISIS.[76] In 2019, the Nigerian military forced the closure of regional offices of two groups, Mercy Corps and Action Against Hunger, for allegedly aiding Boko Haram and the Islamic State in West Africa Province.[77]

The elevation of counterterrorism priorities over health and humanitarian imperatives also seeped into the activities of military and intelligence agencies.[78] The most notorious example was a fake vaccination campaign in the search for Osama bin Laden. In 2011, the CIA was desperate to confirm that Osama bin Laden lived in a certain compound in Abbottabad, Pakistan. One of its schemes was the hiring of a local physician, Shakil Afridi, who was both experienced in vaccination campaigns and known to be ethically slippery, to run a faux Hepatitis B vaccination campaign in the region in the hopes of obtaining blood samples from the children living in the compound. Ruses that disguised its operatives as aid workers, journalists, or Peace Corps volunteers are generally against CIA policy because of their dire ramifications for legitimate and essential activities, but the rules were applied loosely after 9/11.[79] Dr. Afridi, masquerading as a representative of Save the Children, hired community health workers to go house to house, giving injections to children in the region over a six-month period.[80]

The scheme was as harebrained as it was destructive. Bin Laden, who took elaborate precautions to hide, would never have risked allowing blood to be taken from a family member. It would be apparent to anyone with knowledge of vaccination campaigns that it was fraudulent, as it wasn't conducted in accordance with public health principles, had no uniform protocols, and lacked any connection to the local health authorities.[81] Not surprisingly, Dr. Afridi never got blood from the bin Laden children. After the raid that killed bin Laden in May 2011, the CIA urged Dr. Afridi to flee Pakistan for his own safety, but naïvely, he remained. Within weeks after the raid, Pakistani investigators learned of his activities and arrested Dr. Afridi. He was initially charged with treason, but later tried only for an offense unrelated to the vaccination campaign.[82] He was convicted and sentenced to thirty-three years in prison, later reduced to twenty-three years. Leon Panetta, then head of the CIA, along with members of Congress, demanded his release for his assistance in trying to locate bin Laden, to no avail.

Far worse, when news of the fake vaccination campaign emerged, progress in Pakistan toward a global campaign to eradicate polio halted. Pakistan was one of three countries where the virus remains endemic. Even before the Afridi affair, rumors had already circulated widely in Pakistan, encouraged by the Pakistani Taliban, that vaccines were part of a

Western plot or caused sterility. In an instant, the raid sabotaged the painstaking work to counter the disinformation and vaccinate children. Save the Children's foreign staff was thrown out of Pakistan and polio vaccine campaigns were suspended. Later, the Pakistani Taliban issued a *fatwa* characterizing polio vaccination as poison and ordering them to shut down in areas it controlled. Even when campaigns were renewed, many people refused the vaccine as the CIA connection reinforced suspicions about its harms.

Because of the suspensions and resistance, more than three-and-a-half million children missed at least one dose of the vaccine. Polio immunization rates for children in Pakistan declined between 12 and 20 percent compared to earlier times.[83] About a year after the Afridi ruse, a new epidemic erupted in Pakistan: the assassination of vaccinators. By 2015, more than seventy community health workers, the vast majority of them women, and security officials seeking to protect them, in Pakistan had been murdered, mostly by the Pakistani Taliban.[84] Over the ensuing years, vaccination campaigns continued, but often had to be suspended for periods, or were limited in their reach because of violence or threats of violence. The disruptions led to an increase in polio cases that are likely attributable directly or indirectly to the CIA's fake campaign.[85] After a fierce outcry from the public health community, in 2012, the White House announced that the CIA would no longer make operational use of vaccination programs or vaccination workers or seek to obtain DNA through vaccination programs.[86]

For years, humanitarian and health organizations and human rights institutions have raised alarms about the primacy of counterterrorism norms in law, policy, and actions over principles of humanity and the right to health. In 2004, the Inter-American Commission on Human Rights lambasted Peru for prosecuting and convicting a Peruvian doctor of unlawful collaboration with terrorists for having provided medical care to members of the insurgent group Sendero Luminoso, or Shining Path.[87] Since then, though the restrictions have become ever more expansive and draconian, they are still justified without evidence as essential to fight terrorist groups.[88] Frequently heard rhetoric in UN meetings affirming the need to respect human rights and humanitarian law in the context of counterterrorism activities has had no discernable impact in practice.[89] An ever-mushrooming UN counterterrorism bureaucracy that monitors sanctions and addresses policy has been noncommittal on how to reconcile the new regime with humanitarian organizations' missions. The Office of the High Commissioner for Human Rights is the only UN agency that has aggressively opposed counterterrorism laws that hamper access to health care and compromise other rights, but it has been largely marginalized within the UN system.[90]

Some countries have grasped that prohibiting medical activities as part of counterterrorism strategy is irrational, cruel, and counterproductive: irrational, in that there is no evidence that medical care for populations or even terrorists fighters provides any discernible military benefit or enhances the power or capabilities of terrorist groups; cruel, insofar as medical services necessary to reduce human suffering are curtailed while the values of human rights and humanitarian law are ignored; and counterproductive, in providing a boost to terrorist groups to make the case that Western governments care little for people's needs. Some reforms have followed. New Zealand exempted services to alleged terrorists if they are provided solely to meet essential human needs, a position consistent with the principle of humanity. Canada decided not to apply its counterterrorism laws to armed conflict, leaving the Geneva Conventions and the 1977 Protocols as governing law. A 2017 revision to Afghanistan's penal code goes furthest of all in permitting health care without distinction. It states that no necessary medical procedures are to be considered crimes if they are carried out within the technical principles of the medical profession. Surgical procedures in emergencies are specifically exempted from punishment. A categorical protection for humanitarian aid groups was adopted in 2017 by the European Commission, which member states of the EU are required to enact into national law. The exemption does not apply, though, to local health care workers.[91]

Momentum also developed in the governing bodies of the UN to try to harmonize counterterrorism law and practice with the requirements of humanity and dignity as reflected in humanitarian and human rights law.

Through three presidential administrations, though, the United States has largely frustrated and often derailed efforts that might cast doubt on the legitimacy of its expansive approach to material support to terrorism. In December 2018, the United Nations General Assembly adopted a resolution that urged governments to ensure that "counter-terrorism legislation and measures do not impede humanitarian and medical activities or engagements with all relevant actors as foreseen by international humanitarian law."[92] It was the first specific reference to medical activities in a UN resolution on counterterrorism. The language is mild, leaving much ambiguity about its application.

Even so, the Trump administration tried to scuttle the proposal, and when it failed, the U.S. mission to the United Nations in New York, an arm of the State Department, issued a blistering statement condemning it. The statement argued that the resolution was an "unfair and thinly veiled attack against U.S. material support law."[93] Beyond expressing pique, the statement engaged in misdirection, characterizing the resolution as allowing "unrestricted delivery of humanitarian aid or other assistance to terrorist groups or individual terrorists." When it finally addressed the substance of the resolution, the statement claimed that governments had an obligation to prevent support for terrorism "even in the absence of a link to a terrorist act," and regardless of whether it was meant to advance goals of the terrorist organization—a likely allusion to the *Holder* case. That meant that support for aid and medical care groups that communicated with organizations deemed to be terrorist in nature or worked in territory controlled by these organizations should be forbidden. The statement in an international forum amounted to a repudiation of a hundred-and-fifty years of law that has required care for wounded and sick combatants, no matter who they are, what they have done, and regardless of the label placed on them, and outlawed punishment of those who offer it. In doing so, the United States government followed policies of Turkey in the 1980s, Serbia in the 1990s, and rogue security forces ever since.

The Trump administration may have lost in the General Assembly debate, where it was easily outvoted. The General Assembly resolution, though, was not binding; that authority rests with the Security Council. A few months later, the council considered a resolution on curbing the financing of terrorism. France and other countries pushed for an exemption similar to the one in the resolution adopted by the General Assembly. The Trump administration joined Russia in opposing the idea.[94] It threatened to veto the entire resolution if the provision was included. After difficult negotiations, a compromise was reached that was sufficiently weak and meaningless to gain its agreement. The resolution urges states to enact laws that are "consistent with" international humanitarian law and human rights law, and to "take into account the potential effect of" counterterrorism measures on "exclusively humanitarian activities, including medical activities, that are carried out by impartial humanitarian actors in a manner consistent with international law."[95] The phrase "consistent with" is not defined and resembles the vague and general language about complying with international humanitarian and human rights law in prior resolutions that had little impact on counterterrorism laws and practices. The phrase "take into account" imposes no specific obligations at all beyond reviewing potential impacts. The monster continues to devour. A statement by the president of the Security Council on the twentieth anniversary of the post 9/11 Security Council resolution mandating expansion of counterterrorism law repeated the same vague, nonspecific pablum it had recited for years, that counterterrorism measures should comply with international human rights and humanitarian law. It did not call for the end of criminalization of health care or severe restrictions on humanitarian aid that counterterrorism law imposed.[96]

# 4

## HEALTH CARE AS A
## STRATEGIC TARGET

———

### Syria

T HE REGIME OF President Bashar al-Assad was not the only one in the past half century to target hospitals and health workers as a strategy of war or repression. When Mozambique gained independence in 1975, the Apartheid regime in South Africa saw the country's multiracial, socialist government as a threat. As Mozambique had prioritized develop-ment of a responsive health system, South African-supported armed groups destroyed almost two hundred health posts and health centers, looted almost three hundred others, and murdered at least twenty health workers and kidnapped dozens more.[1] During El Salvador's civil war in the 1980s, government forces and armed groups viewed health services as a form of logistical or moral support to the opposing sides and ferociously attacked clinics and the medical community.[2] The trend continued in the decades since. In the civil war in South Sudan, the pattern of government-sponsored violence against health care suggests it was used a political mes-sage.[3] The Tatamadaw's conduct in Myanmar is yet another case.

None of these wars compare, however, to the sustained, ruthless, and relentlessly destructive campaign that ravaged hospitals and health workers in Syria beginning in 2011. From the start of the Arab Spring protests, Assad's security and intelligence forces assaulted regime oppo-nents, including in hospitals, and arrested and tortured doctors who clandestinely provided care to them. When Assad's repression led to war, the regime bombed and shelled hospitals, including makeshift field hospitals. In 2015 Russia joined in the attacks, which numbered more than six hundred by 2021. A doctor working to provide medical care in what would become opposition-controlled territory told me, "Working in a field hospital is like death."[4] This chapter traces the savagery of the strategy and the hand-wringing paralysis of the UN and the Obama administration in the face of atrocities that allowed them to continue, which was followed by indifference to war crimes by Donald Trump.

## SYRIAN SPRING

As throughout the Middle East, the Arab Spring protests in Syria began with peaceful demands and hopes for democratic reform that had already migrated from Tunisia to Egypt to Yemen. In Syria, the protests were fueled by police state oppression, the subjugation of the Sunni majority by the minority Alawite regime, severe sectarian tensions, rising economic inequality, declining agricultural productivity, and the movement of impoverished people to urban areas.[5] President Bashar al-Assad responded to the protests with ferocious repression by the notorious *Mukharbat*, the military intelligence agency that reports directly to the president, along with other security forces. They tortured teenage boys who scrawled anti-government graffiti on walls and shot and killed peaceful protestors. After some advisors urged Assad to be conciliatory, he went through the motions of meeting with reformers, but his strategy remained the use of lethal force against nonviolent protestors.[6] Six months into the demonstrations, the UN reported that the regime had already killed three thousand demonstrators.[7] By the end of 2011, the number killed reached five thousand.[8] Many thousands more were arrested, many of them tortured to death.

It quickly became apparent that protestors suffering gunshot wounds had to avoid hospitals. Regime snipers shot at the injured as they tried to enter civilian hospitals. If wounded people made it inside, security forces often beat patients in emergency rooms; intruded into surgical suites and intensive care units, where they ripped out IV and oxygen tubes and disconnected ventilators; and forcibly removed and arrested patients from the facilities.[9] They were often sent to military hospitals, notorious for their use of torture.[10] In one reported case, doctors had to beg the security forces to allow them to close a patient's abdominal cavity before he was taken away. Police demanded that hospital medical staff provide information on patients, sometimes beating nurses and doctors to get it.[11] Many health workers fled, sometimes leaving hospitals with severely depleted staff.[12] Proregime health workers, contemptuous of the protesters, often denied them treatment or joined in the abuses against patients.

To respond to the needs for emergency care and surgery, doctors who were either opposed to the regime or appalled by the assaults on the wounded began clandestine efforts to provide care. It was a dangerous choice. The regime's pervasive intelligence apparatus summoned health workers suspected of treating protesters for questioning at police stations or intelligence agency offices, where they risked arrest, detention, and torture.[13] In the hidden clinics, care remained challenging, not just because of the need for secrecy but because of the difficulties and risks in obtaining equipment and supplies. The nation's blood banks were run by the Ministry of Defense, so the makeshift clinics had to obtain blood on the black market. Even so, an underground medical network grew quickly.

Dr. Tayseer Alkarim was one of the leaders of this effort. He was four years into a prestigious oncology internship when the demonstrations began. Like many young Syrians, he thought political change was essential, and was now possible. He joined the nonviolent movement for Syrian democracy while participating in the medical response. His group, Doctors Coordinate of Damascus, was the largest of the medical relief organizations springing up in response to the crisis.[14] Now living in Paris, Dr. Alkarim told me that he and his colleagues improvised surgical suites in doctors' offices, clinics, and nonmedical spaces, including homes. In some private hospitals and clinics, Doctors Coordinate of Damascus paid for services in cash and sought to protect sympathetic staff by not revealing the patient's name. But at the major oncology center in Damascus where Dr. Alkarim was interning, the supervising physicians strongly identified with the regime and, he said, "were aggressive against all students who provided services to demonstrators."

The clandestine locations for medical care proved no match for Syria's ubiquitous security services. In August 2011, one of Dr. Alkarim's physician friends was captured by the regime and forced to reveal the names of medical colleagues offering care to the protestors. Word got back to Dr. Alkarim that he had been named. His wife immediately left Damascus for Turkey and he went underground, moving from house to house while still working as a physician and managing the work of other doctors and health care providers. Just before Christmas, however, after leaving a meeting of medical coordination groups, he was arrested, blindfolded, and put in a car, where he was beaten and kicked. Dr. Alkarim was among more than 250 doctors arrested early in the protests for treating wounded demonstrators, according to a local coordination committee. In Aleppo, Homs, Idlib, and Latakia, doctors were disappeared after they had treated injured protesters.[15] Dr. Alkarim was brought to Branch 15, the military intelligence detention facility that would soon become infamous for mass torture and killing. His clothes were taken away and he was interrogated about his medical colleagues. Dr. Alkarim tried to stall so that colleagues who had not yet been apprehended could have time to escape. The interrogators, onto his strategy, repeatedly beat him on the chest, head, legs, and back. He eventually was brought to a cell the size of a small bedroom, measuring about 3-by-3 meters, stuffed with about 40 other prisoners, and later moved to a larger room, 12-by-15 meters, but containing more than 120 prisoners. Doctors, 6 others, and 17 children were among them, the youngest child around 7 years old. For about two more months, Dr. Alkarim was repeatedly moved and finally brought before a military judge, who sent him to a military prison. During his incarceration he got seriously ill but was repeatedly denied any treatment.

At the time in Syria, only the highest ranked students got into medical school, but Dr. Alkarim's membership in an elite profession offered no protection. On the contrary, interrogators told him he was a traitor to the nation. "You studied for free," he was told, "and you stab us in the back." The corruption that was endemic to the regime saved him, as a lawyer bribed a judge to secure his release on bail. The judge told Dr. Alkarim to remain in his house pending further proceedings, but his lawyer advised him that if he wanted to stay alive, he should flee. For twenty-eight harrowing days, repeatedly switching cars and walking to avoid checkpoints and soldiers, he made it the mere hundred kilometers to the border with Jordan. Jordan's security forces wanted to send him back, but Dr. Alkarim told me that they saw how traumatized he was and allowed him to remain. After spending months recovering in Amman, he worked with humanitarian organizations to support medical care for Syrians who had also escaped. He then moved to Turkey to help organize the medical response in opposition-controlled areas of northern Syria. In 2014, he was advised that he was in danger and managed to make his way to Paris.

To formalize the basis for his and others' arrests, in 2012 the regime adopted a new law that defined terrorism as including any act to "disturb public security" by use of particular weapons or "by means of any tool that serves the same purpose."[16] Under that law, anyone who participated in demonstrations against the regime or provided medical services to protestors was deemed a terrorist, which had the effect of criminalizing all medical care in opposition areas. As I was writing this book, I learned that one of my own students at Johns Hopkins had been a victim of these same policies. Mohammad Darwish followed the path of both of his parents and began medical school in Syria well before the protests began. In March 2011, while still a student, as Arab Spring protests were taking place elsewhere, he organized a demonstration promoting democracy in Libya in front of its embassy in Damascus. The police did not interfere, but on March 16, when he and a half dozen other third-year medical students participated in a demonstration promoting reform in Syria, he was arrested. Blindfolded and handcuffed, he was brought to what he later learned was a military airport.

There he was forced onto his knees in a corridor and put in an excruciatingly painful kneeling position, where he remained on and off for four days. Periodically guards beat and kicked him. His captors denied him food and water for two days. When they learned he was a medical student, they demanded the names of others involved in demonstrations. Not wanting to implicate his colleagues, Dr. Darwish falsely denied knowing any other medical students involved in protests. His refusal led interrogators to employ electrical shocks on his elbows and knees that he told me "were like an explosion in my body." The pain was so intense that he "was not even able to scream." It was difficult to breathe. "I smelled flesh burning." Because of the beatings, he could barely walk and asked to see a doctor. When his request was finally granted, the doctor slapped him, saying something like, "Does that make you feel better?" When finally put into a tiny cell with eleven others, he felt lucky to be out of the corridor and away from the arbitrary beatings.

Dr. Darwish learned from a cellmate that his medical student colleagues had been released and, along with his parents, were frantically looking for him. They had also started a campaign for his release, resulting in Amnesty International including him in its list of protesters whose release it sought.[17] The campaign apparently succeeded, as after four weeks in detention Dr. Darwish was released, though not before the general in charge of the detainees showed Dr. Darwish his gun and said, "You will not be arrested again." After his release, Dr. Darwish completed his schooling while clandestinely participating in medical care for wounded protesters. After graduation he was hired by the Syrian affiliate of the Palestine Red Crescent Society (which mostly served Palestinian refugees in Syria). Its association with the international Red Cross/Red Crescent movement offered a modicum of protection from arrest. He remained with the organization until 2016, when a routine stop at a checkpoint almost led to his arrest. He knew he had to leave the country. Like Dr. Alkarim, he navigated a frightening route out of Syria and shortly began employment with the Lebanon branch of the Palestine Red Crescent Society. In response to the catastrophic war in Syria, Michael Klag, then dean of the Johns Hopkins Bloomberg School of Public Health, established a scholarship program for Syrians to come to the school to study toward a master's degree in public health. The first scholarship was awarded to Dr. Darwish.

During his studies and subsequent research position at Johns Hopkins, Dr. Darwish never spoke to me of his arrest and detention until it came up by chance in a conversation. He just didn't think it was important to share the story but was not reluctant to convey his experience. He seemed remarkably unscarred by his torture, perhaps an example of the resilience often observed among some survivors of torture with strong political or ideological commitments.[18] Maybe his easygoing personality helped too. Many other Syrian physicians were, however, deeply traumatized by the sudden turn in their lives from enjoying prestigious careers to being labeled as criminals subjected to arrest and torture, and experiencing the bombing of hospitals where they worked. In 2014, I traveled to Gaziantep, Turkey, to speak with twenty-five health workers who were based in opposition-controlled areas of northwest Syria to learn about their experiences trying to practice medicine while under assault. I had been invited by Dr. Zaher Sahloul, then-president of the Syrian American Medical Society, who I had gotten to know because of his advocacy to protect health workers and civilians in Syria. Dr. Sahloul and his colleagues had transformed the organization from what once had been essentially a social club for expatriate Syrian doctors in the United States into a major humanitarian aid and support organization for health care in opposition-controlled areas of Syria. These expatriate Syrian physicians, along with medical colleagues who had emigrated to Europe, offered training and telemedicine consultations and came to Syria to work side-by-side with colleagues who remained. It was one such training that brought the health workers and me to Gaziantep.

Gaziantep, a thriving and modern city of around two million people, is about sixty miles from Aleppo, and in 2014 was already home to more than a quarter of a million Syrian refugees. Because of its proximity to Syria, it quickly became the base for most humanitarian organizations serving opposition-controlled areas of northwestern Syria. The hotel where I stayed, with its generic décor and function rooms in various shades of beige, could have been plucked out of any city in the United States. Syrian influence in the city, though, was everywhere. At the Topkapi restaurant, a gathering place for Syrians in Gaziantep, Arabic was the dominant language. Syrians told me that Gaziantep's old city, with its labyrinthine market and multicultural architectural styles dating back more than a thousand years, reminded them of Aleppo. The Gaziantep region produces the world's best pistachios, the central ingredient for its baklava, and produces 90 percent of the delicious pastry made in Turkey. More than a hundred stores in the city sell it. But there was an undercurrent of menace in Gaziantep because of its proximity to the Syrian border and an active commercial airport that made it a transit point for young men and women seeking to fight for the Islamic State. The hotel's laconic guard, ineffectual metal detector, and the busy cafes next to and across the street, suggested, though, that local residents and Syrian refugees were either indifferent to or refused to be daunted by the potential danger. And it was certainly an oasis compared to Syria, having a bountiful supply of reliable electricity and ample food—which were by then luxuries in northwest Syria.

The twenty-five Syrian health workers with whom I spoke were mostly young, as by then the most experienced doctors opposed to the Assad regime had the resources to leave the country. Six of the men I interviewed (only a handful of women were at the training) had been arrested and tortured; others had narrowly escaped. Two were detained because they had participated in demonstrations, and another because he had carried a sign with the names of other doctors who had previously been arrested. Others were incarcerated because they had or were suspected of having worked in makeshift field hospitals to provide care to wounded protesters. A pharmacist who established first-aid clinics in Idlib was deemed to be a terrorist. The men were subjected to beatings, electric shocks, and terrifying threats. A thoracic surgeon (I did not record their names for security reasons) told me that after he was arrested in 2012, interrogators demanded to know whether he moonlighted from his public hospital job in one of the clandestine facilities. Their suspicions were correct, but he refused to admit to the truth, even under torture that included electric shock and forced standing for twenty hours. "They told me that if I didn't admit to working in a field hospital, they would torture me more," he said, "but I did not for fear they would kill me." He felt fortunate that his supervisor at the public hospital protected him when questioned, and he was released. Another health worker arrested at a checkpoint reported similarly: "The most important thing was not to reveal my role in medical work."[19]

The health workers reported other close calls. A dentist reported that Syrian Air Force soldiers raided a field hospital where he worked and killed ten patients and two health workers. He luckily survived shots to his leg and hand. He was arrested and brought to a detention facility, where he was held for five months. He told me that what saved him was that the huge but fragmented security apparatus didn't coordinate its agencies well. "The Air Force group that arrested me didn't communicate with the interrogators, so the interrogator didn't know that I had medical training," the dentist explained. In still another case, the director of a field hospital escaped after being warned by a friendly soldier of his impending arrest. Security forces learned of the tip and killed the soldier. Human rights investigators heard similar stories.[20]

## HOSPITALS IN GUNSIGHTS

"We are under great danger of being killed or injured any time," the director of the Idlib Health Directorate, which coordinated services in opposition-held areas of the governate, told me during my trip to Gaziantep in 2014. "All the time and any time: in the morning, in the evening. You don't know if you are going to wake up or not," he said. He was speaking of the regime's missile attacks on and bombing and shelling of hospitals. They began in August 2011, even before the prodemocracy movement had led to armed conflict. In Hama, in western Syria, where protests were strong, Assad's military forces fired missiles at al-Hourani Hospital, destroying the intensive care unit.[21] As the regime's violence against protestors continued, groups began taking up arms against it. They were initially composed of individuals seeking political reform, but over time other groups, including jihadist organizations and the Islamic State, entered the conflict. Gulf countries, Iran, Hezbollah, Russia, the United

States, and others provided weapons, funds, and in some cases military forces, pursuing their own objectives and increasing the lethality of the war.

Syrian missiles, shelling, mortar fire, and bombings of hospitals soon become a barbaric routine in contested regions of the country. The Assad strategy was executed on a vast scale, never before seen. He attacked eight hospitals by the end of 2011, and ninety more in 2012.[22] The World Health Organization reported at the end of 2012 that 78 percent of ambulances had been damaged and more than half were out of service.[23] By fall 2013, an independent commission established by the UN Human Rights Council found that "deliberate targeting of hospitals" is "one of the most alarming features of the Syrian conflict."[24] When I came to Gaziantep in October 2014, Physicians for Human Rights, which had begun tracking attacks on hospitals, had documented 194 attacks on 155 separate hospitals, almost all by the regime.[25] In mid-2014, the World Health Organization reported that only 40 percent of public hospitals were fully functioning (and that included hospitals in regime areas, where hospitals were mostly intact).[26]

The Syrian military by then had added barrel bombs to its arsenal. These consisted of oil-drum sized containers filled with explosives, bolts, and other metal objects, often dropped from helicopters hovering directly above the target. The blast force of this primitive but powerful weapon forced shrapnel deep into every area of the body, and often severed limbs. The regime used barrel bombs thirty times in attacks on hospitals by mid-2014. Through 2016, more than seventy-five hundred Syrians had been killed by barrel bombs, almost all of them civilians, and more than a quarter of them children.[27] The regime also obstructed health care in opposition-controlled areas. After an outbreak of polio, the regime neither organized vaccination campaigns in those areas nor provided vaccines to groups organizing immunization programs. By 2014, vaccination coverage dropped from 83 to 52 percent, with almost all of the difference accounted for in opposition-controlled areas.[28]

The regime had also begun sieges of some areas held by the opposition, severely restricting movement of food, medicine goods, and supplies, and attacking aid convoys. Around the time of my 2014 interviews, the UN's humanitarian office estimated that more than two hundred thousand people were trapped in eleven besieged areas, facing malnutrition and even starvation.[29] One doctor I interviewed was caught with medical supplies in his car in a besieged area, an act deemed a crime by the regime, and only saved by bribery and good fortune. He knew of twenty-eight others who were arrested for carrying medicines. In one of the besieged areas, Eastern Ghouta, in the summer of 2013, the regime launched a chemical attack that killed more than fourteen hundred people, including more than four hundred children. Hundreds more chemical attacks were to follow. Around the same time, some radical groups had begun kidnapping and murdering Western journalists and aid workers, forcing international aid organizations to withdraw staff, leaving Syrian health workers bereft of outside personnel resources.

The combination of war and the destruction of the health system caused a health crisis. Diseases that were once rare, including typhoid fever, measles, and leishmaniasis, reappeared. Chronic malnutrition became widespread. The use of explosives in civilian areas led to more than six hundred thousand people suffering traumatic injuries, a figure that would soon rise to more than a million, even as hospital capacity for surgery plummeted.[30] To address the crisis, Syrians in opposition-controlled areas responded with purpose and alacrity. They set up ad hoc administrative structures to manage health care services. By 2014, these had evolved into directorates that, to a greater or lesser extent, coordinated services. Another indigenous Syrian organization, the Assistance Coordination Unit, with support of international and Syrian NGOs, created a Polio Control Task Force to organize a vaccination campaign in opposition-controlled areas in response to the outbreak. Although initially hindered by a lack of access to vaccines, the campaign managed to reach a million children in opposition-controlled areas, including places ISIS governed.[31] Even so, tensions among directorates and other entities claiming responsibility to coordinate services added to the burdens afflicting health care.[32]

One of the most successful of the health directorates in organizing services was in the rural areas of the Idlib governate (the regime controlled the city of Idlib). In Gaziantep, I spoke to its director about the challenges he and his colleagues faced. An orthopedist originally from Aleppo, he coordinated the work of thirty-eight hospitals, many of them field hospitals opened in schools, municipal buildings, houses, and even chicken coops. The ad hoc health system included ten primary care centers and more than a hundred medical posts that offered basic services, a blood-bank system, and an ambulance service. He also coordinated distribution of medication and supplies and established protocols for practice at the facilities. His work was a valiant response to the health crisis that enveloped opposition-held parts of Syria, but also a precarious one. The once-several-thousand-member medical staff in the area had been reduced to 250 health workers to serve a population that was then of more than 2,000,000 people, 750,000 of whom had been displaced from other parts of Syria. Electricity for the facilities came only from generators, and fuel often ran short to support surgery for the thousands of traumatic injuries a month. Appropriate medical instruments were lacking. The entire directorate had no intensive care unit and insufficient numbers of incubators for high-risk newborns. Doctors told me that more babies were dying from complications from the increasing number of home births, as women feared either getting killed en route to hospitals, or dying in an attack after arriving there.[33]

His most wrenching challenge, though, was coping with the regularity of air and missile strikes on hospitals in the governate. He told me that more than a third of the hospitals in the region had been attacked in the year before we spoke, some of them multiple times. He was present during two attacks, one of them inflicted on a new orthopedic center on the very day it was scheduled to open. "One of the staff was standing in the door of the orthopedic center, and he died that day," he said. Months later, the same facility was attacked again, closed for a week while repairs were made, and then reopened. Transporting patients was also dangerous, he told me. "There were many cases when ambulance drivers have been attacked, especially at night in the dark," where aircraft monitoring the area "see the lights of the ambulance and attack." Ambulances were so vulnerable from sniper attacks, he said, "You get used to it."

But not really. The health workers, working long and exhausting shifts, coping with complex injuries and shortages of supplies, staff, and medication, and in constant danger, suffered a huge toll physically and psychologically. The crushing workload of too many injured people needing attention from too few staff led to tensions with their families because of low (or no) pay and exposure to violence. They also suffered what bioethicists call moral distress, where health providers know what the medically appropriate and ethical course of action is, but because of external or internal constraints cannot take it.[34] "You are not doing what you should," the orthopedist said. As a result, "we are demoralized and burned out." He personally felt vulnerable because of his role in developing a health system outside government control. He never traveled alone anymore. Despite his accomplishments in organizing a functioning health system, the director told me, "I am thinking of leaving."[35] He did not. Remarkably, six years later, when Idlib became the epicenter of the conflict, he was still running the directorate, having built it into a large and sophisticated operation.

At the time of my interviews, the needs, burdens, and risks of providing care in opposition-controlled areas of Aleppo were even greater than in Idlib. During the first half of 2014, Syrian government forces launched 650 impact strikes in areas of Aleppo controlled by nonstate armed groups, frequently with barrel bombs.[36] More than 1,200 children there were killed by them.[37] Six doctors and a surgical assistant I interviewed had each been present when their facility was attacked. Some of the hospitals were destroyed; others suffered major damage. One surgeon told me he had to move from one hospital to another as each was damaged or destroyed. Two of his colleagues had been killed in an attack on an ambulance two weeks before we spoke. Hospitals had become so dangerous that many patients either wouldn't come for treatment or sought early discharge before they were medically ready. One doctor told me, "Lots of people don't dare to go to the hospital, because they know that the hospital has been targeted by the bombardment—five, six times. It's only those who are in grave need who will go to the hospital."[38]

Even as the attacks damaged hospitals, the staff was deluged by the medical needs. The Aleppo Medical Council reported that its five main field hospitals treated more than seventy thousand people in 2013 and performed ten thousand surgeries.[39] The complexity of the injuries and the shortages of staff and supplies added to the burdens. Clinicians' emotions as well as skills were overwhelmed by the injuries they saw, especially those from barrel bombs. One doctor told me, "I have seen ruptured spleens and shrapnel the size of a human hand." Another surgeon said, "I have never seen such injuries." Still another recalled his own sense of horror: "I saw a mother and daughter whose bodies were blown apart, but their hands were still clasped together."[40] The disruptions from the bombing, meanwhile, radically interfered with already difficult operations even when a hospital was able to keep functioning. One doctor told me that while he was operating on a patient, a barrel bomb hit the hospital, shattering windows, breaking doors, and ripping bricks off the façade. The generator needed for the operation stopped, but "twenty minutes later, we got the generator going and I returned to the operation."[41] Parts of Aleppo had no running water, many pharmacies had closed, and dialysis centers could only operate with dramatically restricted hours as there was only limited fuel for electricity. Only about two dozen general or orthopedic surgeons remained, and anesthesiologists and vascular surgeons were gone. Dentists often stepped in to learn surgery on the job.[42] Armed groups in the area often added to the tension, pressure, and moral distress of hospital staff by demanding priority care for their troops, often threatening doctors and nurses with death if they didn't get it.[43] I found it hard to grasp how they persevered.

Like those in Idlib, doctors in Aleppo were traumatized. No security measures or international support could alleviate the demoralization, fear, overwork, and feelings of inadequacy in not being able to do the jobs for which they had been trained. David Nott, a British surgeon who volunteered in Aleppo in 2014, was aghast at the injuries he saw from the barrel bombs and other ordnance. His expertise in complex war surgery often proved futile. His searing six weeks there led to a breakdown when he returned to London, marked by fits of crying, staring at the ceiling, and lying in a fetal position.[44] Many Syrian doctors, nurses, and other health workers spent years working in these conditions. They rarely received any psychological support.[45] As in other protracted conflicts, they coped through religious faith, professional commitment, a sense of solidarity with the communities they served, practical measures to enhance their own security, and improvisation in the face of lack of supplies and staff.[46] Over time, factors that have been found elsewhere to contribute to higher morale, such as training and increased availability of better supplies, helped.[47] Mostly, though, they simply endured and persevered despite their trauma.

Why were hospitals and doctors targeted? "In Syria," the Idlib health director said, "the best students go to medical school, which then gives them a kind of social status. That status is what makes the regime concerned about them. And with the regime's goal of destroying the areas that are not under its control, the doctors are targeted more than others." Other Syrian doctors shared that view: as leaders in the community, they were singled out. No doubt there is truth in that explanation. There are other likely reasons for the regime's repeated targeting of hospitals and doctors. The Human Rights Council's independent commission on Syria identified one: that "the pattern of attacks indicates that Government forces deliberately targeted hospitals and medical units to gain military advantage by depriving anti-Government armed groups and their perceived supporters of medical assistance."[48] Without hospitals and doctors, people couldn't survive the shelling and the bombing and unending traumatic injuries. The destruction of hospitals and health services also was likely part of a strategy to demonstrate the futility of supporting opposition forces, to compel local populations to move, and to demoralize armed groups seeking to try to maintain services in areas they controlled. These purposes were also reflected in the grotesque, persistent war crimes the regime committed to destroy the opposition and their supporters, including bombing and shelling markets, using "double-tap" tactics that targeted rescuers after an initial attack, employing chemical weapons, encircling highly populated areas that led to starvation, and detaining and likely torturing more than one hundred thousand people, thousands of them to death. Through 2018, more than one hundred thousand civilians in opposition-controlled areas in Syria were killed by the regime, mostly from bombing and shelling. They represented more than 70 percent of all violent deaths in the war and included at least thirteen thousand children. Three-quarters of the deaths from explosive weapons were in dense, urban areas.[49]

At the time of interviews in Gaziantep in 2014, neither the doctors with whom I spoke, nor I, imagined then that the war, and the assaults on civilians and hospitals, would grind on for many years to come. The following year, as Syria's military capacity was wearing out, Russia entered the conflict to stave off the possibility of defeat and contributed to the carnage. In the final regime assault on opposition-controlled areas of Aleppo in the second half of 2016, the regime's air force and Russian planes attacked hospitals seventy-three times. Health care in Aleppo deteriorated further.[50] Only eleven ambulances remained in the city. Means of transporting people to hospitals were nearly impossible to find.[51] Doctors who had struggled for five years to serve the people of Aleppo had to flee. By then, the correlation between airstrikes on hospitals and military strategy had become even clearer, and would be repeated in campaigns for eastern Ghouta in late 2017 and 2018 and offensives in northwest Syria in 2019.[52]

In June 2017 I returned to Gaziantep, this time as part of a collaboration among Johns Hopkins, the Syrian American Medical Society, and the International Rescue Committee to help health workers respond to the impossible ethical challenges they faced in the extreme circumstances in which they had to work.[53] Some of the health workers were now refugees from Aleppo; others had again come to the city from Syria for training. Many of them had now been practicing 6 years under duress and assault. By then Syria, with help from Russia, had launched more than 450 attacks on more than 300 medical facilities and killed almost 800 medical personnel. In 2016 and 2017, they attacked ambulances more than 200 times, most using air-to-surface missiles or shelling. Almost 150 of these involved double-tap attacks.[54] To increase their safety, Syrians had moved almost 100 field hospitals to basements, underground, and even into caves in the side of a mountain.[55] Syria and Russia responded with "bunker buster" bombs that could penetrate below the ground to reach fortified and underground hospitals.[56] Two months before my trip to Gaziantep, Syria had launched a chemical attack in the town of Khan Shaykhun, in the Idlib governate. It was the largest such attack since 2013. A UN investigation determined that on impact, a chemical bomb from a Syrian airstrike released sarin, a highly toxic but odorless nerve agent.[57] It killed almost 100 people and injured more than 500 others.

Gaziantep in 2017 was much safer than it was in 2014. The Islamic State was being pushed back from the territory it had controlled in Syria and Iraq, so the city was no longer a major transit point for its fighters. It was Ramadan, and each night the group went back to the Topkapi restaurant for a long celebratory evening meal, full of Syrian delicacies, and to enjoy a momentary respite from the violence and deprivation so close at hand. But the trauma the health workers had endured was obvious. One of the doctors, middle-aged, distinguished-looking, and calm, and with seventeen years of experience, was an anomaly among his peers in having stayed inside Syria until the fall of Aleppo. He had been very well-off before the war, living in an upscale area of Aleppo, and had owned a farm and an expensive car. In 2011, as the regime ratcheted up its violence against demonstrators and doctors who treated their injuries, he had joined many of his colleagues in leaving for Turkey. But he didn't stay long. "I was confused for three days," he recalled, "should I start the job or not start the job [in Aleppo]. If yes, it would be a risk." But he decided that someone had to help. "There are people facing [death], and there is no one to help them. You have to decide if you can do anything or not do anything," he said. "I decided that in fact I lived in this country, I studied in it and lived in it twenty years as a doctor . . . I must do something." He moved back to Aleppo where, from the first day, he saw large numbers of people with severe injuries. He helped organize the Aleppo Medical Council. Until the 2016 battle for the city, cross-border aid provided hospitals with much-needed supplies and equipment such as ultrasound and CT scanners, and a blood bank was functioning. He learned cardiac surgery and received training from medical NGOs in Turkey in dealing with complex traumatic injuries. Some other specialists returned to Aleppo to help. As more women feared going to hospitals to give birth, more community midwives were trained to deal with complications in childbirth.[58]

The need to make wrenching decisions continued. The doctors adopted grim triage standards, emphasizing survival chances, not the traditional standard of prioritizing those with the most severe injuries. He said, "You can't help forty war-wounded at the same time, you provide aid for cases you can help," he said. "You are a doctor, you want to save as many people [as] you can. . . . It was the hardest and most painful moment to feel you have to let people die because you can't serve all in need." He faced distraught parents who begged for surgery for their severely wounded child. All too often, he had to refuse them. "We didn't have the resources or staff to save them," he said. Another doctor told me of a time when he needed to tell a distraught father that the fuel for a generator to power an incubator to save his premature baby had to be used for other patients. He remained haunted by it years after the fact. The doctors also had to weigh seemingly bizarre choices: whether patients were better off staying in the hospital to recover properly, or being discharged to avoid the chance of being bombed, despite the risks of going home before medically indicated.[59]

The strain took an ever-greater emotional toll on the doctors and their families. The surgeon took painkillers to sleep, as he was haunted by the injuries he saw and his inability to save so many of the wounded. He also had to make decisions about how much risk he should take, and how his decisions about taking those risks affected his family. "I pulled my children from home and brought them to the countryside in order [to] not be at risk," he said. As they begged him to leave the hospital, family relations became strained. By 2016, he and his colleagues were bereft of any glimmer of hope. They just continued to work. He said, "You have to go on, many times as I was in the operating room, the hospital was bombed, and we resumed working." His work in Syria didn't end until the regime began its final assault on opposition-controlled eastern Aleppo. Like other doctors and hundreds of thousands of others, he finally fled to Turkey.

The despair the health workers conveyed was pervasive. A physician told one of my colleagues on the project, "I am subjected to constant punishment and self-lashing continuously without interruption. I am actually doing humanitarian work and helping the wounded and save the lives of people, but the situation continues. Every day someone dies—we cannot save lives because there is no possibility." He tried to convey the unfathomable burden of the years of strain. "We have been living in this state for many years. Sometimes I think really, how do I eat, drink, and live, and think about the bombing and the people who died, with the sense that my mind will explode. . . . When a wounded [person] dies and his family starts weeping on him in the hospital, I feel guilty, sometimes I feel that I killed him because I could not help."[60] Female health workers had to cope with additional pressures, such as needing accompaniment for travel in rural areas and prohibitions on touching a male patient, denial of equal salaries and appointment to senior positions, and lack of respect for their professionalism. One woman said that the prevailing attitude was that "female doctors do not know as much as male doctors."[61]

The doctors had also been deeply affected by their fellow physicians' experience in trying to cope with a chemical attack in April 2017 in the town of Khan Shaykhun in southern Idlib. After I returned from Gaziantep, my colleague Diana Rayes interviewed five health professionals who had been at the site of the attack about their frustrating and painful efforts to respond. At the time of the interviews, they were also still reeling from the recent death of one of their colleagues, Dr. Ali Darwish, an orthopedic surgeon, in Latamnah Hospital, which was built into the side of a mountain in Hama, a half-hour's drive from Khan Shaykhun, as a result of another chemical attack. A bomb with sarin detonated at the hospital entrance. The cave's ventilation system was not adequate to prevent it from seeping deep into the hospital. Dr. Darwish wanted to complete an operation but lost consciousness as he worked, and later died from the exposure.

A pharmacist who responded to the Khan Shaykhun chemical attack told Diana that it had been preceded by airstrikes on targets in the town. When he arrived in Khan Shaykhun, he said, "nobody was in the street, and it smelled like death." A surgeon whose family lived in the town rushed to try to help. When the surgeon arrived in Khan Shaykhun, "it was like a city of ghosts, a very emotional scene, people were frightened, afraid to leave their homes. . . . Everyone was afraid of a second chemical attack." He stopped at hospitals in the region where victims were taken, one of which had been mostly destroyed a few days before, but whose emergency department was reopened to try to help victims. The scene at one of the hospitals was chaotic. The only masks available were designed for dust, not chemical agents. A pharmacist told Diana that damage to another hospital from the airstrikes and sarin forced it to suspend operations. At another, he said, "We found that the staff escaped the hospital, you can still see the smoke getting out of the hospital, no one is there. Some of the hospital staff got injured and they received urgent care."

The surgeon distributed medications at each hospital. By then, however, many of the victims had already died, and some emergency responders who came to help and had no protective equipment were themselves injured by breathing the toxic gas.[62] He told the story of a woman and six children found dead in their basement. They showed signs of the cause of death and indications of their suffering: suffocation and bruising, foam coming out of their mouths, prominent pupils. The surgeon explained what likely happened. "They were near the attacked area so they took shelter assuming it was a standard air strike. People in this town, especially in the northern district, are used to air strikes and they usually go hide in the basements when the air strike starts." It was a sensible, but fatal decision. He said that as sarin is heavy, "people hiding in the basements die first; this is what happened with that family we found."

Much of the medical effort proved futile. One doctor explained, "I think that medical providers barely saved 1 to 2 percent of the chemical attack victims. We have no prior training, medical staff, or equipment to deal with it. I believe that what we were able to provide was too little."[63] The chemical attacks demoralized the medical community even further. The surgeon who worked in a cave hospital said, "It had a big effect on creating a hopeless environment. . . . We fear being victims of the attack and not finding anyone to rescue us." Another surgeon, who had worked throughout the war, said the fear and, with it, loss of hope, reached new depths. Another doctor said, "Although we have a lot of experiences with bombs and other aerial weapons, we never had to stop working, thank God. We lost all hope when chemical weapons started being used. . . . we no longer felt safe in the cave." Many felt abandoned. One said, "death has become normal to the rest of the world, no one is reacting." Diana was shaken by these interviews, later recalling "the devastation in their voices, the apathy they felt toward the international humanitarian system, and above all, their unwavering faith in God and the destiny he had ordained for them." In the aftermath of the attack, NGOs and international agencies provided more protective equipment, antidotes, and training to respond to chemical attacks. But the psychological trauma suffered by the doctors and other health professionals persisted.

Meanwhile, the years-long siege of Eastern Ghouta, just a few miles outside Damascus and home to four hundred thousand people, continued. The regime repeatedly blocked humanitarian convoys, including medical supplies, and obstructed UN efforts to gain access; between November 2017 and the end of February 2018 only one convoy reached the city. Throughout the war, the UN often deferred to the regime's decisions on access to besieged areas, allowing itself to be manipulated and undermined, to the detriment of the health of hundreds of thousands of people in dire need.[64] In December 2017, Dr. Imad Al-Kabbani, director of health for opposition-controlled parts of Damascus and rural Damascus, perhaps best expressed the overwhelming despair doctors felt. In an appeal to the director general of the World Health Organization, he wrote, "Once, we were family doctors, pediatricians, specialists . . . now we are specialists in war trauma, chemical attacks, and siege-induced starvation." He continued, "We are facing an intolerable situation, artificially created by the Syrian government as a collective punishment for all civilians. The siege of Ghouta, together with systematic attacks on healthcare and the attendant silence of the UN, threaten not only our patients' lives but also our hope for our patients, our mental health, and our profession."[65]

In 2018, the regime launched a new offensive against Eastern Ghouta, dubbed "Operation Damascus Steel," which included what Amnesty International called "war crimes on an epic scale."[66] It sent more than 130 air strikes, along with barrel bombs, missile attacks, and artillery fire against the city. The assaults hit twenty-five hospitals. With remaining facilities overwhelmed and undersupplied, often operating while damaged, a doctor was quoted as saying, "The word 'catastrophe' can't describe what's happening."[67] Late that month, the UN Security Council called for a thirty-day humanitarian pause to allow supplies to enter, but the regime continued to obstruct and delay, allowing a few trucks in but removing medical supplies from them. The end came in April, after more attacks including chemical weapons. Two months later, a UN investigative commission reviewed the events of the siege and found pervasive war crimes and crimes against humanity, including deliberate starvation of the population and systematic targeting of health facilities.[68]

## GLOBAL PARALYSIS

Assad's regime, devoid of institutions that could restrain his depredations, and characterized by the arrest and torture of any critics, meant that concerted international action alone had any hope of curbing these violations. With military support from Russia and Iran, and having diplomatic protection through Russia's veto power at the UN Security Council, other nations' condemnations and economic sanctions had little effect. Only some form of sustained support for protection of civilians or direct military action against him might have curbed his atrocities. Still, from the start, Bashar al-Assad recast himself as a victim. During the period of peaceful protests seeking reform, he asserted that the demonstrators were not prodemocracy but part of a foreign conspiracy. He soon adopted the rhetoric of counterterrorism, labeling his opponents terrorists. In 2019, his ambassador to the UN acknowledged that the regime attacked some hospitals, but only because they had been "taken over by terrorist groups" as military posts, prisons, and arms depots, and were thus no longer functioning as hospitals. He also claimed that terrorist groups targeted hospitals.[69] All the evidence contradicted those claims.[70] Atrocities in Syria were documented contemporaneously as in no previous conflict. In addition to testimonial evidence, international and Syrian NGOs, investigators from the media, and the UN and flight trackers relied on real-time video, satellite imagery, analysis of soil samples, apps for data collection, and even cockpit transmissions. Courageous Syrians smuggled out hundreds of thousands of photos of men tortured in Syrian detention facilities. The UN General Assembly established a special unit to collect evidence of war crimes and crimes against humanity for possible prosecution.

The overwhelming evidence provided ample foundation for international action to protect Syrians from the worst of the horrors inflicted on them. When we returned from the 2014 Gaziantep trip, Dr. Sahloul and I wrote an op-ed that we managed to place in the *New York Times* recounting the health workers' experiences.[71] Like other efforts to stimulate action to protect Syrians from the ongoing atrocities, it was to no avail. The increasing global knowledge of what was taking place in Syria led to outcries by human rights organizations and investigators, but by then atrocities in Syria had become so common that the ones we reported were just added to the list. One of the doctors I interviewed in 2014 had asked me, "Why do nations abandon us?"

Certainly, global mechanisms had been established in the years before the war in Syria to address mass atrocities. In 1998, the International Criminal Court was created, and four years later it started work after sixty governments ratified its governing statute. Russia, though, vetoed every attempt to refer Syria to the court. Out of fevered discussions in the years after genocides in Rwanda and Bosnia, an international consensus on a "responsibility to protect" doctrine emerged that imposed a global obligation to protect people against war crimes and crimes against humanity. The new doctrine, adopted by a 2005 UN world summit, placed primary responsibility on governments to prevent atrocities in their own countries. But it also recognized the international community's obligation broadly to prevent mass atrocities and, where necessary, to use diplomatic, humanitarian, economic and, in extreme cases, military means, to prevent or stop them. The new doctrine was seen as a true breakthrough. The UN special advisor on responsibility to protect, Edward Luck, said that the doctrine was an answer to the longstanding problem in which "the capable have stood by as the slaughter of civilians unfolded. . . . They have looked for excuses not to act rather than for reasons to intervene."[72] The doctrine inspired efforts to prevent atrocities, including the Obama administration's creation of the Atrocities Prevention Board to promote concrete actions to prevent and stop the crimes.

The military dimension of attempts to stop atrocities was given the awkward name "humanitarian intervention." President Bill Clinton engaged NATO to conduct airstrikes against Bosnian Serb forces after the Srebrenica massacre in 1995 that contributed to ending the war. A few years later, without UN Security Council authorization, NATO initiated an air campaign against Serbia for its systemic assaults on ethnic Albanians in Kosovo. Military action as a means of stopping atrocities generated intense controversy among humanitarians, human rights advocates, and political scientists, and even more so after President George W. Bush invoked human rights abuses as a rationalization for his 2003 invasion of Iraq. Still, in 2011, the UN Security Council authorized coercive military action against Muammar Gaddafi's attacks on civilians in Libya. It was the first time in the UN's history that the Security Council specifically authorized military means to protect civilians over the opposition of the affected government. Russia and China, though expressing concern about authorizing the use of military force, did not exercise their veto power to block the move. The resulting six-month air campaign, though, boomeranged. It may have protected some civilians, but it also empowered competing rebel groups and led to the grisly execution of Muammar Gaddafi and a protracted war. The persistent political chaos, instability, and ongoing humanitarian crisis diminished support for the responsibility to protect.

Intervention required geopolitical stars to align, but that never happened in Syria. The Libya intervention enabled Russia to rationalize its opposition to initiatives to protect civilians in Syria. In 2011, Vitaly Churkin, Russia's ambassador to the UN, said, "The situation in Syria cannot be considered in the Security Council in isolation from the Libyan experience."[73] Eight times over the next six years, Russia vetoed Security Council attempts to compel the Syrian government to stop the assaults or face consequences if it did not. It blocked referrals to the International Criminal Court. The most it allowed was cross-border humanitarian aid into

Syria without the permission of the Syrian government, but it ended that commitment in 2020 even in the midst of the COVID-19 pandemic. Syria became such a toxic subject at the Security Council that pragmatists among governments sought to avoid discussion of Syria altogether during debates on violence against health care in conflict.

The question remained whether the United States would act outside the Security Council, as Bill Clinton did in Kosovo, and provide leadership to stop atrocities. Unlike in Kosovo, though, there was never sustained pressure on President Barack Obama. Syria never became a cause for activists and students as Darfur had been, with rallies on the National Mall and "Save Darfur" signs outside churches and synagogues exhorting action. The administration faced few political demands to act beyond those from human rights and humanitarian groups, editorialists, and Syrian expatriate groups and their allies in congress. One group that did lobby for protection of health care in Syria was the Syrian American Medical Society (SAMS). Dr. Sahloul organized lobbying trips to Congress, spoke around the country and to the media, and recruited a senator, Dick Durbin (D-Ill.), to the cause of protecting health care and civilians in Syria. He became a trusted source of information for then-U.S. ambassador to the United Nations, Samantha Power, who had written *A Problem from Hell: America and the Age of Genocide*, the definitive book on the failure to act in the face of mass murder.

In July 2013, SAMS wrote a letter to President Obama urging him to establish a no-fly zone to protect civilians and humanitarian aid, creating safe areas inside Syria for humanitarian operations and a medical airlift program. Under international humanitarian law, safe zones for civilians are only established with the consent of the parties to the conflict, but the Security Council had the authority to establish them under the UN charter.[74] No-fly zones, such as had been employed in Iraq in the aftermath of the Gulf War of 1990–91, amounted to a threat of force if the Assad regime did not keep its aircraft away from designated areas.[75] The idea for such a zone in Syria, even without Security Council approval (made impossible by Russia's likely veto), was promoted by influential senators including Carl Levin, then chair of the Senate Armed Services Committee, and

John McCain, the highly influential ranking member. It was opposed by the Pentagon, which was concerned about the logistics of managing hundreds of planes and risking live shooting that could drag the United States into the war. In May 2013 President Obama ordered the Pentagon to consider options for a no-fly zone.[76]

SAMS gained an audience with President Obama. Dr. Sahloul recalled that apart from urging Obama to save lives and meet medical needs, he bluntly appealed to Obama's legacy. He argued that Obama would be remembered for what he did or did not do in Syria. It turned out, though, that President Obama had a different legacy in mind, which was not to engage in another war in the Middle East. When, in August, Syria launched the massive chemical weapons attack on Eastern Ghouta that killed fifteen hundred people, including three hundred children, the president was confronted with a decision. Assad had crossed Obama's asserted "red line" of not employing chemical weapons, and Obama seriously considered direct military action to take out suspected chemical weapons sites. But in a meeting of his top advisers, Obama said that a president shouldn't start or get involved in one conflict after another, citing Afghanistan, Iraq, Libya, Yemen, and Somalia. According to Ben Rhodes, an Obama speechwriter and national security assistant, the president said, "It is too easy for a president to go to war."[77] Obama believed—probably correctly—that there would be no public support for intervention.[78] As a result, during a meeting in Russia, Obama agreed to a proposal by Russian President Vladimir Putin for Assad to remove his store of chemical weapons in lieu of U.S. airstrikes. Obama's decision is widely recognized as a turning point, signaling to the world that the Syrian people would be left to whatever befell them.

The continuing atrocities, though, led to anguish within the administration about the millions of Syrians at risk. In early 2015, a group of senior former State Department officials and others urged President Obama to establish three zones to provide a safe place for civilians in northern Syria, with the support of U.S. air power. The idea remained controversial among foreign policy analysts, with some arguing that guarantees of protection could escalate the war and create potential risks to American soldiers, while others urged that the risks were worth taking. Though she had supported military action against Assad in 2013, National Security Advisor Susan Rice agreed with Obama's reluctance to order no-fly zones. "If we set up a no-fly zone or safe zones on the ground," she later wrote, "we were buying a costly, dangerous, lengthy, and uncertain military commitment" on top of U.S. engagement in wars in Iraq and Afghanistan.[79] Opponents also argued that a no-fly or safe zone could lead to greater harm to civilians, though the refusal to act led to much more carnage. By 2015, however, the debate had become sterile. Though ratcheting up humanitarian assistance, Obama had not changed his thinking about a military response in Syria except to fight the Islamic State there. Assad faced no consequences for bombing hospitals. When Russia entered the war in 2015, the absence of a no-fly zone or safe zones left it, too, unrestrained by any need to avoid open military conflict with the United States. It joined Assad in the assaults on hospitals. Shortly after Donald Trump took office in 2017, he retaliated against Syria's use of chemical weapons in Khan Shaykhun by firing missiles on Syrian airfields. The response, however, was a one-off. There was no follow-up or any change in a hands-off policy. A year later, after another chemical weapon attack, Trump again launched missiles targeting chemical weapons stockpiles. Again, there was no follow-up. Journalist Dexter Filkins, an acute observer of Middle East wars over two decades, wrote that Obama and Trump carried out a policy that amounted to "risking nothing, losing nothing." Its price was the enduring calamity of Syria.[80]

In April 2018, at a loss to secure protection by the international community for their hospitals, twelve medical humanitarian groups, with encouragement from the UN's humanitarian agency, proposed to risk sharing the coordinates of sixty health facilities with Russia, by way of the UN. The process of sharing coordinates is an element of a process called "deconfliction," an odd term that was a holdover from efforts to avoid "friendly fire" among troops of the same army. The hope was that, with the information on hospital locations, Russia would pressure Syria to refrain from further attacks on hospitals. Sharing location information was of course extremely risky, as it could help Russia and Syria target hospitals.

The medical groups agonizingly debated the risks and benefits of participating in the deconfliction process. The Syrian American Medical Society reluctantly joined the process but showed no confidence in its success, characterizing its participation "as a last-resort decision" and assumed that "such attacks are likely to continue."[81]

Their skepticism turned out to be justified. By September, six hospitals identified in the deconfliction list were attacked. UN officials tried to show optimism, saying that only a few of the 120 health facilities hit by heavy weapons in 2018 were on the deconfliction list.[82] They encouraged groups to add more facilities to the list.[83] By then, though, medical groups had lost faith in deconfliction, as there were no consequences to the perpetrators in targeting a hospital on the deconfliction list. They concluded that the only purpose for the list might be for later accountability, as the perpetrators of attacks had been put on notice of the location of health facilities.[84] That remote possibility didn't justify further cooperation, as sharing coordinates made attacks that much easier.

In the spring of 2019, Russia and Syria began an assault on Idlib, the last holdout of opposition forces. In May alone, in one twelve-hour period, Russia bombed four hospitals.[85] It employed bunker-busting bombs again. Nine of the hospitals hit were on the deconfliction list.[86] By the end of July, the UN gave up on deconfliction. Mark Lowcock, the UN under-secretary-general for humanitarian affairs, told the Security Council, "I have come to the conclusion that in the current environment deconfliction is not proving effective in helping to protect those who utilize the system."[87] The UN Secretary-General launched an official board of inquiry into the breaches of the deconfliction commitment, focusing on seven of the airstrikes in 2019, four of which were on medical facilities. Its mandate was limited, though, as it was instructed not to draw any conclusions on potential legal liability. The UN high commissioner for human rights announced that by September the number of medical facilities damaged in attacks had grown to fifty-one.[88] Using different combinations of photographic and video evidence, weapons identification, satellite imagery, testimony, and cockpit recordings, analyses by the *New York Times*, Amnesty International, and Human Rights Watch meticulously documented five, eighteen, and eighteen attacks on health facilities, respectively, and determined that they were committed by Syria and Russia. There was no evidence of military objectives in the vicinity of the attacks.[89] One of the attacks, on the Ariha Surgical Hospital, killed at least fourteen civilians and wounded sixty-six others.[90]

While the UN board of inquiry proceeded, the Syrian assault on Idlib continued. By the end of February 2020 almost a million people, many of them previously displaced, were forced out of their homes, 80 percent of them women and children. Hundreds of thousands of people were stuck in informal camps with little access to sanitation, shelter, schools, or health care. Some people living in the camps burned old clothes to gain some warmth.[91] Health facilities had to suspend operations. Thirty-one of them relocated closer to the Turkish border. The pressures on remaining facilities, operating far beyond their capacity, led to mayhem.[92] Lowcock by then described the situation as having "reached a horrifying new level."[93]

In April 2020, the secretary-general's board of inquiry found that Syria and its allies were responsible for attacks on all three of the health facilities it investigated that were on the deconfliction list (the fourth health facility was not on the list); for unexplained reasons, it declined to name the allies to which it referred, particularly Russia.[94] Two months later, Russia withdrew from the deconfliction process altogether. As the hospital attacks during the war climbed toward six hundred, and the deaths of health personnel approached one thousand, former WHO Director General Margaret Chan's question from years before—whether attacks on health care were the new normal—gained a depressing urgency. Some asked whether the principle of humanity and its incorporation as law in the Geneva Conventions remained alive. The more pressing question concerned the willingness of the international community to exert effective pressure to put a stop to atrocities committed by those who showed contempt for the law.

There will always be butchers in the world. There was no prospect of internal reform given Assad's single-minded focus on preserving power and his indifference to human rights. Outside pressure, though, was thwarted at every turn. The structure of the Security Council, allowing any of its permanent members to veto action, was the biggest obstacle, but not the only one. The governments that could have protected civilians from Assad issued futile condemnations but declined to act beyond imposing economic sanctions. At the end of 2019, Susan Rice acknowledged that "the human costs of [Assad's] slaughter stung our collective conscience" and that "the gap between our rhetorical policy and our actions constantly bedeviled U.S. policy making." She nevertheless excused nonintervention as "the right choice for the totality of U.S. interests."[95]

As the conflict approached a decade in length, a million displaced people were living in the cold and mud outside Idlib, where children died of hypothermia. The health directorate was still functioning even as a radical Islamic group ruled the region. Between November 2019 and February 2020, the UN Human Rights Council's independent commission reported that Russian and Syrian and related progovernment forces launched twenty-five air and ground strikes against hospitals in Idlib and western Aleppo, including a maternity hospital and a hospital in a cave. The commission found that in western Aleppo, the assaults included "an apparent effort to erode the viability of the last functioning medical facilities in the town of Atarib and its environs."[96] The hospitals that survived were desperately short of fuel to run generators. Resources to address the COVID-19 pandemic were inadequate and living conditions for the displaced people promoted transmission. As had happened so often before in Syria, health workers were exhausted, demoralized, and psychologically scarred. In March 2020, German Chancellor Angela Merkel called for a no-fly zone in the region. Her remarks amounted to whistling in the dark.

On September 20, 2020, almost ten years after Dr. Mohammad Darwish was arrested and tortured in Syria, intelligence agents in the city of Homs arrested his mother, Basma Khaldy, an ob-gyn, for allegedly offering treatment to wounded demonstrators in 2011. She was later transferred to military intelligence headquarters in Damascus. With the help of connections and bribes, Dr. Khaldy was released on October 11, but intelligence agents continued their harassment, coming to her house to question her. After months, and more bribes to obtain a passport, she and her husband, also a doctor, were among the 70 percent of the country's health workers who fled the country. More than nine hundred of the health workers who remained during the war had been killed.

Around the time of Dr. Khaldy's departure, the International Rescue Committee released a survey of 74 health workers and 237 residents of northwest Syria. Two-thirds of the health workers reported that they had been in a hospital when it was attacked and almost half had lost colleagues to injury or death during the violence. Almost all of them experienced psychological trauma from the violence. About half of the residents, including 59 percent of the women questioned, said they feared going to a health facility because of the danger of attack. They, too, along with their children, had suffered psychological trauma, including feelings of hopelessness, loss of sleep, nightmares, and depression, that they attributed to attacks on health facilities.[97]

March 2021 marked the tenth anniversary of the start of pro-democracy protests that were greeted with brutality and led to war. By then, more than thirty-three hundred health workers had been arrested, detained or disappeared. On March 21, artillery shelling of a major surgical hospital in western Aleppo killed seven patients, among them a twelve-year-old boy, and injured fifteen others, including five medical staff. It went largely unnoticed in the international media. Some governments initiated investigations of war crimes in Syria under principles of universal jurisdiction, and convictions were obtained in Sweden and Germany. None of the cases involved violence inflicted on health care. Referral of Syria to the International Criminal Court remained as distant as ever.

# 5

## RECKLESSNESS

---

### The Saudi Assault on Yemen

I N NOVEMBER 2016, DR. FOUAD Othman returned to his native Taiz, often considered Yemen's cultural capital, and the country's third largest city. Dr. Othman had just completed his doctoral degree in community medicine and public health in Cairo after practicing medicine and teaching at the medical faculty in Taiz from 2004 to 2011. By the time he returned, a cruel war launched by Saudi Arabia and its allies in March 2015 had devastated the city. Only two hundred thousand people were left, just a third of its prewar population. People were fearful of walking on the streets. As a result of attacks on hospitals, foreign nurses and local health workers had fled, and fuel, drugs, oxygen, and medical supplies for hospitals were running short. Incubators, dialysis machines, and other critical equipment were badly damaged. As a result, only a few of Taiz's hospitals were functioning, and those only barely.

One hospital had bullet holes in the walls of the cardiac, intensive care, and maternity units. In another, Dr. Othman said, two floors were closed because of snipers, and "inpatient and outpatient trauma care and the renal dialysis center couldn't function." Armed groups, mostly Houthi, a Shiite-related tribe based in northwestern Yemen along Saudi Arabia's border, had set up military posts around, and sometimes in, hospitals, and they used their proximity to steal from and attack ambulances. As in many conflicts, fighters scoffed at rules of medical triage designed to give priority to patients most in need, instead demanding attention, terrifying the staff in the process. Around the time Dr. Othman arrived in Taiz, a surgeon was forced to operate on a wounded fighter at gunpoint. One emergency room physician told MSF, which by then was supporting four hospitals there, "Do I feel safe working in the hospital? I never feel safe. There is no respect for health facilities. Our hospital has been targeted and shelled many times." One emergency room supervisor said, "We are frustrated and depressed because we cannot save our patients' lives and we watch them die in front of our eyes."[1]

Even as the health system reeled, the need for medical care increased. Doctors were confronted with gunshot wounds and injuries from airstrikes, blasts, shelling, and landmines. The high price of food and water shortages led to rapidly escalating health crises for pregnant women, babies, young children, and people with chronic diseases. Doctors and nurses saw an upsurge in respiratory tract infections, acute diarrhea, intestinal parasites, skin diseases, viral infections, and severe malnutrition. Ironically, though, in the midst of the crisis, Dr. Othman had trouble finding a medical position, as health workers in Taiz, as elsewhere in Yemen, were not getting paid. After three months of looking for paid work, he found employment with NGOs to help address the health catastrophe resulting from the war.

His first opportunity came in February 2017, when Dr. Othman took a position with an international NGO, Mercy Corps, to monitor a nutrition project in a nearby area where the primary health care system was still intact. Even before the Saudi offensive even began, half of Yemen's children under the age of five experienced chronic or acute malnutrition, and 47 percent of all children suffered from stunted growth. Half the population already depended on some form of humanitarian aid. Almost a third of the country's twenty-five million people lacked access to basic health care.[2] The Mercy Corps project itself was in part a response to the high price of food, a result of the Saudi blockading of ports and its obstruction of internal transport due to the war. By the beginning of the year, three times as many Yemenis were acutely malnourished as the year before the war.[3]

Later that year, Dr. Othman went to work for the World Health Organization to help its response to a cholera epidemic that had broken out in the fall of 2016, likely a consequence of the bombing of water and sanitation facilities by Saudi Arabia and its coalition. The first cases were concentrated in and around the capital, Sana'a, in the west, and spread eastward from there. Cholera is a bacterial disease transmitted through contaminated water or food and leads to severe diarrhea and dehydration. It can be fatal if left untreated. Treating cholera requires detection, verification, and rapid response. The collapse of Yemen's health system undermined its capacity to respond quickly.[4] As of the summer of 2017, the vast majority of cases and deaths were in areas controlled by the Houthis, which had fewer resources and whose water and medical infrastructure had been subjected to bombing by a coalition led by Saudi Arabia.[5] Two years later, the disease had sickened more than two million people and killed thirty-seven hundred of them.[6] By comparison, before the outbreak in Yemen, there had not been as many as six hundred thousand cases worldwide in any of the past twenty years.[7]

## BIN SALMAN'S WAR

Saudi Arabia's new defense minister (and later, crown prince), Mohammed bin Salman, never expected that the war would still continue into the fall of 2016. He had assembled a coalition of ten Gulf and Middle Eastern states and troops loyal to Yemen's former president, Abdrabbuh Mansur Hadi, to seek to dislodge the Houthis, who had ousted Hadi. The Houthis had long been marginalized in the politics of Yemen and resented Saudi efforts to counter potential Iranian Shiite influence in the country. During 2011, the Houthis participated in Arab Spring demonstrations against the three-decade rule of Ali Abdullah Saleh. As the protests and political turmoil continued, Saleh was forced to step down, and was replaced by Hadi. A national dialogue led to an agreement for a new constitution. In 2014, though, the Houthis rejected the agreement and, along with forces loyal to former president Saleh, took up arms. In the fall, they captured the capital, Sana'a, and dissolved parliament, leaving Hadi to flee to Saudi Arabia.

Bin Salman said the war was essential because the Houthis had ousted a legitimate ruler, were a threat to his southern border and, more dubiously, that they were proxies for Saudi Arabia's enemy, Iran.[8] He believed that the massive airpower in the possession of Saudi Arabia, the United Arab Emirates, and other partners, combined with an embargo on goods coming into Yemen, would bring rapid victory. He launched the offensive in March 2015. It was a disastrous misjudgment, as he could not defeat the Houthis, and the war threw the people of the poorest country in the region into displacement, disease, and despair.

Though a close ally of the United States, the Saudis gave the Obama administration only a few hours advance notice of its war plans. They nevertheless requested weaponry, intelligence, targeting, and midair refueling assistance, as well as political support from the U.S. Many defense and diplomatic officials in the U.S. government were dubious about the war. General Lloyd Austin, head of the U.S. Central Command (and later secretary of defense in the Biden administration), which is responsible for U.S. military action in the Middle East, said, "I don't currently know the specific goals and objectives of the Saudi campaign."[9] Others were even more blunt, characterizing the war as misguided and with little chance of success.[10] Nevertheless, as Robert Malley and Stephen Pomper, two senior national security officials of the Obama White House, explained in two *mea culpa* analyses years later, the administration, though skeptical about the war, felt it had no choice but to support it. It wanted to support Hadi, who officials saw as a legitimate leader. Saudi Arabia was a key ally, and the administration was concerned about jeopardizing an already frayed relationship with the Saudis. They were still furious with the U.S. abandonment of Egypt's President Hosni Mubarak during the Arab Spring protests and strongly opposed the then-imminent agreement with Iran over its nuclear weapons. Moreover, Malley and Pomper noted, the Obama administration was so focused on its ongoing campaign against al-Qaeda in southern Yemen that it did not appreciate how unpopular President

Hadi had been.[11] As the war began, the White House issued a press release justifying the Saudi attack as a legitimate effort to restore the government of President Hadi and protect its borders. The administration quietly approved the Saudis' request for advanced weapons and other forms of military assistance. European nations did as well.

Middle East experts who understood the regional dynamics believed the war doomed and dangerous. Robert Jordan, former ambassador to Saudi Arabia, suggested that the Saudis' war would alienate the Yemeni population.[12] Others noted that the Saudis exaggerated the Houthis' allegiance to Iran while underestimating their military prowess. If military and political analysts were unimpressed by the Saudi aims and strategies, global humanitarian and health agencies were terrified at the prospect of a major war in Yemen. It was apparent to them that war waged with advanced airpower against an enemy entrenched in urban areas would bring still more suffering to people who were already ill-fed and beset with the worst health status in the region. Its ratio of doctors to the population was about the same as Afghanistan, which had been at war for decades. Yemen also had a history of poor patient-provider relations that led to an unusually high prevalence of patient- and family-inflicted interpersonal violence on health providers.[13] Health organizations dreaded the consequences of even greater insecurity.[14] They worried, too, that a war would threaten the fragile progress the country had made in the preceding years in reducing the deaths of children under the age of five.

The Cassandras were correct. On the first day of the campaign, at least eleven civilians were killed by coalition airstrikes in Sana'a, the country's capital, and one of the major Houthi-controlled cities. Four days later, an airstrike hit a displaced persons' camp housing more than ten thousand people, killing twenty-nine civilians and wounding forty others, including fourteen children. Within the first three days, a hundred civilians had died. At the same time, the Saudis began their blockade of the major ports through which the country's fuel and 90 percent of its food was imported. In the second month of the war, coalition airstrikes began to hit hospitals. Three hospitals were hit in April alone, two of which were destroyed.[15] Dozens more airstrikes were to follow.

From March through June 2015, the World Health Organization's grim, weekly situation reports expressed ever greater alarm at the dire consequences of airstrikes and the blockade on health care, clean water, and electricity. A month into the war, the UN Security Council put the humanitarian concerns aside and adopted a resolution that legitimized the Saudi campaign. With no mention of coalition conduct and only a glancing reference to the already deteriorating living conditions of Yemen's people, the resolution condemned the Houthis and imposed a tough arms embargo on the group and an asset freeze and travel ban on its leaders. U.S. officials, suppressing their private doubts about the war's rationale and the prospects of Saudi success, echoed the Saudi line that the resolution was essential to curb Iran's allegedly nefarious purposes in Yemen.

The resolution was not wrong to point to the brutality of the Houthis. Kate Kizer, a Yemen analyst, has noted that, with their in-your-face slogan, "God is great, Death to America, Death to Israel, Curses on the Jews, Victory to Islam," the Houthis vacillated between "incompetence and malevolence," combining "human rights violations with administrative ineptitude and political intransigence."[16] Early in the war, the Houthis captured Taiz, Dr. Othman's home city. After anti-Houthi forces, supported by the Saudi-led coalition's airpower, eventually recaptured large sections of the city, the Houthis responded with a siege and regularly shelled the city and its hospitals mercilessly from the surrounding hills. It shelled Al-Thawra hospital, which was treating about fifty wounded people a day, from those hills at least a dozen times in the first three months of the war. The hospital kept operating, but the emergency room, medical wards, burn center, dialysis center, and gynecological and obstetrics departments were all damaged, along with water pipes throughout the building, all of which impeded its ability to treat those wounded in war.[17] The siege also led patients to die in hospitals because of shortages of medical supplies, fuel to run generators, oxygen tanks, dialysis machines, and medicine.[18] As the war continued, human rights investigators from NGOs and the UN consistently found that the Houthis wantonly attacked civilians, used hospitals for military purposes, blocked humanitarian access, and engaged in other serious infringements of human rights.

Yet Saudis' and, to a lesser extent, coalition partners' modern air power caused the most deaths and destruction. They rarely appeared to target hospitals and other civilian structures, but neither did they abide by their legal obligations to distinguish between civilian and military objects and to take precautions against harming civilians when targeting military ones. Failure to do so can be a war crime. A month into the war, the UN's humanitarian affairs office, desperate to protect civilians and the hospitals, schools, housing, and infrastructure from coalition bombs, began a deconfliction process. As in Syria, aid organizations submitted the names, coordinates, and other information about facilities and operations to the UN, which in turn provided them to Saudi military planners to take steps to ensure that they were not subjected to airstrikes. The U.S. Central Command established an additional deconfliction system and, later in 2015, the U.S. Agency for International Development compiled its own list of additional critical infrastructure, including factories and commercial facilities needed for a functioning economy. The International Committee of the Red Cross and MSF established their own deconfliction procedures with the Saudis. The lists extended to movements of humanitarian convoys. Ultimately thirty thousand sites were placed on a no-strike list. Aid groups notified the coalition of more than thirty thousand movements of humanitarian supplies, convoys, and personnel.

As in Syria, the deconfliction process failed. Coalition bombs continued to fall on structures on the no-strike list. The Saudis brushed aside criticism, claiming that they were committed to and respected international humanitarian law, that all their targets were military ones, and that any civilian casualties were the product of proportionate responses to a major military threat. "We are very careful in picking targets," the Saudi foreign minister said a few months later. "We have very precise weapons. We work with our allies including the United States on these targets."[19] Meanwhile, the humanitarian crisis deepened, and civilian casualties increased. By July, just four months into the war, more than fifteen hundred civilians had been killed and more than thirty-six hundred wounded.[20] The World Health Organization moved Yemen to its highest level of crisis, the same as Syria. By late summer, almost a million and a half people had been internally displaced, and 80 percent of the population needed humanitarian aid. A third of the population faced hunger.[21]

In September, an airstrike hit a wedding party, killing at least 130 people. Then-UN Secretary-General Ban Ki-Moon condemned the airstrikes and other assaults on civilians, saying it demonstrated "disregard shown by all sides for human life."[22] The first week of that month, the coalition launched eighteen airstrikes in Sa'dah, leading health workers to hide inside hospitals.[23] In October, the coalition bombed the Haydan Hospital in Sa'dah, the only advanced medical facility in the region, which had treated thirty-four hundred people wounded in the war during the preceding months. The toll would have been worse had most of the staff and patients not run out of the hospital, including the maternity ward, after the first strike.[24] In December, in at least the twentieth airstrike on a health facility, the Saudi-led coalition bombed an MSF mobile clinic in Taiz, right after MSF had urgently called on the coalition to avoid its clinic during an ongoing air attack against targets in the city. The hospital was on the no-strike list, had a logo on the roof, and MSF had shared its coordinates with the Saudis. When airstrikes hit the neighborhood of the hospital, MSF contacted its Saudi military liaison to seek to prevent an attack on the clinic, without success.[25] By September, the UN High Commissioner for Human Rights reported that 60 percent of civilians killed to date in the war had died in airstrikes.[26]

The attacks, fighting, and blocking of medicine and medical supplies had, in less than half a year, led Dr. Ahmed Shadoul, the World Health Organization's representative in Yemen, to conclude the worst. "The health system is on the brink of collapse," he announced.[27] He said that at least a quarter of health facilities were not functioning at all, and staff and patients feared coming to hospitals that were still operating. Facilities that had not been attacked faced shortages of medical staff and supplies.[28] Additionally, the coalition hit desalinization plants and water bottling facilities, which contributed to outbreaks of malaria and dengue fever. The Yemen Ministry of Public Health and Population, with support from the UNICEF, the Global Alliance for Vaccines and Immunization, and humanitarian partners, made heroic efforts to continue child vaccination campaigns, conducting five rounds of vaccinations, but they reached only about a third of Yemen's children. UNICEF estimated that nearly ten thousand children under the age of five may have died in the first year of the war from preventable diseases because of a decline in immunizations and primary care to treat diarrhea and pneumonia.[29] Moderate to severe anemia in children, stunted childhood growth, and mothers' deaths in childbirth all increased.[30] The UN humanitarian agency, meanwhile, reported that the violence had forced the majority of Yemenis into destitution.[31]

Like health workers in Syria, Yemeni doctors and nurses had to treat gruesome injuries, and contend with increased malnutrition and disease, shortages of supplies, overwork because of the flight of many health staff, the deaths of their colleagues, stresses of dangerous travel, economic worries about providing for their families, and the shame and moral distress of not being able to meet patients' needs. All the while they suffered fear and anxiety from the threat of violence against them. And as the Syrians did, Yemeni health workers found ways to continue to carry out their jobs through religion, fatalism, and a sense of duty, while also experiencing feelings of helplessness, inadequacy, and despair.[32]

Even as the debacle was unfolding it was becoming increasingly clear that the Saudis' war was going nowhere. In early 2016, the International Crisis Group concluded that the war had "become a bloody stalemate" and "no side is close to a decisive military victory." It found, too, that Western political and military support facilitated the war's continuation and impeded the possibility of compromise.[33] Others expressed concern that the coalition campaign was working at cross-purposes with U.S. interests, empowering the al-Qaeda affiliate in southeastern Yemen that the United States was fighting with drone strikes and other military actions.[34] The strategic concerns were accompanied by ethical and legal ones. In the summer of 2015, International Crisis Group analyst April Longley Alley described the crisis as "catastrophic" and that the "the scale of the humanitarian crisis poses a stark ethical challenge to the Saudi-led Coalition and its supporters, including the United States and the United Kingdom."[35] Four years later, with the war continuing, Malley and Pomper reflected that "however indirectly the U.S. might be culpable for the calamity befalling Yemen, it is culpable nonetheless." It had gotten "into a car with a reckless driver" and "never got out of the car."[36]

## ENABLERS

Officials of the Obama administration and the British government, the largest and second-largest suppliers of arms to the Saudis respectively, were acutely aware of the ethical, policy, and legal concerns growing out of their political and military support for the Saudis. At the start, Obama had ordered weapons sales and military support for defensive purposes only.[37] Within the first couple of weeks of the war, though, that constraint evaporated. The administration expedited previously committed arms deliveries to the Saudis and the United Arab Emirates, sent additional weapons, and expanded intelligence sharing. Twenty-five U.S. military personnel assisted a joint planning cell in the Saudi operations center.[38] Within months, U.S. weapons sales to the Saudis and its partners exceeded $8 billion. Between 2013 and 2017, arms sales to the Saudis and Emiratis represented more than 25 percent of all U.S. weapons exports.[39] The French and German governments also increased arms sales, though far less than the British, whose export licenses for military goods to Saudi Arabia grew from £83 million in 2014 to £2.9 billion in 2015.[40] By early 2018, the value of its arms exports licenses reached £4.7 billion.[41] It also supplied more than eighty Royal Air Force personnel and six thousand contractors to assist in targeting, train pilots, maintain aircraft, and supervise the loading of bombs and other functions.[42]

Both countries had laws restricting the sales of arms to abusers of human rights and humanitarian law, but both governments interpreted them to permit the transfers to the Saudis.[43] Beyond these arms transfer laws lurked an even more serious concern: Was their military support of the Saudis and their coalition aiding and abetting war crimes? Documents obtained by Reuters under the Freedom of Information Act revealed that some State Department officials "had their hair on fire" over the sloppy targeting and lack of precautions in the air campaign and worried about potential U.S. liability for the attacks. By August 2015, the documents showed that these concerns were raised in National Security Council meetings. Later that year, State Department officials discussed options to limit U.S. exposure.[44] The next month, Representative Ted Lieu urged the chair of the joint chiefs of staff to cease American support for the airstrikes until the Saudis demonstrated that they had instituted proper safeguards to prevent civilian deaths.[45]

Some mid-level administration officials urged halting support of the coalition war effort, but senior officials told me that they never seriously considered that option. The administration also stood by the Saudis in their efforts to prevent investigations of its conduct. In September 2015, the Netherlands proposed a resolution at the UN Human Rights Council to establish an independent investigation of violations of international law during the conflict. Many European countries supported the proposed resolution, but the Saudis and their allies fought hard against it. The United States delegation, whose support for the resolution might have ensured its passage, stayed on the sidelines, and the proposal died.[46] It took two more years of pervasive human rights violations before the council was able to establish an independent group of experts to examine the conduct of the war.

The British government was less reticent about its support for the war, pushing back hard against pressure from well-organized citizens, especially the Campaign Against the Arms Trade, an NGO dating to 1974 and sustained by churches, trade unions, and peace groups. In the summer of 2015, when evidence of the coalition's indiscriminate bombing deaths had become alarming, Foreign Office Minister Tobias Ellwood answered questions from a member of parliament, saying, "We have received explicit assurances from the Saudi Arabian authorities that they are complying with International Humanitarian Law. We have not seen any credible evidence that suggests that the coalition has breached the law."[47]

Over the next year, two parliamentary committees issued reports concluding that the arms sales violated British law. Officials offered contradictory responses. In February 2016, then-Foreign Secretary Philip Hammond denied any violations by the Saudis: "We have assessed that there has not been a breach of international humanitarian law by the coalition." Hammond later said, "The [ministry of defense's] assessment is that the Saudi-led coalition is not targeting civilians; that Saudi processes and procedures have been put in place to ensure respect for the principles of international humanitarian law; and that the Saudis both have been and continue to be genuinely committed to compliance with international humanitarian law." Five months later, the statements had to be corrected since no such assessment had been made.[48] In November, in a report submitted to parliament, the government argued, on the one hand, that the government engaged in "robust case-by-case assessments" on arms export applications. On the other hand, it said, "We are not acting to determine whether a sovereign state has or has not acted in breach of [international humanitarian law]" and pleaded ignorance of the facts needed to make such a judgment. It claimed deference to coalition members, who, it said, "have the best insight into their own military procedures and will be able to conduct the most thorough and conclusive investigations."[49]

The Campaign Against the Arms Trade and other groups filed a lawsuit alleging violation of the country's arms transfer law, which prohibits arms sales if there is a "clear risk" that they will be used to violate international humanitarian law. In response, the government claimed that Saudi processes and procedures ensured respect for international humanitarian law and that its leadership was genuinely committed to compliance. The government also asserted that it had engaged in a rigorous review of the airstrikes but lacked sufficient information to determine whether they constituted violations of international humanitarian law. Despite all the legal obfuscation, in public pronouncements the government revealed why it sought to cast objections to the sales aside. Saudi Arabia was by far the largest customer for its weapons in the world, and these sales were both lucrative and a potential source of British influence in the Middle East. Then-Prime Minister David Cameron visited a defense plant in early 2016, a week after the parliamentary committee called for suspension of arms sales to the Saudis and the same day the European Parliament called for an arms embargo. He touted the "brilliant things" it was selling the Saudis.[50]

One of the initial justifications for supporting the Saudis was, as Malley and Pomper explained, was to be a moderating influence on the Saudis.[51] The Obama administration and the British government privately urged the Saudis to be careful in their targeting in Yemen and pressed to resolve the conflict. Neither government, however, used the powerful leverage created by the arms sales to put meaningful pressure on the Saudis. Instead, the Pentagon sent a contingent of experts on international humanitarian law to train the Saudis on the requirements of the Geneva Conventions. Of potentially greater consequence, in October, the State Department sent Larry Lewis, an expert on avoiding civilian casualties in military operations, to Saudi Arabia to help its military understand why they persistently hit nonmilitary targets. An unassuming and cerebral defense analyst, Lewis nevertheless was passionate about protecting civilians in war. He had written reports for the Pentagon that assessed why civilians were killed in U.S. military operations in Iraq and Afghanistan and offered recommendations on how to limit civilian casualties in the future. To perform that task, he reviewed details of how military operations were conducted, determined why they went awry, and based on his analysis proposed operational changes that could avoid or ameliorate harm to civilians.[52] In some cases, he found that the target was misidentified. In other cases, he suggested a need for "tactical patience" before releasing a bomb or missile against a military target in a densely populated area. He told me, "If you have a target but don't need to engage immediately, take more time. Look from different angles at the situation on the ground. Can you anticipate a better time?"

Lewis was in a weak position with the Saudis, though, because of his subordinate role in the U.S. government. He was then based in the State Department, not the Pentagon, and in the human rights bureau, a division with little political clout. The Defense Department kept its distance both from coalition conduct and from Lewis's work in order to insulate it from any claims of U.S. responsibility for, or complicity in, the conduct of the air war. Within his own bureau, officials were skeptical that technical support for the coalition would change its behavior and worried that providing it could encourage continued airstrikes and war crimes and deepen the humanitarian crisis. Thus, far from the assignment representing a major commitment by the Obama administration to monitor how the weapons it provided were used, Lewis lacked diplomatic, military, and political support.

He nevertheless went to the Saudi military headquarters, where he reviewed data on airstrikes, consulted with targeting officers and others, and reached a conclusion: many of the errors were a product of the extensive use of "dynamic strikes." These were bombing runs that lacked a planned target; instead, pilots attacked a site based on information conveyed to them while flying from spotters on the ground. As the Saudis and partners quickly ran out of military installations, weapons depots, and other fixed military targets to attack, 90 to 95 percent of all bombing runs were dynamic strikes, while the working definition of what constituted a target became ever more elastic, including the presence of fighters in or around a civilian structure. These dynamic strikes were made possible by the midair refueling capability provided by the United States that allowed planes to fly around looking for targets. Lewis noted that planned airstrikes are subject to rigorous preflight procedures including review of intelligence, identification of civilian objects near targets, population density in the area, the nature of the weapons employed, and the likely direction of destruction. Because dynamic strikes lack these safeguards, the U.S. military subjects its own dynamic strikes to strict rules and rigorous procedures for approval. It also trains spotters to ensure that an appropriate target is hit and on how to avoid preventable civilian casualties.

Even with stringent safeguards, dynamic strikes have a high potential of going awry. In October 2015, just as Larry Lewis's assignment began, a U.S. A-130 ground attack aircraft from Bagram Air Base in Afghanistan bombed a large MSF trauma center in Kunduz, Afghanistan, destroying it and killing forty-three people. It was the largest trauma hospital in the north of the country. In 2014 MSF treated twenty-two thousand patients in the hospital, and between January and August 2015 performed more than three thousand surgeries.[53] The A-130 is equipped with sophisticated sensors and navigation systems and its flight crews are trained in targeting procedures and international humanitarian law. Yet a Pentagon review of the airstrike found a litany of errors: the calling in of an airstrike without proper approvals; the lack of mission briefing and no-strike list review for the crew before takeoff; geosensors on the aircraft that were not accurate from the range where the crew fixed on the target; and lack of confirmation from the crew's base that the target was not on the no-strike list. Darkness prevented the crew from seeing the identification of the trauma center as a hospital. Once the attack began, despite frantic calls by MSF staff to U.S. and NATO contacts in Afghanistan and the Pentagon, the assault continued for a half hour without the crew realizing that they were repeatedly attacking a functioning hospital.[54]

If the potential for error in dynamic strikes was high in sophisticated U.S. air operations, it was astronomically greater for the coalition conducting airstrikes in Yemen with inexperienced crews, loose procedures, and untrained spotters. Consultation of the no-strike list in dynamic strikes was not required.[55] As a result, U.S. military advisors helping Saudi military planners in the operations planning cell in targeting assessments were irrelevant. Additionally, the Saudis "had a very weak team," Lewis told me, "doing graduate level problems." Andrew Exum, a Defense Department official at the time, later wrote from a broader perspective: "The deficiencies in the Royal Saudi Air Force at the operational level were glaring. Decades of U.S. training missions had not produced a Saudi military capable of independently planning and executing an effective air campaign that minimized collateral damage."[56]

Lewis's analysis found that the Saudis repeatedly misidentified civilian structures such as hospitals as military targets. Even when a military target was identified, no proper assessment was made of the presence of civilians. Lewis shared his analysis with Saudi military planners and diplomatically explained that the U.S. military itself made mistakes and had developed a process not to cast blame, but to understand and correct them. Lewis suggested that the Saudis create a formal review process for assessments of mistakes in targeting, and from that analysis operational adjustments could follow. The Saudi officers agreed. They called the mechanism a Joint Incidents Assessment Team (JIAT), composed of individuals from Saudi Arabia and coalition allies Kuwait, Yemen, Qatar, Bahrain, and the United Arab Emirates. He also recommended specific changes in practice, including consultations with the no-strike list and tactical patience. Lewis was optimistic about the officers' receptivity. "I walked away thinking that they were doing what they were supposed to do," he told me. He also found modest improvements in practice after he shared the results of his reviews.

At higher levels, though, there was little interest in reducing harms to civilians, only to escape accountability for them. This stance first became evident as the new process was moving forward. In June 2016, the UN special representative on children in armed conflict prepared her annual report, to be issued by the secretary-general, on grave violations of rights of children in armed conflict. Each year, the special representative prepares an annex to the report identifying state militaries and nonstate armed groups that commit recurrent violations of grave violations including lack of respect for schools and hospitals. It is commonly referred to as the "list of shame." Once placed on the list, the party is supposed to develop an action plan to remedy the violations. Changes in targeting practices could have been a part of such a plan. She recommended that Saudi Arabia be listed in the annex.

Typically, the secretary-general accepts the proposed annex and includes it in his report. When officials in Saudi Arabia learned of the recommendation, though, they threatened to cut its substantial financial contribution to UN humanitarian operations if Saudi Arabia were included on the list. Under that pressure, then-Secretary-General Ban Ki-Moon removed the country from the annex. After an outcry by NGOs and media coverage of the removal of Saudi Arabia from the annex, Ban held an extraordinary, unprecedented press conference in which he acknowledged that he changed the annex, explaining that "I also had to consider the very real prospect that millions of other children would suffer grievously if, as was suggested to me, countries would defund many UN programs." Even as he yielded, though, he expressed frustration at the extortion, saying, "it is unacceptable for member states to exert undue pressure."[57]

Meanwhile, a cease-fire in the war was in place for peace talks led by Secretary of State John Kerry. The talks broke down in August 2016, and the coalition renewed its air campaign with a vengeance. On August 15, a coalition airstrike hit an MSF hospital in the north, killing twelve people and wounding twenty others. Additional airstrikes hit a food factory, a school, and a bridge on the no-strike list that was essential to the passage of humanitarian aid. The same month the *Guardian*'s analysis of airstrike incidents collected by the Yemen Data Project, an independent group tracking the conduct of the war, revealed that fully a third of airstrikes hit civilian targets, including fifty-eight hospitals.[58] Obama administration officials finally started speaking publicly against the indiscriminate air attacks. UN Ambassador Samantha Power tweeted, "Strikes on hospital/school/infrastructure in #Yemen devastating for ppl already facing unbearable suffering & must end."[59]

The renewed bombing in August coincided with the first report of the Joint Incident Assessment Team. Instead of a public release of the report, the Saudi Press Agency purported to summarize its findings and recommendations. What it released instead was a whitewash. It misrepresented facts and falsely claimed that the victims of the strikes were responsible for the deaths and injuries. In two cases concerning MSF-operated facilities, for example, the press agency falsely claimed that MSF had not properly identified the facilities as medical ones.[60] In 2018, an expert panel appointed by the UN Human Rights Council to investigate human rights and humanitarian law violations in Yemen found that the public summaries raised questions about whether JIAT methods were flawed, whether it engaged in proportionality assessments, and whether its conclusions about nonresponsibility of the coalition for civilian casualties had any basis. It also received reliable evidence that, at times, the JIAT's findings were substantially altered by the Saudi Ministry of Foreign Affairs.[61] A year later, the panel reached similar conclusions about the JIAT's lack of independence, methods, legal analysis, impartiality, and conclusions.[62]

In this tense environment of renewed bombing and Saudi hardball, Lewis returned to Riyadh in September 2016 with additional recommendations to senior Saudi military officials to end the now-pervasive mistargeting. The officials he met with included General Abdulrahman bin Saleh al-Banyan, chief of the joint staff of the Defense Ministry. Lewis told me that the general did not engage, appearing uninterested in the findings and on what should be done. Others in the Obama administration saw a similar pattern: receptivity to reform by mid-level officers but resistance and rejection by those at the top. Jeremy Konyndyk, then head of the Office of Foreign Disaster Assistance and responsible for overseeing the humanitarian response for the United States government, put it simply: "The Saudis at highest levels didn't really care who they bombed." Recognizing the lack of commitment at the top to avoiding civilian casualties, the State Department ended Lewis's assignment and he departed.

A few weeks after Lewis's departure, on October 6, the Saudi-led coalition bombed a funeral held in the Great Hall of Sana'a, one of the largest public halls in Yemen, with more than a thousand people attending. It killed at least 137 men and injured 671 men and 24 boys. The airstrike put the war on front pages around the world and elicited furious condemnations. The Obama administration, frustrated and angered by Saudi intransigence, issued a statement about the "troubling series of attacks on Yemeni civilians" and warned that "U.S. security cooperation is not a blank check." It announced a review of its support for the war "so as to better align with U.S. principles, values and interests."[63] Bin Salman responded that Saudi Arabia would investigate the incident and said that the team would include a U.S. expert who had previously worked with JIAT, a clear reference to Larry Lewis. The statement was untrue. The Obama administration, by then unimpressed with Saudi assurances of reforms in targeting or responsiveness to help, and not wanting to be seen as complicit in Saudi conduct, declined to send Lewis or anyone else to assist the Saudis in conducting an investigation.

Even then, the former senior administration officials told me, the option of withdrawing all military and arms support for the Saudis was not on the table. The policy review meandered into December, ending with a tepid decision only to stop selling precision-guided weapons to the Saudis. That decision left the vast majority of arms sales and military support in place, including the in-air refueling that facilitated dynamic attacks. The decision to refrain from new sales of precision weapons, though, reflected the uncomfortable truth: the Saudis problem was not the use of imprecise weapons, but misidentification of targets.

The British government's response to the ongoing carnage from the air was less critical, even after the Labour Party sought to curtail support for the Saudi-led coalition until an independent inquiry was conducted on whether the air campaign violated international law. In late October, then-Foreign Minister Boris Johnson claimed that the UK was "monitoring the situation minutely and meticulously." At the same time, he argued that arms sales were central to Britain's influence. He claimed that if it declined to continue them, "we would at a stroke eliminate this country's positive ability to exercise our moderating, diplomatic and political influence on a crisis where there are massive UK interests at stake." Instead, he contended, other countries "with nothing like the same compunctions or criteria or respect for humanitarian law" would fill the gap.[64] In fact, the government's flaccid response to the violations amounted to a license to continue the crimes.

In January 2017, Donald Trump became president and was, like the British prime minister, more concerned about arms sales than avoiding civilian harm. His first foreign visit was to Saudi Arabia, where he touted, indeed vastly exaggerated, new arms sales to the regime. On the eve of his visit, Trump also notified Congress of his intent to reverse Obama's decision to end sales of precision-guided weapons, which was subject to Congressional review. The only feint of concern about the bombing was that renewed sales were linked to technical assistance and training for the Saudis in targeting and in the law of armed conflict.[65] These steps had been tried before and proven ineffective in changing Saudi attitudes or conduct. Nor did they then. Airstrikes against hospitals, the killing of civilians, and the ongoing destruction and suffering in the country continued into a third year. Political opposition to arms sales and military support for the Saudi-led war began to gain traction. In 2017 a procedural vote in

Congress to move forward a resolution of disapproval of arms sales only failed by a few votes. The Saudis were no longer able to thwart a resolution at the UN Human Rights Council for an international investigation of alleged violations of the law of war. The same year, now-UN Secretary-General Antonio Guterres included Saudi Arabia in the "list of shame."

Saudi officials, meanwhile, continued their aggressive public relations offensive, often wrongly citing the JIAT's work. They issued a glossy report in English that celebrated Saudi Arabia's justification of the war, its humanitarian spending and activities, and its purported efforts to avoid civilian casualties. The report denied well-documented facts about attacks on hospitals and other civilian structures.[66] The Saudi Ministry of Media later claimed that "airstrikes carried out last year were in accordance with international law and many of the alleged strikes were falsely attributed to the Coalition."[67] Its campaign yielded some successes. In 2018, the UN secretary-general again removed Saudi Arabia from the list of shame, despite his report showing that nineteen schools and hospitals had been attacked.

Meanwhile, the war continued its grim course. In March 2018, the UN deputy high commissioner for human rights reported dramatic increases in civilian casualties.[68] According to the Yemen Data Project, by mid-2018 more than 30 percent of sorties were directed at nonmilitary entities such as schools, markets, hospitals, factories, and farms.[69] The coalition also launched a campaign, now supported by ground forces and artillery, to retake the port of Hudaydah, a step that threatened to reduce even further the importation of humanitarian goods. In August, the UN Human Rights Council panel established the prior year issued its first report, finding that it "identified no significant changes in the Coalition's *modus operandi*," and that the coalition, including Saudi Arabia and the United Arab Emirates, "may have conducted acts in violation of the principles of distinction, proportionality and precaution that may amount to war crimes."[70] It also found that the Houthis may have committed war crimes. UN officials were running out of strong language to describe the war. Mark Lowcock, the undersecretary-general for humanitarian affairs, said in January 2018 that the "Yemini people face what looks like the

Apocalypse."[71] More than four million Yemenis had now been displaced.[72] Later that year, Robert Worth, a *New York Times* journalist, visited a hospital in Sa'dah that had survived the war. He was overwhelmed by the smell of "old food, sweat, urine and medicine." There was vomit on the floor, and mothers with their malnourished children and skeletal bodies on cots or on the floor outside the hospitals because there was no room for them inside. The health minister told him that birth defects were increasing, apparently a result, he thought, of toxic residues from bombs and other ordnance. The health disaster was extending beyond vulnerable children and the elderly, as kidney dialysis was not available, and a quarter of a million people with diabetes were at risk because necessary medications were not available.[73]

As political pressure and consequent congressional and parliamentary disquiet grew, American and British officials continued to obfuscate. Nikki Haley, Trump's UN ambassador, wrote a February 2018 op-ed that blamed Yemen's humanitarian crisis on the Houthis and said not a word about coalition bombing.[74] The next month, General Joseph Votel, commander of the U.S. Central Command, testified in the Senate, mimicking the British line that refueling, intelligence, and other support gave it "access" and "influence" with Saudi Arabia. He alluded to Larry Lewis's past work, testifying that "sharing our own experiences" was helpful in avoiding civilian casualties, despite the lack of any evidence that the Saudis had acted on the advice. General Votel even obliquely referred to the moribund JIAT, testifying that Saudi Arabia was following the U.S.'s lead in establishing the "architecture to investigate civilian casualties."[75] In the same hearing, though, General Votel pleaded ignorance on whether U.S. munitions were ever used in airstrikes that went awry.[76]

The following month, Robert Karem, the assistant secretary of defense for policy, testified before the Senate Foreign Relations Committee on Yemen. When asked about civilian casualties in the Saudi-led coalition's air campaign, he repeated the claim that U.S. influence had led to improvements in targeting practices, the use of the no-strike, and midair refueling by the U.S. He testified that "aerial refueling allows Coalition aircraft to spend more time in the air, thus giving our partners more time to validate targets, practice tactical patience, and reduce the risk of civilian casualties."[77] By this time, of course, it was well known that civilian casualties were often a result of dynamic attacks, which in turn were enabled by mid-air refueling. His reference to tactical patience alluded to Larry Lewis's work, but the statement otherwise contradicted Lewis's findings. When pressed on whether he had confidence that civilian casualties were actually reduced, he could only cite confidence in an improved process.[78]

Later that month, General Joseph Dunford, chairman of the joint chiefs of staff, again told the Senate Foreign Relations Committee of the "positive impact" of U.S. advice that "will allow them to conduct strikes while mitigating civilian casualties. . . . So, it's a long, plodding process . . . but I think it's paying dividends over time."[79] None of the witnesses at the two hearings mentioned that the State Department abolished Larry Lewis's position a few months after Donald Trump took office. Lewis left the government and there hadn't been any American involvement in the JIAT for eighteen months. Meanwhile, the Trump administration revised the government's internal arms transfer policy, which had prohibited them where the United States has knowledge that they will be used to conduct attacks against civilians. The revision restricted the policy to only those attacks intentionally directed against civilians.[80] Indiscriminate attacks that dominated in the war were excluded.

In August 2018, in another horrific airstrike of the now three-year-long war, coalition planes struck a bus filled with school children, killing forty of them along with eleven adults. Fragments of bombs manufactured in the United States were found at the site. The Trump administration condemned the attack but, like its predecessor, distanced itself from any responsibility. Secretary of Defense James Mattis said, irrelevantly, "We do not do dynamic targeting for them."[81] The Pentagon told a journalist that as it was not a party to the conflict, and that it would not perform an investigation of the attack.[82] Congress was not impressed. A bipartisan amendment to the National Defense Authorization Act prohibited in-flight refueling unless the secretary of state certified that the Saudis and the United Arab Emirates were permitting humanitarian access and taking demonstrable actions to avoid disproportionate harm to civilians and civilian infrastructure. Soon thereafter, Secretary of State Mike Pompeo issued the certification. Parts of the memo accompanying it reads as though it had been written by staff to reach an opposite conclusion. It acknowledged that the Saudi-led coalition's campaign brought civilian casualties at a rate that remained "far too high," and that "recent casualty incidents indicate insufficient implementation of reforms and targeting practices. Investigations have not yet yielded accountability measures."[83] To justify his certification, Pompeo cited the same commitments the Saudis had been making, and violating, for years: improved rules of engagement, training on the law of war, utilization of the no-strike list, and investigations by the JIAT.[84] Refueling assistance and arms sales continued.

The war in Yemen burst out into greater public consciousness in the United States through an act that had nothing to do with the war: the murder of *Washington Post* journalist Jamal Khashoggi in October 2018 by Saudi operatives working for Bin Salman. In November, under greater pressure than ever, the Trump administration ended refueling assistance to the Saudis, and the following month the Senate voted to cut off U.S. military assistance to coalition. Finally, in early 2019, the House of Representatives, now with a Democratic majority, followed. Trump vetoed the bill. Congress, however, did employ its power to put a hold on billions of dollars of arms transfers to Saudi Arabia, particularly precision-guided weapons. In May, however, Pompeo issued an emergency certification waiving Congressional review on the ground that the arms were essential to counter Iran in Yemen, thereby permitting the sales to proceed. A later review by the State Department's inspector general found that the certification "did not fully assess risks and implement mitigation measures to reduce civilian casualties and legal concerns associated with the transfer of the precision-guided weapons.[85] By then, Germany, Finland, Norway, and Denmark had ceased their arms sales, but American and British sales continued.

During this period, the British government, too, was subjected to increasing domestic political pressure. It continued to resist. Jeremy Hunt, the British foreign secretary, while acknowledging the dire humanitarian situation in Yemen, cited his work toward a peace agreement and archly claimed the moral high ground of the power of "influence" in continued arms sales and military support to the Saudis. Like the American generals, he asserted that "curbing such support" would "surrender our influence and make ourselves irrelevant to the course of events in Yemen." He argued that the alternative was "to leave the parties to fight it out, while denouncing them impotently from the sidelines. That would be morally bankrupt."[86] In mid-2019, though, a British appellate court held that the government had not made the determination required by law regarding whether the Saudis were violating international humanitarian law or not. It also rejected the argument that Saudi Arabia's expressed desire to adhere to international humanitarian law sufficed as a substitute for a determination of compliance or noncompliance with the law. The court noted, too, that the Ministry of Defense had not reviewed dynamic strikes.[87] The government was forced to suspend arms sales. In July 2020, the government filed its report on the required review. It said that its analysis did reveal "patterns, trends of systemic weaknesses" in Saudi compliance, but that any violations of international humanitarian law "occurred at different times, in different circumstances and for different reasons. The conclusion is that these are isolated incidents."[88] It ended the suspension of arms sales.

During this long tale of reckless coalition conduct and equally reckless Western complicity, there were ample opportunities to prevent destruction of the country and its fragile health system. The Saudis and their allies could have restricted dynamic strikes, instructed flight crews to consult the no-strike list, assessed civilian presence near targets, learned from prior errors, and supported mid-level officers who sought to comply with the law. What is especially telling about coalition conduct was that the internal dynamics were the reverse of the usual pattern. Military leaders who express a genuine belief in the centrality of adhering to the Geneva Conventions too often don't operationalize them. They don't establish rules designed to forbid their troops from attacking or interfering with health care and sufficiently train mid-level officers and frontline troops in the rules. They don't provide sound guidance on proper targeting, offer education in the laws of war, or hold soldiers accountable. Here, though, mid-level Saudi officers were receptive to means to prevent civilian casualties. Larry Lewis told me that many of them were even offended by offers of training in the Geneva Conventions, as they considered themselves to be a modern military force familiar with and committed to compliance with the laws of war. The problems were, rather, with their superiors at command and political levels who were indifferent to those norms and laws. For them, the legal and moral issues arising from the airstrikes were merely a public relations matter. At every turn, the leadership engaged in manipulation, dissembling, spin, and intimidation. It kept its arms suppliers at bay through rhetoric that would please them and accepting technical support that made little difference to their conduct.

Its arms suppliers had the means to change the coalition's calculus. The arms sales were an essential part of the war effort. The supplying governments should have begun by calling acts by their proper name. Reckless and indiscriminate airstrikes are war crimes, as multiple reports from the UN and human rights organizations showed. Despite their arrogance, Saudi leaders were very sensitive to diplomatic pressure and global opinion, demonstrated by their investment of financial and political capital to try to derail human rights investigations and criticism from global institutions. Yet when condemnations might have made a difference, two U.S. administrations and the British government went out of their way to avoid calling out coalition violations of international humanitarian law, much less to identify them as likely war crimes. Instead, they hewed to the line that they were a moderating influence on the Saudis, when the evidence was that they were, instead, enablers. In the absence of a change in practice, they should have ended arms sales.

Former Obama officials Rob Malley and Stephen Pomper called the tale of U.S. entanglement in the war "a painful story" that included a combination of unwillingness to challenge the partnership with the Saudis, wishful thinking, and expediency. Their analysis devotes most attention to the initial decision to support the Saudis and only later mentions what they call the "limited and belated" step in late 2016 to halt the sales of precision weapons to the Saudis.[89] The prospect of not supporting the Saudis was never considered. Some proponents of continued support cited the original justification of limiting Iranian influence in the region.[90] In my research, though, I was told that another former senior official said, in essence, "The relationship with the Saudis was seen as too valuable, and too fragile, for that. . . . I don't think anyone who had any influence in the administration argued we should just completely walk away. . . . They are our partners. We have many other interests with them. And this would have been basically telling them to go to hell." Even if one agreed with the former official's point about the important and fraught relationship with the Saudis, it survived many other severe crises, from the engagement of Saudi nationals in the 9/11 attacks, to the contentiousness over the Iran nuclear agreement, to U.S. support for Arab Spring reformers. More importantly, loyalty to an ally cannot begin to excuse the years-long enabling of the assaults on innocents with impunity.

There is another flaw in the official's defense. My conversation with the former national security officials confirmed, once again, that the willingness of governments to try to stop gross human rights violations committed by other states is often tempered by diplomatic, national security, economic, and geopolitical considerations. Yemen, however, was not simply a case where commitments to human rights were constrained by other perceived national interests. The U.S. and British governments were not passive bystanders. Their fighter jets, bombs, missiles, and mid-air refueling enabled the Saudis and its partners to conduct the war as they did. At least two dozen coalition airstrikes killed civilians with these weapons.[91] American and British leaders were thus morally and, arguably, legally implicated in aiding and abetting coalition conduct.[92] The Geneva Conventions go even further. They direct its signatories not only to obey their provisions but to "ensure respect" for them. While the reach of that rather opaque requirement is controversial, at a minimum it requires entities that sell weapons and provide technical support to other combatants to ensure that the Geneva Conventions are not breached.[93]

In August 2019, the expert group appointed by the UN Human Rights Council released another lengthy report based on its comprehensive investigation of human rights and humanitarian law violations in Yemen. As other reports on the conflict by UN human rights agencies it was thorough, comprehensive, and credible. It made for sickening reading. It found all parties had committed serious violations of international humanitarian law, including that "Individuals in the Government of Yemen and the coalition, including Saudi Arabia and the United Arab Emirates, may have conducted airstrikes in violation of the principles of distinction, proportionality and precaution, and may have used starvation as a method of warfare, acts that may amount to war crimes." It determined that there had been no adequate investigation of or accountability for the violations. It also found that states that provided arms to the parties to the conflict "may be held responsible for providing aid or assistance for the commission of international law violations," and noting specifically that "the legality of arms transfers by France, the United Kingdom, the United States and other States remains questionable."[94] A year later, its conclusions were even more emphatic, that "states transferring arms to parties to the conflict in Yemen in blatant disregard of the documented patterns of violations of international law and human rights law . . . may amount to aiding and assisting international wrongful acts in contravention of international law."[95]

American and British policy in Yemen is in some respects paradoxical. Each had a record, however imperfect, of championing adherence to the Geneva Conventions and investing heavily in inculcating its values in training its own troops and those of other countries. Each supported a 2016 resolution at the UN Security Council demanding an end to violence against health-care workers and institutions in war. Yet the refusal to take responsibility for the behavior of proxies, allies, or arms customers in warfare also has a long history. In the 1980s, the United States provided continued assistance and training to military and police forces in Central America that it had ample reason to know were committing war crimes. In recent years, the use of proxy forces in Syria and Iraq, Afghanistan, Nigeria, and elsewhere have raised compelling questions about U.S. responsibility for the conduct of its partners in killing civilians.[96] The experience in these wars has led Congress to require the Pentagon to help its partners and proxies develop capacities to better protect civilians in their operations.[97] NGOs have proposed better assessments of partner capabilities and risks, advisory and mentoring support in combat operations, feedback loops on operations in the field to improve protection, robust investigations of violations, and ensuring accountability.[98] Whether their efforts to persuade supporters of proxy and partner wars remains to be seen. Regardless, legal accountability for complicity in others' conduct remains essential, including for enabling activities through arms sales.

Those arms sales are growing globally. In 2017, the global arms trade was valued at around $94 billion, with the United States, Russia, France, Germany, and China the leading suppliers.[99] The transfers grew by 23 percent from the first to the second decade of this century.[100] As in Yemen, there is strong evidence elsewhere that weapons sales tend to escalate the level of conflict.[101] According to a UN panel, for example, in South Sudan, these weapons supplies were "instrumental in prolonging and escalating the war" and had "a devastating impact on civilians and on the overall security situation in the country."[102] In the Central African Republic, one of the poorest countries in the world, armed groups obtained powerful assault rifles, machine guns, rocket-propelled grenade launchers, and ammunition from Sudan.[103] In 2014, an international arms trade treaty that regulates sales and prohibits transfers to entities that violate human rights or international humanitarian law went into effect, but the United States, Russia, and China have not joined it. Without restrictions on arms sales, and sellers' taking responsibility for the way weapons that they transfer are used, there is little hope of stopping assaults on health care by entities that care little for the harm they bring to hospitals, health workers, and patients.

As the war continued, Dr. Othman continued his work with the World Health Organization in Yemen, coordinating agencies engaged in the health response, and joined the faculty of Taiz University. He said that the health situation gradually improved as violence decreased, especially once the Houthis were pushed out of the area where he works. More supplies came in, but obstruction of access continued. Even as some hospitals are being rebuilt, the health system was far from recovering at the time the COVID-19 pandemic struck Yemen, adding more misery and death to a deeply suffering population. As of late 2020, 40 percent of the population was projected to face acute malnutrition. Lisa Grande, then-UN humanitarian coordinator for the country, estimated that, because of the destruction of the health system and the vulnerabilities of the population, the death toll from COVID-19 could exceed those from airstrikes, hunger, and disease during the war.[104]

When Joe Biden took office as president in 2021, he immediately paused arms sales to the Saudis for offensive operations in Yemen. Meanwhile, while the threat of COVID-19 alarmed global experts, Yeminis and health workers were more overwhelmed by malnutrition, cholera, diphtheria, dengue fever, unsafe childbirth, and a potential famine.[105] The Houthis controlled territory in which 70 to 80 percent of the people of Yemen live.

# 6

# OBSTRUCTION

---

## The Israel-Palestine Conflict

HENRI DUNANT'S CRUSADE to limit suffering in war originated in what he saw on the battlefield: wounded soldiers left to suffer alone, without solace, much less medical evacuation. As the Geneva Conventions developed, his concern about abandonment remained central, obligating combatants to attend to the wounded and sick "to the fullest extent practicable and with the least possible delay."[1] Yet timely evacuation during active combat and passage of ambulances in chronic conflicts remains hugely problematic, obstructed by military bureaucrats' rules, frontline soldiers' indifference, and commanders' neglect. It may be the case that disallowance of medical evacuation and passage through checkpoints are responsible for more deaths than spectacular incidents of violence. The conduct, however, remains largely invisible, and incidents are rarely tracked.

The tragedy is that timely, safe passage of first responders and ambulances in conflict zones need not be problematic. Straightforward operational mechanisms and procedures, enforced in the field, can reconcile the need for rapid access to care while preventing their misuse for military purposes. In the early 2000s, spurred by outside pressure and misgivings within the Israeli military at the number of first responders killed by its soldiers, Israel initiated reforms that led, for a time, to greater safety for emergency responders and the wounded. It could be a model for other militaries. As the Israeli-Palestinian conflict ground on, though, and the politics changed, Israel's commitment waned and its interference, often violent, with ambulances became a chronic feature of the conflict.

## INTIFADA: DON'T SHOOT THE AMBULANCE

In March 2002, during the height of the second Intifada in the Occupied Palestinian Territory, I led a group of medical investigators from Physicians for Human Rights to Israel, Gaza, and the West Bank. In just a two-week period, Israel Defense Forces (IDF) soldiers shot and killed six Palestinian emergency medical responders as they sought to evacuate Palestinians wounded during active fighting in the West Bank. Among the victims were Dr. Khalil Suleiman, the director of the Palestine Red Crescent Society (PRCS), part of the international Red Cross/Red Crescent movement, in the West Bank town of Jenin, and Dr. Ahmad Othman, the director of a hospital near Bethlehem. The Israeli human rights group B'Tselem reported that on March 4, Dr. Suleiman, three crew members, and another physician were traveling in a PRCS ambulance to come to the aid of people injured in the fighting in Jenin. Before entering Jenin, the ambulance had been inspected for weapons by IDF soldiers and cleared in accordance with a procedure where the ICRC acted as intermediary to expedite medical evacuation.

The Geneva Conventions rule is that ambulances mut be protected and respected provided they are not used, outside their humanitarian function, to harm the enemy; it applies in occupied territory as well.[2] To ensure they are not misused by acts such as the transport of weapons or fighters, combatants are permitted to inspect ambulances for weapons or other improper uses and approve their passage, but they may not unduly delay passage or arbitrarily invoke potential misuse to deny urgent medical evacuation.[3] The Israel Defense Forces affirm the obligation, and the Supreme Court of Israel has recognized the duty to "do everything possible, subject to the state of the fighting, to allow the evacuation of local inhabitants that were wounded in the fighting."[4] The IDF did not dispute that it had approved the passage of Dr. Suleiman and Dr. Othman, as well as others in ambulances its soldiers attacked.[5] In the case of Dr. Othman, the IDF spokesperson said that the shooting was an accident as Israeli soldiers had not been informed about approval and fired at the vehicle when it did not stop.[6] In the same two-week period, from February 28 to March 13, though, Israeli fire wounded ten other PRCS emergency responders, destroyed two ambulances, and damaged ten others.[7] Because of its role as a confidential interlocutor between parties to a conflict and to preserve the neutrality of its own humanitarian activities, the ICRC rarely issues public statements criticizing a party to a conflict force by name. The multiple breaches of agreed-to procedures, and the resulting deaths, however, so angered the ICRC that its country director, René Kosiernick, issued a stinging press release that the ICRC felt "betrayed by the behavior of the IDF, which has willfully and brutally trampled on the rules of the Geneva Conventions."[8]

The second, or Al-Aqsa, Intifada began in September 2000 after the then-opposition leader Ariel Sharon provocatively visited the Temple Mount, a Muslim holy site. His visit triggered Palestinian demonstrations and soon a cycle of violence and terrorism, marked especially by more than 140 suicide bombing attacks by Palestinians until the Intifada had run its course in 2005. The bombers targeted shopping malls, restaurants, discotheques, buses, and other places central to urban life. Terrorists also launched rocket attacks and gunfire at Israeli settlements. The attacks killed hundreds of Israelis. Another four hundred planned attacks were likely foiled.[9] The bombings put people on edge. Sandrine Tiller arrived in Jerusalem shortly after my delegation left to be ICRC liaison to the PRCS, and Magen David Adom, the Israeli ambulance service. Years later, she still recalled the tension and fear in Jerusalem: "Suicide bombs going off everywhere. Everyone was so wound up." She said that a mother told her, "'I'm sending my kids to school on two different buses. Do you know what that's like?' It was pure fear that you were under attack at any moment."

Israeli security forces were severely challenged by the Intifada. The IDF initially responded to the attacks by arresting and detaining thousands of Palestinians, imposing travel restrictions in the West Bank and Gaza, and loosening rules to authorize shooting of suspected terrorists. As the number of terror attacks escalated, in February 2002 it took a more dramatic step, launching what would become a three-week Israeli military incursion into West Bank refugee camps. Designed to dismantle terrorist infrastructure, it was the largest military operation in the West Bank since the 1967 war. For Palestinians living in West Bank towns, the Israeli soldiers, tanks, and other heavy military equipment created an intimidating presence. Israel restricted movement of Palestinians and imposed curfews. Tiller told me, "Palestinians were very tense because they were living under curfews, having incursions in their neighborhood. The kids were crying all the time; there was domestic violence in the houses, and incredible tension. Then the curfew was lifted for a whole hour, people would run out to do shopping and then would be abused by soldiers." In Gaza, too, tensions were high. The IDF had launched airstrikes into Gaza to target militants. Dr. Eyad Saraj, an internationally known psychiatrist who founded and ran the Gaza Community Mental Health Programme, told me at the time that the attacks traumatized not only children but had deeply affected him. "It is so horrific," he said. "I couldn't sleep at night I was so terrified. When I walked out, I thought Gaza would be flattened."

I felt the fear and tension when we arrived in Jerusalem. As I walked by bus stops, I found myself quickening my step. The guards armed with automatic weapons stationed in front of restaurants and our hotel were more a reminder of risk than an assurance of safety. One day, while meeting with the International Committee of the Red Cross on the other side of Jerusalem from our hotel, I heard the sound of an explosion—another bomb. The circuitous route my taxi driver took back to the hotel was nerve-wracking. I checked to make sure everyone was accounted for but was shaking when I called the PHR home office to let them know we were all okay.

The intense fighting in the West Bank generated an urgent need for medical evacuation of the wounded. ICRC negotiated and managed a process for these evacuations with the civilian-military coordination unit of the IDF and the Palestine Red Crescent Society. It was supposed to work as follows: when PRCS received a request to come to the aid of a wounded person, it contacted ICRC, which forwarded the request to the IDF civilian-military coordination unit. The civ-mil unit contacted commanders in the field to request clearance, and when it received a response, the unit conveyed it to ICRC. If it was positive, the ICRC gave the go-ahead to PRCS. The multiple rounds of calls required made the process awkward and time-consuming at best, and given the tension stemming from clocks ticking with human lives at stake, emotionally fraught. "What would happen is that I'd get a call from the PRCS ops room," Sandrine Tiller explained, describing how she might be told of an unconscious baby in a certain neighborhood. She would then call the Israeli civil liaison office and request the ambulance and be told to wait until they called her back. "And then you would just wait and wait and wait and think about the unconscious baby," she said. The PRCS would call back, anxious to come to the rescue, saying something like, "What the hell is going on, we've got to get out there." As liaison, she would call the Israelis asking if they had given the greenlight. She recalled often saying, "'It's really urgent.' But they would say no, standby, and then call back in a few minutes and say yes you have the green light."

Even when the IDF granted permission, the tensions didn't cease. Palestinian medics and drivers were proud of their work and reputation. They were committed to professionalism and impartiality, as were Israeli health workers. Dr. Jonathan Halevy, director general of a Jerusalem hospital, the Shaare Zedek Medical Center, told our delegation, "Politics stops at the front door. We treat people, not beliefs." The PRCS medics resented Israeli demands to search PRCS ambulances, which the law permits, and their humiliating treatment by IDF soldiers, which it does not. Once Tiller was meeting with a Palestine Red Crescent staff member to review financial matters when he described his experience going to work that day with his son. An Israeli soldier forced him to kneel before him, just to humiliate him.

The process often did not work as intended. IDF responses to requests for ambulance passage were too often very slow, or did not come at all.

Tiller became deeply frustrated by both the failing system and her sense that the IDF was resisting taking steps to fix it. Once, she said, she met with the district IDF civil liaison staff and presented a list of cases where the IDF had prevented passage of ambulances, including cases of people in a medical crisis such as obstructed labor. The civil liaison staff responded with vague and noncommittal answers. She said that the officers were "always a bit doubtful" about the facts presented or reverted to the mantra that "you know they always carry bombs in ambulances." She was angry that "there was no accountability" and "their response was not humanitarian."

The attacks on emergency responders in March made the evacuation of the wounded even more fraught. Dr. Hossam Elsharkawi, then operations director for the PRCS, told me later that "It was a moment of extreme anger and frustration and pure rage within the organization, that despite the organization trying to do its best to conduct its medical mission with maximum integrity, they were still attacked again and again despite the green light." The uncertainty and violence also affected its labor relations. "It was a difficult time for senior management for us in PRCS," he said. "There was almost a revolt among rank and file, with frontline medics saying, 'these bullshit principles and IHL [International Humanitarian Law] and we still die.' Their families were showing up at headquarters, furious." The head of the ICRC's office in Gaza told me that medics there were "completely terrorized." PRCS was also under pressure from patients' families, who screamed about delays in their loved ones receiving urgent aid.

Israeli soldiers, for their part, were anxious and suspicious because they were both the targets of suicide bombers and held responsible for preventing terror attacks. For an IDF soldier, any Palestinian might be a terrorist. They were deployed to volatile areas of the West Bank in relatively small numbers, while the local populations angrily chafed at the restrictions and controls they faced. The soldiers often became hypervigilant when they saw a vehicle, even an ambulance, moving during long curfews. At the time of our visit, there had been no reported incidents of ambulances carrying weapons or combatants. Peter Lerner, then a captain and later a lieutenant colonel (and now retired) in the IDF, who had been engaged in coordinating work between the IDF and the ICRC since 1992, told me later that the IDF had intelligence at the time to confirm their suspicions that ambulances were transporting weapons. A week or so after our team left, the IDF discovered an explosive belt in an ambulance.

Lt. Col. Lerner personally experienced the tragedies resulting from systemic failures in medical evacuation. In November 2002, Iain Hook, manager for a UN Relief and Works Administration (UNRWA) project to rebuild the Jenin refugee camp in the West Bank, was shot by an IDF sniper in the UN compound during a gun battle between the IDF and Palestinian militants. UNRWA officials called an ambulance and invoked the liaison process. "At the time I was in the planning process of an operation taking place in Bethlehem," Lerner recalled. He had no cell phone and was disconnected from outside communication, which he needed for his work as civ-mil medical liaison. "This guy was trying to get hold of me while I was in this discussion with the generals. And when I came out of it, I'd seen he'd looked for me when I tried to call him back." By then it was too late. IDF soldiers had refused ambulance access to evacuate Hook, delaying medical intervention, and Hook died before reaching a hospital. UNRWA officials expressed outrage.[10] The international media covered Hook's death. UN Secretary-General Kofi Annan issued a damning statement, and the Security Council considered a resolution condemning Israel. I later spoke to Lerner's superior, then-Major (and later lieutenant colonel) Daniel Beaudoin, deputy head of the foreign relations branch of the Coordinator of Government Activities in the territories for the IDF. He acted as chief liaison between Israel and humanitarian organizations, including the ICRC. He told me that even though the mistakes made by Israeli soldiers in the Iain Hook case were understandable, they should not be condoned.

A study of American soldiers' behavior at checkpoints in Iraq helps explain the Israeli soldiers' conduct and the systemic failures underlying them.[11] Thomas Gregory, the author, reviewed more than 150 declassified incident reports where American soldiers killed Iraqis in the vicinity of checkpoints in 2006–7. The incident reports revealed that the soldiers shot at civilians despite evidence that they had not engaged in threatening behavior. Victims had been driving in the wrong lane, holding an object, or driving fast. Thomas notes that at first glance the shootings look like simple mistakes in a highly volatile environment. The soldiers' accounts, however, suggested that their anxiety, unease, and assumptions about Iraqis may have led them to misinterpret innocent movements for indications of hostile intent. To compound the problem, the rules under which the soldiers operated were broad and subjective, allowing them to infer hostile intent when observing any behavior by someone approaching a checkpoint that seemed somehow out of the ordinary. Gregory concluded that tighter rules designed to promote decisions based on facts rather than fears, training on how to distinguish real from imagined threats, and accountability to the rules could have avoided the tragic killings without jeopardizing soldiers' safety.

In an eerie parallel to the American experience in Iraq, the IDF had loose rules about what constituted an imminent threat to Israeli soldiers, and commanders failed to train soldiers about the need to allow ambulances cleared for passage to move safely to evacuate wounded people.[12] Additionally, the clearance coordination system for ambulances was understaffed and inadequate to perform its function. The six deaths in March 2002 were the latest incidents in a larger pattern. From 2000 through early 2002, IDF soldiers wounded 134 PRCS emergency responders and damaged 174 ambulances.[13] After the March shootings, Lt. Col. Lerner recalled, the IDF realized that system-level problems in medical evacuations needed to be addressed. "One of the most significant things that stuck out to me was the image of an ambulance being flattened by our tanks. It was clear that something had to change," he said. The first problem was staffing. Lt. Col. Lerner had only three other soldiers to assist him in the liaison process. With "just one person on the phone at the time and they have to answer for six operations that have taken place simultaneously," errors were inevitable. Compounding the problem, Lt. Col. Lerner said, Israeli soldiers would see "all of these different types of emergency vehicles traveling around," many without apparent authorization. Lerner also pointed out that many ambulance services and international organizations attempted to travel in nonemergency vehicles during the curfew, an especially dangerous time.

After our delegation's discussions with Israeli and Palestinian health workers and administrators, military officials, the ICRC, members of the Knesset, human rights groups, and others, the delegation sent a letter to the minister of defense. One of our major recommendations was to reform policies and procedures to ensure safe passage of ambulances to evacuate the wounded.[14] Around the same time, in early April 2002, the Israeli NGO Physicians for Human Rights Israel (which is not affiliated with the U.S.-based group), filed a petition in Israel's High Court seeking an order for the IDF to cease violations against Palestinian emergency medical responders, citing fourteen recent incidents of obstruction and violence against ambulances and their personnel. Israel's judicial system was unusual in permitting challenges to military practices to be adjudicated in court, though it had a reputation for deferring to the IDF.[15]

The government responded that the IDF recognized that it was bound by the rules of international humanitarian law, "not only because these rules are binding under international law, but also because they are required by morality itself, and even due to utilitarian reasons."[16] The government cited the potential for bombs in ambulances but acknowledged that it nevertheless had a duty to permit legitimate and inspected ambulances safe passage. It stated, somewhat misleadingly given the shortages, that the IDF allocated resources for liaison and humanitarian aid in combat zones. On April 8, the court issued its decision. It did not address the specific allegations about particular incidents set out in the petition but acknowledged that the alleged violations were "on the face of things, severe." It went on to say, "We see fit to emphasize that our combat forces are required to abide by the rules of humanitarian law regarding the care of the wounded, the ill, and bodies of the deceased. The fact that medical personnel have abused their position in hospitals and ambulances has made it necessary for the IDF to act in order to prevent such activities but does not, in and of itself, justify sweeping breaches of humanitarian rules."[17] The court required the IDF to "instruct the combat forces, down to the level of the lone soldier in the field, of this commitment by our forces based on law and morality . . . through concrete instructions which will prevent, to the extent possible, and even in severe situations, incidents which are inconsistent with the rules of humanitarian law."[18]

The government committed "to allow all medical vehicles quick and safe passage without exception."[19] Changes were slow in coming, though, perhaps complicated by a dramatic escalation in terrorism and Israel's military response. On March 27, a few days after we left Israel, a suicide bomber attacked a dining room in a resort hotel in Netanya, outside Tel Aviv, where a large group of Israelis were celebrating Passover. The attack killed 19 people and wounded more than 170 others. The same week the IDF said it found a suicide bomber's explosive belt in a Palestinian ambulance. On April 8, the day the court ruled, then Prime Minister Ariel Sharon ordered a second, and far more aggressive reoccupation of West Bank refugee camps and cities, including Ramallah, Nablus, and Bethlehem. Infantry, assault helicopters, and tanks entered the Jenin refugee camp. Palestinian fighters booby-trapped the area and ambushed Israeli forces. The IDF responded with armored bulldozers that leveled large parts of Jenin. At the same time, the IDF imposed even more draconian restrictions on humanitarian movement in the West Bank. The ICRC wrote to Sharon, saying that the severity of the restrictions on its movement would compel it to leave. Francois Bellon, a highly experienced ICRC hand, who arrived in Israel two months later to lead its delegation, told me that 2002 was the low point for the organization's work in the region.

Eventually, reforms in coordination and movement of ambulances to evacuate the wounded from places of combat proceeded. Sharon asked the ICRC to stay and assured the organization that it would be able to do its job. Reforms in the clearance process and respect for ambulances focused on command leadership and increased staffing for the coordination process, and established clear procedures and better communication in the field. In 2003 the IDF instituted a mandatory training for soldiers on medical evacuation in combat. Lt. Col Lerner said that liaison staff spoke to soldiers at volatile locations, which he described as a "huge leap." For its part, the Palestine Red Crescent Society, with support from the ICRC, repainted its ambulances to tangerine reflective orange to make it easier for IDF soldiers to identify them. The ICRC also distributed booklets to frontline soldiers with pictures of the PRCS ambulances, the major provider of emergency medical evacuations in the West Bank, and the uniforms the staff wore.

PRCS also submitted a request through the ICRC to import flak jackets and helmets for its emergency medical teams. At first, Israel refused, deeming them to be military equipment prohibited in the West Bank. But the PRCS used its contacts to arrange a confidential meeting with the IDF. Dr. Elsharkawi said, "They heard us out. It was a practical conversation." One of the Israelis expressed appreciation for the PRCS's professionalism and policy against misuse of ambulances and recognized that any cases of misuse were not representative of the organization's stance. "These guys had level heads," he said. "They knew that a single case does not represent the hundreds of medics and the organization. At the end they allowed import of flak jackets for Gaza and the West Bank. A certain rapport was established. They trusted that PRCS would conduct itself in a principled manner."

Though slow to develop, the reforms had positive results. By late 2003 and into 2004, the ICRC's Francois Bellon agreed with the IDF's Beaudoin and Lerner that medical evacuation in periods of active conflict improved. The reforms also punctured some commonly accepted myths about asymmetrical warfare, where a conventional military faces armed groups that use unconventional tactics including those that contravene the laws of war, such as terror attacks. One myth is that in asymmetrical warfare, conventional forces are compelled to choose between fulfilling obligations of humanity and law and duties to prevent terrorist attacks, such as those perpetrated through bombs in ambulances. Bioethicist Michael Gross argued that in the asymmetrical conflict between the IDF and Palestinians, these duties can't be reconciled. He claimed that the conflict of obligations "upended traditionally honored guidelines for passage of ambulances" and created "dilemmas for which international law and custom offer no ready solution."[20]

As the experience during the Intifada and the reforms undertaken showed, there is no dilemma or conflict of obligations. Adopting appropriate procedures, implementing and staffing them properly, and training soldiers can fulfill the requirements of expeditious medical evacuation while protecting against misuse of ambulances, placing soldiers at needless risk, or disrupting military operations. Firing at ambulances did not pit medical and humanitarian needs against the prevention of terrorism. Instead, it represented a failure of military doctrine, training, practice, and accountability. With the impetus of pressure and internal soul searching, the IDF showed that the problem could be solved when leadership and implementation mechanisms were put in place. The politics of achieving the change was difficult, but no military considerations were sacrificed in the process. As the Israeli-Palestinian conflict continued, however, the reforms proved fleeting.

## CHECKPOINTS: THE RECURRING NIGHTMARE

Checkpoints within the West Bank and Gaza and between the occupied Palestinian territory and Israel have long been a dreary fact of life for Palestinians. For women in labor and people in need of treatment for chronic diseases, routine care, or medical emergencies, traveling to health facilities has been at best a grim chore and at worst a nightmare that sometimes ends in death. Even in the absence of active fighting, harassment and delay of Palestinians needing to pass through checkpoints has been a source of anguish and anger over decades of occupation. In 1996 and 1999, human rights groups brought cases in the Israeli courts alleging unwarranted checkpoint delays for Palestinians urgently in need of medical care. In response to the 1996 case, the IDF committed to revising its procedures to expedite passage through checkpoints of people in need of emergency care. In the 1999 case, the High Court found that even though the IDF had drafted new procedures, they had neither been disseminated nor implemented.[21] As a result of the 1999 case, in January 2000 the IDF announced that it would alert all the soldiers staffing checkpoints to the policy. The court ordered its implementation by the end of the month.

The policy hinged on what constituted a medical emergency. According to the new rules, emergency was defined to include imminent birth, bleeding and burn injuries, and other medical conditions as determined at the discretion of the checkpoint commander. It also required the commander to check with medical personnel if time permitted, and to give the benefit of any doubt to Palestinians. For nonemergency cases, the patient was supposed to get advance permission from a district coordination office after supplying documentation of medical need. The policy mandated that delays for inspection and approving passage be limited to thirty minutes in nonemergency cases. The rules and procedures, especially for people with chronic conditions needing regular treatment such as dialysis, however, were cumbersome and highly bureaucratic. Aside from the time-consuming steps, Palestinians frequently had to supply records that were not readily available. Nonetheless, if the policies had been effectively implemented, they could have ameliorated some of the harms to patients and emergency responders. But many of the agreed-to measures were not put into practice.[22]

During the second Intifada, accessing medical care became even more complicated and fraught for Palestinians. The IDF created more than a hundred new checkpoints within the West Bank and Gaza and erected hundreds of unstaffed roadblocks that prevented cars from traveling from one place to another in the West Bank.[23] B'Tselem reported in 2001 that at least twenty-seven Palestinians died because soldiers prevented or delayed the passage of people with medical needs through a checkpoint.[24] In March of that year alone, a cancer patient in need of an operation was prevented from reaching a hospital in Ramallah for two days. An eleven-year-old child with a high fever died after her family, which was bringing her to a hospital in Nablus, was delayed at a checkpoint. The Palestine Red

Crescent Society told Israel's High Court of another 121 cases of delays in transporting the sick and wounded in a period of less than five months at the end of 2000 and the beginning of 2001.[25] Our delegation learned of a case where a man bleeding from three gunshot wounds didn't reach a medical facility because the IDF obstructed the ambulance's passage through a checkpoint. We received repeated reports that in Ramallah a dozen medical personnel were detained and three ambulances confiscated at checkpoints.

Naomi Chazan, then deputy speaker of the Knesset and a peace activist, told me at the time that Palestinian friends regularly called her about tragedies stemming for obstruction and delays, including two mothers who lost babies at checkpoints. "It's absolutely the kind of thing that keeps you up at night," she said. She wrote to the prime minister to protest, without effect. In the summer of 2002, a UN report by Catherine Bertini, the personal humanitarian envoy of the UN secretary-general, found that thirty-nine children were born at checkpoints and the teams of one NGO were turned back half the time. As a result of similar obstructions and road blockages, some Palestinians gave up seeking needed health care. Far more mothers gave birth at home, increasingly without skilled attendances, and stillbirths in the West Bank increased by more than 30 percent. The blockages also forced UN mobile clinics to shut down. Hospital admissions reflected the decline in access. The report also stated that St. Luke's Hospital in Nablus experienced a 49 percent decline in general practice patients, a 73 percent decline in specialty services, and a 53 percent decline in surgeries.[26] Roads in the Nablus area were closed entirely for varying periods of time in 2003, preventing ambulances from entering the city. Overall, utilization of health care in the West Bank declined by about 60 percent. The obstruction of medical passage was just one element of the IDF soldiers' conduct. Many engaged in what became routine humiliation of and violence against Palestinians at checkpoints and indifference to their needs of travel. In 2001, the outrages led a group of Israeli women to create *Machsom*, Checkpoint Watch, to monitor the conduct of the IDF at the checkpoints, try to persuade the soldiers to act more humanely toward Palestinians, and document harassment and delays.[27]

Francois Bellon, the ICRC delegation head at the time, told me that even as IDF reforms increased the safety of medical evacuation in areas of active conflict in late 2002 and 2003, chronic checkpoint problems persisted. Human rights investigators found that soldiers at checkpoints delayed passage and sometimes turned back ambulances even in medical emergencies and did not consult with medical officers as required.[28] In a 2004 statement, the government agreed that it had a moral as well as legal obligation to permit medical passage notwithstanding the need to be on guard for the possibility of ambulances transporting bombs or fighters. It acknowledged that it had received more than three hundred complaints at checkpoints, which it labeled "inquiries," about "health matters," but did not set out any plan to address them.[29]

The unresolved problems at checkpoints led a group of Israeli anthropologists and conflict experts from the Hebrew University of Jerusalem to embark on a study of the checkpoints.[30] The researchers interviewed dozens of frontline soldiers, military commanders, government officials, and Palestinian academics and activists, and reviewed rules, documents, and media reports. They found that, contrary to IDF claims, violence by soldiers against Palestinians at checkpoints was common. It was not unusual for soldiers to damage vehicles and verbally abuse, hit, or kick Palestinians, or threaten them with weapons. The research group also confirmed that the Palestinians' experience at checkpoints was typically humiliating, demeaning, arbitrary, and degrading. Those findings were consistent with a prior survey of 150 soldiers by a former IDF psychologist that revealed high numbers of self-reported acts of violence against Palestinians.[31] Later studies contained similar findings.[32] Among the reasons for the misconduct, the Hebrew University team found, included the lack of standardized rules—in fact, they were ever-changing—and lack of training and discipline of soldiers regarding abuse of Palestinians. Commanders' assessment metrics for the soldiers' conduct were limited to strict security criteria, such as stopping Palestinian aggressors, and collecting intelligence. Soldiers understood that they were unlikely to be held to account for mistreatment of Palestinians.

The Hebrew University group also looked at the soldiers' perceptions about their assignment to and experience at checkpoints as a contributing factor. The interviews revealed that soldiers found their work at checkpoints to be boring, demeaning, and a low-status job for a combat soldier. The culture at checkpoints included distrust and dehumanization of Palestinians. At the same time, the soldiers had little guidance in making difficult decisions about who was dangerous and who was not, which contributed to their anxiety and aggression. Oded Na'aman, an Israeli philosopher who served in the IDF during the second Intifada, illuminated the impossible choices soldiers faced at checkpoints, how Palestinians suffered from those choices, and the moral distress the soldiers experienced as a result. Minute to minute, hour to hour, he wrote, soldiers were expected to determine which Palestinians might be threats, but "there are no principles or rules to tell him a terrorist from a harmless citizen." As a result, soldiers felt constrained from giving Palestinians the benefit of the doubt: "If you let everyone through who comes with a kid and a fractured arm, you'll be letting terrorist[s] through before you know it." Na'aman wrote that the soldiers' minds inevitably focused on the potential danger:

> As you stand at the checkpoint, you must constantly consider the various ways in which you may be attacked: Where are they going to come from? What will their strategy be? Is that child as innocent as he seems, or is he smuggling a weapon? Is that ambulance really rushing a woman to the hospital to give birth, or are there enemies hiding inside? Is that old man harmless, or is he deliberately diverting your attention from something that is happening behind your back? You have to get into their minds. They are creative, and they have already exploited our naivety and good will in the past. They can come up with anything, and you have to come up with it first.[33]

Command instructions added to the propensity to abuse. To guard against terrorists manipulating their way through checkpoints, Na'aman wrote, commanders told soldiers to "demonstrate presence" through an unofficial policy of instilling fear in Palestinians through the use of arbitrary force.

At first, he said, soldiers might be conflicted about intimidating and threatening Palestinians without attempting to distinguish whether they were innocent or hostile. The soldiers initially worried about not acting in accordance with their values by adopting a stance of "moral indifference" to the humiliation and violence inflicted on all Palestinians. Soldiers often began by resisting temptation to abuse, but day by day they "can no longer feel the distinctive moral shock [they] felt when [they] first arrived at the checkpoint" and found only validation through the respect fellow soldiers showed for severe treatment of Palestinians.[34]

The Hebrew University group recognized that the IDF took some steps to respect humanitarian needs at checkpoints. These included placement of more experienced reservists as "humanitarian officers," and the establishment of administrative complaint mechanisms for Palestinians. But the researchers found that, in the absence of command leadership and standards of conduct and accountability, these efforts were insufficient. They found that some senior officials in the Israeli military recognized the "high moral price" the country paid for the treatment of Palestinians at checkpoints. The future minister of defense, Moshe Ya'alon, who was IDF chief of staff from mid-2002 to mid-2005, said, "I am worried by the fact that even if we do win this war, in the end, we will not be able to look at ourselves in the mirror."[35]

Political scientist Samy Cohen added another perspective to the understanding of the harsh practices and obstructions at the checkpoints. He noted that Israel was at first slow to respond to the terror attacks during the second Intifada, but in 2002 began to respond far more aggressively, engaging in collective punishment, targeted killings, and demolitions of the houses of families of Palestinians suspected of violent acts against Israel. He said it took no corresponding steps to impose military order and discipline, once a hallmark of the IDF, thus opening the door to abuses by IDF soldiers.[36]

The conduct of Israelis soldiers in denying or obstructing passage of ambulances and other vehicles carrying the wounded and sick at checkpoints was little different from that of other militaries. Israel is unique only in the extensive reporting of its checkpoint practices by human rights and civil society groups over the course of decades. Other countries also typically lack clear policy, doctrine, rules, and training and disciplinary practices to facilitate ambulance passage at checkpoints. According to data collected by the ICRC from twenty-three countries in 2012 and 2013, of the almost eight hundred acts of violence against medical transports it found, almost a quarter of them were at checkpoints.[37] The true number is likely much higher, because most incidents are not reported. In Afghanistan and Iraq troops often misidentified people at checkpoints as an enemy.[38] Throughout the war in Colombia, ambulances were among the more frequent targets of violence, including robbery, extortion, kidnapping and physical attacks on crews.[39] In eastern Ukraine, thousands of people a day, most of whom are over the age of sixty, seeking to cross the contact line between government and insurgent troops for medical care routinely faced hours of waiting, even in freezing weather.[40] In South Sudan's civil war, all sides have obstructed passage of vehicles carrying people needing emergency care, stolen medical supplies, and even abducted and killed health workers and others seeking passage.[41] In Yemen, roadblocks and checkpoints have become pervasive, severely delaying passage of humanitarian supplies, health workers, and ambulances, and providing an opportunity to extort funds from medical and aid groups.[42] In Somalia, checkpoints complicate the ability of health workers to reach the facilities where they practice.

The chaos at the checkpoints, the moral distress it caused among soldiers, and the dissatisfaction at high levels of command at the arbitrary practices added to the political pressure generated by *Machsom* and human rights organizations for reform. In 2004, then-Prime Minister Ariel Sharon appointed a retired major general, Baruch Spiegel, to head a group to examine the humanitarian and "fabric of life" issues for Palestinians, including at checkpoints. Spiegel found what others had reported before: lack of clear rules; lack of discipline and accountability for soldiers; fatigue, stress, humiliation, and anger among frontline troops; and infringements of human rights of Palestinians.[43] He recommended distinguishing "envelope checkpoints," designed to manage Palestinians' travel within the West Bank, and "closure" checkpoints, between the

Israel side of the new separation barrier and the West Bank and East Jerusalem.[44] Especially at closure checkpoints, he recommended the use of technology and physical infrastructure comparable to machinery employed at international borders. Spiegel sold the changes as a major humanitarian reform and authorities portrayed the system as rational, humane, and service oriented.[45] He was so successful in marketing his proposals that the United States provided $50 million to Israel to fund the checkpoint infrastructure, which imposed permanent restrictions on Palestinian movement.[46] Additionally, over time, in the name of professionalization and improved service, checkpoint operations were increasingly outsourced to private security companies, keeping IDF soldiers mostly at arm's length from daily interaction with Palestinians.[47]

The new system in some respects regularized procedures for people in need of medical care and the passage of ambulances. Yet it largely replaced one form of arbitrariness and access limitations for another. Israel vastly expanded its permit system for passage and the bureaucratic requirements that accompanied it. Health facilities in the West Bank and Gaza were ill-equipped to provide medical care for cancer, eye and kidney diseases, and orthopedic and pediatric conditions, or offer nuclear medicine and MRIs. These services, among others, were provided by the six major Palestinian hospitals in East Jerusalem that are located on the Israeli side of the separation barrier. To access this care through the closure checkpoints, tens of thousands of Palestinians had to obtain a permit. To get one, they had to present medical documents with evidence of their condition, their appointments at specific times, and other information. The permits were time-limited. In some instances, women anticipating childbirth in an East Jerusalem hospital could only get a permit for two days; if labor didn't begin, the women had to apply for another permit. Additionally, West Bank patients needing emergency care in East Jerusalem had to transfer to another Palestinian ambulance based in East Jerusalem. The process, known as "back-to-back," required complicated authorization procedures that were often medically contraindicated and delayed care.

To improve ambulance transport from the West Bank to the East Jerusalem hospitals, in 2005 the ICRC negotiated a memorandum of understanding among Israel, the PRCS, and the Israeli ambulance service, Magen David Adom, that included a provision allowing PRCS West Bank ambulances to enter East Jerusalem. Israel at first declined to implement the agreement. In 2011, six years after the agreement was signed, an independent monitor found that West Bank ambulances were allowed to make the entire trip to East Jerusalem hospitals without the need for patient transfer. He noted, though, that the approval procedures for passage "are complicated, time consuming and vulnerable to disruption," and a source of "consternation and disappointment."[48] Later, Israel returned to the back-to-back process, which it applied to 93 percent of PRCS transport cases from the West Bank to East Jerusalem.[49] At the end of 2019, fourteen years after the agreement was signed, the International Conference of the Red Cross and Red Crescent adopted a resolution expressing "strong disappointment that after nearly 14 years the MoU is not yet fully implemented and particularly noting the recent difficulties, delays and limitations by Israeli public authorities on the licensing of PRCS ambulances to operate in East Jerusalem and noting the potential related negative humanitarian consequences."[50]

The permit system and other checkpoint barriers led to decreased access to care for Palestinians. A study conducted in 2005 found that almost 20 percent of more than two thousand patients traveling to two hospitals in Nablus and one in Bethlehem experienced checkpoint delays. Those who were delayed were significantly more likely to be admitted to the hospital than those who were not. That finding suggests either that the delays in transit worsened the person's condition or that people having to cross checkpoints known to be sources of delay postponed seeking care until their condition had deteriorated.[51] Outpatient visits at Makassed Hospital in East Jerusalem declined 30 percent after the permit system went into effect.[52] About 20 percent of applications from the West Bank patients for care in East Jerusalem between 2011 and 2013 were denied or delayed, a percentage that persisted through 2019.[53] Individuals living in Gaza had even more difficulty gaining a permit to travel to East Jerusalem or elsewhere, and had far lower approval rates. In 2017, Israel denied exit permits for Gazans altogether. Although that decision was overturned by the courts as an illegitimate means of putting political pressure on Hamas, Israel still denied or unduly delayed action on almost 40 percent of applications for permits for medical treatment outside Gaza.[54] Israel also required PRCS staff and hospital employees who lived in the West Bank but worked in East Jerusalem to renew their own permits every three months (for some people, the period was later extended to six months). The delays in renewal processing led to the shutdown of the East Jerusalem ambulance service for weeks at a time and the inability of hospital employees to get to work.[55]

Within the West Bank, Israel vastly increased the number of "envelope checkpoints" as well as unattended physical barriers, and movable or "flying" checkpoints. By September 2006, there were more than five hundred physical obstacles to travel within the West Bank, a 40 percent increase from a year before. In a single week in December 2006, the UN reported 160 flying checkpoints were in use.[56] In mid-2007, there were eighty checkpoints, forty-seven of them within the West Bank, plus an additional fifteen in Hebron, and the number increased in the years since.[57] Ambulance delays and violence and harassment of ambulance drivers and medics at checkpoints continued.[58] Just as in 2002, the Israeli practices took a toll on Palestinian ambulance crews because of the dangers they faced, the uncertainty that dominated their work, and the moral distress caused by not being able to reach people in need, stress that pervaded their personal as well as professional lives.[59]

Facilitating Palestinians' access to health care in routine circumstances could have been resolved without compromising security. No doubt it would have taken effort to design an effective system to meet Palestinians' medical needs while protecting Israel's security, but that course was certainly feasible, as the government had previously acknowledged to the courts. Israel took a different course and succeeded in restricting access to medical care without much political pushback. Denials of permits and delays at checkpoints were not obvious and visible in the way the killings of medical responders in 2002 were. The very bureaucratization of checkpoints created an image of rational procedure. In addition, the Israeli government and its right-wing allies adopted a strategy that extended beyond rebutting human rights reports on denials of Palestinians' access to care and other violations of Palestinians' rights. They campaigned aggressively to delegitimize the groups that criticized Israel's treatment of Palestinians and deny them access to sources of funding.[60] What is so tragic about this story is that in 2002, Israel was a leader in reforms in ensuring safe access of ambulances during active conflict. In the much less fraught circumstances of crossing checkpoints, it instead imposed greater and more damaging restrictions on access to care. Checkpoint and permit policies became an element of broader concerns about Israel's responsibilities regarding Palestinians' health needs. When COVID-19 struck, it provided only a small quantity of vaccines to Palestinians in the West Bank and Gaza, despite the requirements of the Geneva Conventions for an occupying power to adopt measures to contain epidemics.[61]

In 2015, and again in 2020, after consultations with more than two dozen militaries around the world, the ICRC published detailed recommendations on improving health access in military operations, including checkpoint procedures that would enable people in need to reach hospitals without undue delay. The proposals were highly practical: map health care providers and ambulance services that may need to travel through checkpoints; liaise with health professionals on medical evacuation; create standard operating procedures for passage at checkpoints, including how to manage passage during curfews, and discuss them with health providers and community leaders; establish liaison and communications mechanisms to notify soldiers at checkpoints that an ambulance is en route; train troops in the procedures; and establish a "lessons learned" system to address and troubleshoot problems. The recommendations also addressed passage of family and other vehicles not identified as ambulances when they needed to pass quickly to expedite care for wounded or sick individuals.[62] Five years later, few militaries had taken any steps toward adopting them. In 2020, the ICRC issued another report on military practice, finding that delays at checkpoints remained among the five most common forms of attacks or interference in health care in armed conflict and other emergencies.

The result of inaction has been continued, pointless suffering.

## GAZA: VIOLENCE AGAINST
## AMBULANCES REDUX

Journalist Lawrence Wright wrote, "Gaza is a place that Israel wishes it could ignore: the territory has long had the highest concentration of poverty, extremism, and hopelessness in the region."[63] He wrote that in 2009, four years after Israel's disengagement from Gaza and two years after Hamas forced its former partner, Fatah, out of a unity government and took exclusive control of Gaza. Hamas fired many doctors and other medical personnel affiliated with Fatah.[64] Hamas refused then, as now, to recognize Israel's right to exist or to renounce violence against it. In the decade since Wright wrote those words, the situation for almost two million Gazans penned into a small strip of land has only worsened. They had already suffered from active fighting earlier in 2009 and two more short, but devastating, wars were to follow. Ten years later, Israel's blockade deprives them of necessities. Hamas's corruption, mismanagement, and tyranny oppresses them. They cannot leave because of Israel's permit policies. Youth unemployment is 70 percent.[65] Those who live in the eight refugee camps in Gaza are squeezed into tiny warrens of deprivation.

The brief but terrifying wars between Israel and Hamas in a period of less than six years are generally known by their Israeli code names Cast Lead (2008–9), Pillar of Defense (2012), and Protective Edge (2014). The responsibility for each of the wars, like almost everything involving the Israel-Palestinian conflict, is hotly contested; suffice it to say that, at the high risk of oversimplifying, Hamas frequently fired rockets indiscriminately into densely populated areas in Israel and Israel employed airstrikes, missile attacks, and ground assaults to seek to destroy terrorist networks in Gaza. The tally from the three wars was thousands of people killed, the vast majority of them Palestinian; the evisceration of Gaza's economy, already weakened by isolation and restrictions on commerce; and a generation of children and adults left traumatized. Over the course of the three conflicts, the IDF damaged 34 hospitals, 105 clinics, and 85 ambulances.[66] Its destruction of water treatment plants, pump stations, and other infrastructure reduced access to safe drinking water for 90 percent of the population.[67] Whether Israel's conduct violated international humanitarian law in these assaults was and remains equally and bitterly contested. Consistent with the focus of this chapter, I consider only the IDF soldiers' shooting at ambulances, killing medics, and prevention of evacuation of the sick and wounded.

The IDF launched Cast Lead on December 27, 2008, after months of tensions with Hamas and the breakdown of a ceasefire. After a week of Israeli airstrikes and assaults by attack helicopters and increased Hamas rocket firings into Israel, the IDF began a ground invasion with tanks and troops, supported by artillery. Hamas responded with more rocket and mortar attacks into Israel. Israel's air and missile strikes hit schools, hospitals, water and sanitation networks, and water facilities. In the three-week war, about fourteen hundred Palestinians were killed, four thousand homes demolished, and seventeen thousand others partially destroyed. Three Israeli civilians and a soldier were killed. Medical evacuation of the wounded and humanitarian access was supposed to be facilitated by an expanded IDF civilian-military coordination unit. But the system broke down immediately, with lethal results as in 2002.

On the first day of the ground invasion, January 3, 2009, the IDF shelled several houses in the Zeitoun area of Gaza City, where it suspected Hamas fighters were operating. The shelling killed many civilians and many more were injured. The ICRC requested access by Palestinian ambulances to retrieve the wounded, but for three days the IDF did not respond. By then alarmed at the suffering of the wounded—at least one of the wounded died the first night—and the terrible delay in reaching them, a PRCS ambulance without clearance sought to rescue them. IDF soldiers refused it entry into the area. Finally, four days after the PRCS's initial request, the IDF permitted it access during a three-hour humanitarian ceasefire. The ambulances arrived at a scene of horror. As recounted in a press release issued by an enraged ICRC: "The ICRC/PRCS team found four small children next to their dead mothers in one of the houses. They were too weak to stand up on their own. One man was also found alive, too weak to stand up. In all there were at least twelve corpses lying on mattresses."[68] In the house next door, the team found fifteen survivors including several wounded people. A third house contained corpses.

As the teams of medics were searching for the wounded, IDF soldiers positioned about eighty meters away demanded that they leave. The ambulance team refused and evacuated eighteen wounded people and twelve others. The head of the ICRC delegation for Israel and occupied territory, Pierre Wettach, said, "This is a shocking incident. The Israeli military must have been aware of the situation but did not assist the wounded. Neither did they make it possible for us or the Palestine Red Crescent to assist the wounded."[69] The outrage extended to the ICRC's headquarters in Geneva, where its president, Jakob Ellenberger, issued a statement demanding unrestricted access for emergency evacuation at all times.[70] A spokesperson for Israel did not explain the IDF's action or the failure of the coordination system, saying only that better channels of communication with the Red Cross were needed.[71] The IDF said it would investigate if a complaint were filed. It did review the shelling of the housing in Zeitoun, but I could find no evidence of an IDF investigation of the refusal to rescue the wounded.

Ambulance access did not improve as fighting continued after the Zeitoun incident. As in 2002, PRCS clearance was delayed, and ambulances and medics were shot at by Israeli soldiers and tanks even after clearance was given. Marwan Hammouda, an ambulance driver for PRCS, told human rights investigators about one incident where he and medics came to evacuate the wounded. The ICRC had coordinated access with the IDF, and medics arrived after fighting in the area had ended. IDF soldiers shot at them and they had to withdraw.[72] IDF soldiers also fired on a convoy of thirteen ambulances cleared for travel to Egypt. Because of the long delays PRCS experienced in receiving a response to its requests for emergency medical evacuation, and feeling responsible to respond to life-threatening injuries urgently, it sometimes sent ambulances to the wounded without clearance. The IDF often shot at them. In a mere three weeks, the IDF killed sixteen Palestinian on-duty health workers and injured twenty-five others, four of them in a single day. Twenty-nine Palestinian ambulances, representing 20 percent of the fleet, were destroyed or damaged.[73]

Years after procedures for medical evacuation in active conflict were supposed to have been resolved, human rights groups again petitioned Israel's High Court for ambulance access and an end to violence against emergency responders. Colonel Moshe Levy, head of the IDF coordination unit, told the court, as his predecessors had represented seven years earlier, that the IDF recognized its duty to allow medical evacuation and was committed to it. Colonel Levy did not assert that Hamas's many violations of international law justified refusal of medical evacuation by Israel, as Israel understood well-established law that breaches by one side do not excuse violations by the other. Like his predecessors, though, Colonel Levy did not address any of the specific allegations in the petition. Instead, he asserted, as they had, that the IDF did not deliberately attack medical personnel who are "genuinely seeking to provide medical assistance," and that incidents were likely a product of "conditions under which the fighting was taking place."[74] To show its humanitarian commitment, the IDF also said that it had established a clinic for wounded people at Israel's boundary with Gaza. The court's ruling, issued a day after a cease-fire ended active fighting, affirmed the IDF's duty to permit medical evacuation of the wounded and not to attack medical personnel engaged in the performance of their duty, so long as they were not engaged in military activities outside their humanitarian function. But as in 2002, the court denied the petition without addressing the facts of the cases, in "view of the statement made to us that a serious effort will be made to improve the evacuation and treatment of the wounded." It added, "It is to be hoped that the humanitarian mechanisms will operate properly in accordance with the obligations of the State of Israel."[75]

It was a forlorn hope. After Cast Lead, Israel's Ministry of Foreign Affairs issued a public report on its conduct of the war. It affirmed a commitment to abide by the Geneva Conventions and said that it instructed soldiers to respect and protect health care facilities, personnel, and vehicles, subject only to limitations concerning their misuse, and cooperation with inspection and clearance procedures.[76] The report congratulated the

IDF for the numbers of requests for ambulance coordination it handled to evacuate Palestinians. It did not, however, address days-long delays in approving emergency evacuations and the consequences for injured people, or the IDF's firing at ambulances after they had been cleared. Nor did it review cases where a Palestinian medic was killed while trying to save the life of a wounded person except to acknowledge one case in which it said a local IDF commander mistakenly concluded that an ambulance had been used for military purposes.[77] It also cast blame on Hamas for allegedly misusing ambulances for military purposes and aspersions on the ambulance teams for incidents where ambulances proceeded for evacuation without clearance.

The IDF also conducted internal investigations of a series of claims of alleged violations of the laws of war during Cast Lead. One of them, led by Israeli Colonel Erez Katz, reviewed complaints about IDF shooting at medical facilities.[78] Colonel Katz reported that his investigation revealed that Hamas made "extensive use of ambulances to transport terror operatives and weaponry." As evidence, he cited only an Italian newspaper article and unspecified "reports" of such conduct, so it is difficult to assess the basis for his conclusion. Israel's ambulance service, Magen David Adom, however, vouched that PRCS had not used ambulances to transport weapons or ammunition or misused the Red Crescent emblem, and a UN investigation did not find evidence of Hamas misusing ambulances.[79] Colonel Katz also cited incidents where ambulances had not received clearance and were driven in a suspicious manner, but did not address whether ambulances that were cleared, properly marked, and traveling with lights flashing, were shot at. Nor did he consider whether ambulance access was unreasonably delayed. Col. Katz also found that, in incidents he investigated, five of seven medical responders wounded were "Hamas operatives." It is not clear on what basis he made this judgment (and he provided no evidence), but if they were affiliated with Hamas they were still entitled to protection, just as IDF medics are, so long as they were not used outside their humanitarian function to commit acts harmful to the enemy. Colonel Katz concluded that the IDF "took extraordinary care" in ensuring the safety of medical evacuation.

The Ministry of Foreign Affairs report also discussed the IDF's rules of engagement, which emphasized minimizing harm to civilians and protection of medical vehicles from attack unless they are used for military purposes.[80] Accounts by soldiers on the ground during Cast Lead, though, paint a different picture of instructions in the field that suggest why ambulances were so vulnerable. The Israeli group Breaking the Silence collected testimonies of the experiences of more than fifty soldiers who participated in Cast Lead. These may not constitute a representative sample of the soldiers who served, but the consistency of their narratives provides insight into the reasons for the shootings. One of the most frequent themes in the testimonies is that instructions from field commanders permitted and even encouraged shoot-on-sight responses to movements of people and vehicles. One soldier said:

> The brigade commander and other officers made it very clear to us that any movement must entail gunfire . . . you don't need to be shot at. . . . You don't only shoot when threatened. The assumption is that you constantly feel threatened, so anything there threatens you, and you shoot. No one actually said, "shoot regardless" or "shoot anything that moves." But we were not ordered to open fire only if there was a real threat.

He added: "As for the rules of engagement, we did not get instructions to shoot at anything that moved, but we were generally instructed: if you feel threatened, shoot. They kept repeating to us that this is war and in war opening fire is not restricted."[81]

Another soldier confirmed, "whatever gets in your way, you do everything to prevent its getting in your way, regardless of the humanitarian implications of such an action."[82] One reported that the message was to have "a light finger on the trigger. You see something and you're not quite sure? You shoot."[83] A number of other soldiers confirmed that they were expected to shoot at anything that looked suspicious.[84] One of them emphasized the instructions were not always explicit, but the message was clear: "We weren't told outright to shoot anything we saw moving, but that was the implication."[85] Another reported, "The issue of civilians became irrelevant as soon as you'd enter combat—the rules change. You shoot. It's war. In war no questions are asked."[86] Another soldier said: "My impression about rules of engagement was that, at least at our level, they were not clear. There were no clear red lines. In urban areas, it's very much at the commanders' own discretion."[87] It is not hard to see how, even with strict official rules of engagement, the quick trigger policies in the field and the breakdown in the coordination system likely contributed to the harrowing and sometimes fatal experiences of emergency medical responders. Unlike in 2002, however, after Cast Lead the IDF did not take a close look at the gross failure of safe ambulance evacuation or what reforms were needed.

Unreasonable delays in approval of evacuation and airstrikes against and firing at ambulances was reported again during the week-long operation Pillar of Defense in 2012.[88] They recurred, too, in the most lethal of the wars, Operation Protective Edge, in 2014. In the fifty-day conflict, an estimated 2,200 Palestinians were killed, with counts of civilian deaths ranging from the Israeli number of 750 to a UN assessment of 1,500. A large number of children were killed. More than a quarter million residents of the Gaza strip were displaced. Israel suffered seventy-one deaths, five of them civilians. Seventeen hospitals and fifty-six primary health care clinics were damaged. Sixteen health workers were killed while on duty, and eighty-three others, mostly ambulance crew members, were injured. Forty-five ambulances were damaged.[89]

As previously, ambulance responses were often seriously delayed for many hours and, in some cases, days.[90] Again, PRCS medics, frustrated by the delays in approval, sometimes went to the rescue without clearance. Yousef Al Kahlout, a paramedic, told a medical investigation team, in words reminiscent of 2002, "We would wait for long minutes, sometimes hours, awaiting coordination, and people kept calling and pleading for evacuation, we could hear them crying for help. We knew they were bleeding, dying . . . so very often we couldn't wait and just went off [to assist them]."[91] According to data collected by Palestinian groups in Gaza, more than five hundred wounded people never reached medical assistance because of ambulance blockage or delays.[92]

As in Cast Lead, the use of discretion by junior officers in the field encouraged hair-trigger shooting.[93] On the night of July 25, 2014, after coordination with ICRC, Mohammed Al Abadla, a PRCS driver, along with a medic, were on their way to rescue a wounded man. Both were in uniform. PRCS told UN and B'Tselem investigators that rubble blocked the road, so they called the ICRC to act as an intermediary with the IDF. The IDF soldiers then instructed the medics to walk toward the injured man while signaling Israeli soldiers with a flashlight. After the medics gave the signal, an Israeli soldier shot Al Abadla in the leg and chest. His medic partner called the ICRC again, which coordinated IDF approval for two more ambulances to come to their aid. Despite clearance, soldiers continued to shoot at the ambulances, delaying medical attention to Al Abadla for another thirty minutes. He died soon after he was finally reached.[94]

In another case, an IDF tank fired at an ambulance staffed by two medics, 'Aaed al-Bura'i and Hatem Shahin, and a driver, Jawad Bdeir. They had received approval to come to the assistance of wounded people in the town of Beit Hanoun near the northern border of Gaza. A tank nevertheless fired and injured all three men. Shahin and Bdeir managed to escape the vehicle before the tank fired again, but al-Bura'i did not. Its shells hit the ambulance once more, destroying it and killing him. To evacuate the two injured men, another ambulance came after receiving IDF authorization. The tank fired at the second ambulance as well, shattering its windshield and wounding two of the medics in the second ambulance.[95]

Gazans were so angry at what they saw as the ICRC's failure to protect them that they accused it of collaboration with Israel. The accusations led to an extraordinary ICRC press release and video denying the charges and sharing its horror at the deaths and injuries. It asked Gazans to "understand the limits of our role and look to the politicians to end this deadly, miserable conflict."[96] In the aftermath of the war, the IDF's military advocate general opened internal investigations of allegations of IDF violations of international humanitarian law, including the killing of Mohammed Al Abadla, the medic who was shot in the chest. Five years later, no decision had been announced. In the case of the killing of 'Aaed al-Bura'i, the medic killed by tank fire in Beit Hanoun, the advocate general differed from human rights groups and UN investigators on whether the first ambulance had coordinated its movement. He acknowledged, though, that the IDF had cleared the second ambulance after ICRC had coordinated the evacuation.[97] In that case, the advocate general said that the IDF unit had received intelligence that a vehicle with a bomb might be approaching the IDF unit. It attributed the shooting vaguely to "gaps in communication between the forces," as a result of which notification of coordination "did not reach the forces in the field." The advocate general concluded that while the medic's death was "regrettable," the "professional discretion exercised by all the commanders involved in the incident had not been unreasonable under the circumstances."[98]

Like the aftermath of Cast Lead, the killings did not stimulate an examination of systemic and command failures, including the gaps in communication cited by the advocate general and field-based rules encouraging fire that may have been a factor in the deaths and injuries. Israeli military investigators had long eschewed consideration of systemic failures and the responsibility of senior commanders to adopt policies, train soldiers in them, and hold violators accountable.[99] At the same time, as with checkpoint practices, pressures for accountability and reform diminished as the political and judicial environment moved further to the right on questions concerning the human rights of Palestinians.

The lack of reform led to continued IDF violence against Palestinian medics and ambulances, and this continued after the wars in Gaza ended. Beginning in October 2015, individual Palestinians engaged in unorganized, apparently random attacks on Israeli police and civilians, mostly around Jerusalem and near the boundary of Gaza and Israel. They used knives and, later, firebombs and other weapons. During a three-month period, the attackers killed more than twenty Israelis and injured many more. Almost ninety of the alleged attackers were immediately killed by Israeli security forces. Thus began a new cycle of violence, accompanied by further restrictions on Palestinian movement. Palestinians demonstrated against the killings, sometimes violently. Israel answered with a hundred additional roadblocks and checkpoints in the West Bank and

Gaza, and twenty-nine cement barriers around eight East Jerusalem neighborhoods, including three around a major hospital. They either prevented or significantly delayed ambulance movement.[100] PRCS operational updates, issued every three days in late 2015, contain dry, clipped accounts of dozens of incidents where Israeli security forces delayed passage or fired tear gas or rubber-coated bullets at its ambulances and emergency responders.[101] The barriers were kept in place until December of that year.

Violence against medics reappeared in Gaza as well, particularly during the "Great March of Return" protests at the Gaza boundary in 2018 and 2019. Hamas used highly provocative and dangerous tactics in the protests, including attempting incursions and launching incendiaries, including flaming kites, into Israel. Other protesters, though, were citizens protesting the despairing circumstances in which they lived, hemmed in, impoverished, and without access to jobs, educational opportunities, and good health care. Israel shot live fire across the Gaza fence, killing more than two hundred and fifty Palestinians and injuring more than thirty thousand of them, with more than seven thousand suffering gunshot injuries. MSF treated about three thousand of the wounded and reported that about half of them suffered open fractures with severe soft tissue injuries. Many others had bones smashed and severe vascular wounds. A large proportion of the wounds became infected.[102] Only 17 percent of the applications of these wounded individuals to leave Gaza to obtain treatment were approved by Israel.[103] During the protests, the IDF killed three medics, all of whom were wearing a paramedic vest or jacket. Through the end of 2018, more than five hundred more medics were injured, at least half of them from live ammunition, rubber bullets, or shrapnel.[104]

Israel and its allies blamed Hamas for the injuries and deaths to protesters and medics. They cited Hamas's history of rocket attacks and, now, incendiaries, directed indiscriminately at Israel's civilians, including children. Tensions over the killing of medics also devolved into pointless arguments about whether bullets hit a medic directly or ricocheted off the ground, and whether medics had associations with Hamas. What was really at stake was the principle that wounded people and first medical responders must remain safe even in this very unconventional and volatile form of conflict. As Israel had demonstrated many years before, safe medical evacuation in the midst of hatred, provocation, and even terrorist acts is difficult, but can be accomplished safely when commanders are committed to it, properly instruct and train their troops, and enforce discipline. In the aftermath of the 2002 killings, medical evacuations became safe without jeopardizing the safety of Israeli troops. When they ignored duty, as other militaries around the world so often do, they put the lives of the wounded and sick and their rescuers in jeopardy.

# 7

## ARMED GROUPS

Threats and Violence by Nonstate Actors

ENRI DUNANT DRAFTED the original Geneva Convention in a European world that pitted armies of nations against one another. Contemporary armed conflicts are very different, mostly civil wars and insurgencies, though they often attract arms, funding, and fighters from outside the countries where they are fought. There were fifty-four of these wars in 2019, the highest number since World War II.[1] The preceding chapters reflect this shift. They focus on the conduct of state security forces, but in every case the enemy was one or multiple armed groups—Chechen rebels, the Kosovo Liberation Army, the PKK, the Karen National Liberation Army and other insurgent groups in Myanmar, the Taliban, the Houthis, and Hamas and other Palestinian groups. More recently, another transformation in armed conflict took place: the number of armed groups in these conflicts competing for power, territory, and resources in conflicts proliferated to more than six hundred in 2020, five times as many as in the previous decade.[2] More than 40 percent of recent internal conflicts involved as many as nine belligerents, and more than 20 percent of them had more than ten armed groups.[3] One consequence is that today's wars last twice as long as they did in 1990.[4]

Most armed groups lack access to the air power that can flatten a hospital, though many obtain advanced weapons. Even without high-tech armaments, in the last decade, armed groups attacked health care in wars in more than twenty countries. They may burn clinics, kill patients and medical staffs in hospitals, loot medical supplies, attack medical transports, kidnap staff, demand priority in care for their own fighters, and control health care services through threats and intimidation. Though largely unreported, these attacks can be ferocious and catastrophic. To cite just one example, in 2017, a militia affiliated with the Democratic Republic of Congo's then president, Joseph Kabila, attacked a hospital in the town of Cinq in a region near the border with Angola. Assailants raped women and girls and set fire to an operating room, trapping thirty-five patients inside. By the end of the onslaught, the group had killed ninety patients and at least two members of the medical staff, leaving "a mountain of bodies."[5]

The objectives of armed groups in attacking health care often resemble those of conventional militaries, for instance, denying care to enemies or gaining a strategic or tactical advantage. Similarly, some of the inducements and pressures that may restrain violence against health care are similar to those that may affect state military behavior. But the drivers of the attacks by armed groups and the incentives and strategy to stop them may differ from those of state militaries. This chapter consists of case studies about some of the logics armed groups adopt to attack health care, and the potential restraints on their conduct in five conflicts: the Liberian civil war, which was characterized by generalized violence against civilians; Afghanistan, where the Taliban sought to take power and show the population it could provide health services; the Central African Republic, where the conflict involving more than a dozen armed groups morphed into a sectarian as well as political and resource-driven fight; Syria and Iraq, where the Islamic State established its "caliphate"; and the Democratic Republic of the Congo, where violence against health care prolonged a major outbreak of Ebola.

## GENERALIZED VIOLENCE AGAINST
## CIVILIANS: LIBERIA

When I met Liberia's minister of health and social welfare, Dr. Walter Gwenigale, in 2010, I saw that, just as with the primary care clinic I had visited in the capital, the ministry's headquarters building had no running water. But just as the clinic was busy treating hundreds of children who suffered from malaria, the ministry was humming with plans to rebuild a health system destroyed in two civil wars. The first war had lasted from 1989 to 1997, and the second from 1999 to 2003. During the wars, Dr. Gwenigale—known to all as Dr. G—ran Phebe Hospital, located in rural Bong county, three hundred kilometers north of the capital, Monrovia. Dr. G sent his immediate family abroad for safety, but felt he needed to remain in Liberia to keep the hospital open and its patients and staff safe from soldiers and marauding, savage armed groups. In both wars armed groups recruited many thousands of child soldiers who were taught to kill without mercy. A quarter million civilians were killed in the first civil war, about sixty thousand in the second.[6] The armed groups burned villages, summarily executed local leaders and citizens, raped and abducted people, and looted whatever people possessed. Rural clinics, doctors, and nurses were not necessarily specific targets but were caught up in violence against civilians generally. During volatile times, Dr. G hid people with war wounds as intruding groups often assumed these patients were enemy fighters and would kill them. He tried to convince the groups that it was in their interest to leave the hospital alone so it could treat their wounded, but his efforts at persuasion were often futile. Worse, he told me that, as power in the area shifted, each succeeding group suspected the medical staff of loyalty to a different set of fighters.

The postwar Truth and Reconciliation Commission cataloged the sickening violence of the war but said little about attacks on health care, as it was simply caught up in the pervasive violence against civilians. Its list of atrocities, though, mentioned the massacre of a hundred people in Phebe Hospital.[7] Dr. G was not present in September 1994 when one armed group, the National Patriotic Front of Liberia, headed by Charles Taylor—who was later convicted of war crimes for murder and rape during the civil war in neighboring Sierra Leone—was about to force another group, the United Liberation Movement of Liberia for Democracy (ULIMO), out of the area. ULIMO warned the hospital staff to leave because the new occupiers would likely accuse them of allegiance to ULIMO. The staff refused, choosing to stay with their patients. When soldiers from the National Patriotic Front arrived, they killed patients, staff, and others in the hospital. Dr. G's mother was among them. Though devastated by the loss, he didn't second guess his decision to keep the hospital open. Dr. G later told an interviewer, "We knew we were taking a risk by staying. Many people did not feel comfortable leaving because we had a job to do. Sadly, what we were trying to prevent happened anyway: we thought that if we left the hospital, it was going to be destroyed and that we would not have anything left at the end of the war. So that is why we stayed."[8]

The toll on health care in those wars was evident in a postwar government assessment. About 95 percent of the prewar health facilities were partially or totally destroyed, and only 10 percent of communities had a clinic left. A mere forty-three physicians and twenty-one nurse-midwives remained in the country.[9] Key health indicators, including infant, child, and maternal mortality were among the worst in the world. Even five years after the war, 40 percent of the population had to walk more than two hours to reach a health clinic. Only a minority of women and children could access services to reduce child and maternal mortality, a national priority.[10] Liberia's major hospital, named after President John F. Kennedy after he committed the funds to build it, lacked rudimentary equipment and services. When peace finally came, the new president, Elaine Johnson Sirleaf, appointed Dr. G to be health minister, but there was barely a health system to run at all. The corrosion of already weak health systems as a result of violence against them is one of the most common features of internal wars: as clinics and health posts close, doctors, nurses and midwives flee, supply chairs collapse, vaccination campaigns wither, and management capacity declines. Women and children are often the worst affected, as maternal and reproductive health care declines.[11] It is no surprise that most of the countries at the bottom of UN indices of life expectancy, child and maternal mortality, and vaccination coverage are places of protracted, multiparty wars.

Dr. G. fearlessly started plans to construct a new health system from scratch. He persuaded the United States and other donors to invest in his plan to train a new cadre of health workers, establish clinics, and hold them all accountable to national quality standards. The donors agreed to pay 80 percent of the costs. They also provided technical support and helped create strong financial accountability systems. As is often the case in health development programs, donor support also brought a tug of war, with donors wanting to orchestrate the plan and Dr. G determined to maintain local control. When I met with him, he ridiculed donors who gave speeches and issued policy papers celebrating their commitment to the local direction of health care systems while trying to micromanage the use of grant funds. His strategy was to charm and resist. He was optimistic about the health reconstruction effort. When I visited clinics and reviewed the plans, I was impressed and wrote about his approach as a model for postconflict societies.[12] By 2010, though major challenges remained, there were measurable increases in capacity, especially for primary care.[13] Still, it was a steep hill given the enormous needs and the weak base. The timetable was long. Four years after my visit, Liberia still remained at the bottom of the UN's human development index indicators for health. Then, in 2014, Ebola struck West Africa. An outbreak in Nigeria, which had more resources and a more developed health system, was contained, but Liberia's capacity to stop such a devastating outbreak was weak. It was only the sustained leadership from NGOs, the Ministry of Public Health, the United States, and, later, the World Health Organization, that ended the epidemic, but not before almost five thousand people died of the disease.

In recent years, political scientists have empirically explored and theorized about strategic, tactical, ideological, social, and political factors, and recruitment practices that may influence why certain armed groups either target civilians or refrain from doing so. Some scholars point to strategic reasons for attacks, such as efforts to overcome the resistance of another group, to gain advantage in an area where the group exercises little or no control, to enforce the loyalty of a population or punish it for allegiance to others (especially where it lacks positive incentives to gain its support), to take control of local resources, to demonstrate its disruptive power, or simply to exact revenge.[14] These considerations can change over time. Political objectives and ideology can also influence behavior. Political scientist Tanisha Fazal showed that armed groups that are fighting for secession are more likely to adhere to the laws of war because they want to be seen by the local population and the international community as legitimate.[15] Another political scientist, Jeremy Weinstein, examined the influence of armed groups' recruitment practices on conduct, finding that rebel groups that bring in members on ideological grounds rather than for pecuniary reasons are less likely to engage in indiscriminate violence against civilians.[16] Other scholars have argued that groups with strong communal ties and ideologically committed cadres may commit violence against civilians more selectively, as do groups in territory they control.[17] The nature of an organization's structure and hierarchy, and disciplinary practices and socialization mechanisms, can influence whether it inflicts violence on civilians.[18] These factors play out in different ways in different contexts and are not always reflective of the best optimum military strategy.[19] Jessica Stanton offers evidence for an alternative theory, that the decision to attack civilians by armed groups (and, she argues, state militaries) is strategic and depends on their relationship with domestic and international constituencies.[20]

In some of these wars, armed groups attack health facilities and health workers for the same reasons they attack civilians, villages, schools, and local leaders, e.g., to control territory or to intimidate, control, or force displacement of local populations. In these cases, health care is just another victim of generalized violence against civilians. In Liberia, for example, the war was characterized by hostility to people not affiliated with the armed group, with violence inflicted on entire communities, and exacerbated by the large numbers of child soldiers. Similarly, in the civil war in South Sudan that began in 2013, armed groups and the government's army (which evolved from a nonstate armed group), repeatedly looted or burned clinics as they attacked villages. Hospitals and clinics became places for opportunistic killing and armed groups denied access to hospitals and clinics as one element of leverage to force population movement.[21] As two MSF staff wrote, "fighting rarely stops at the hospital gate."[22] In some conflicts, health workers affiliated with Western aid organizations may be targeted, just as all expatriate aid workers are, because they are seen as extensions of Western influence and agendas thought of as acting as spies, being corrupt, or competing with them for the allegiance of the population, or suspected of disrespecting local cultural norms.[23] Some of these attitudes can extend to local community health workers conducting polio vaccinations that are viewed as a Western plot.

Frequently, though, the circumstances, motives, and logics creating either vulnerability or safety for health care differ from those affecting civilians generally. Some analysts have indeed contended that violence against civilians may not correlate with violence against health care.[24] Armed groups may refrain from attacks on health care in a quest for legitimacy among the population, which needs access to health services; or they may destroy clinics and hospitals as tangible symbols of a state they want to demolish. In many internal wars, armed groups lack the capacity to provide care for their families or their own wounded combatants, so may be more restrained in violence toward health care than toward civilians generally.[25] On the other hand, this same interest may lead armed groups to coerce health workers to give priority care to their fighters, or punish the medical staff for perceived inadequate care.[26] In wars as diverse as those in Nepal, northern Uganda, and ISIS-controlled parts of Syria and Iraq, armed groups abducted health workers to treat their own fighters.[27] Financial interests can come into play, too, as stolen medical supplies and drugs can be a source of income for groups or individuals. In places where civilians perceive clinics and hospitals as places of refuge, armed groups may respond by attacking them. In an internal review, MSF found that that the five most frequent reasons for attacks on its facilities are: demands for preferential treatment for fighters or denial of care to enemies; retaliation for perceived substandard medical care; looting and violence for economic gain; takeover for military advantage; and attacks on specific facilities that had been set up or are perceived to be places protecting civilians.[28]

The conduct of armed groups can also be affected by the fact that health providers and the communities they serve have agency. They are not necessarily passive victims. They often develop relationships with the groups and engage in negotiations for security and safety. They may have leverage over armed groups, such as by maintaining health care for a group's fighters or offering them first-aid training, and in return demanding adherence to their rules, such as no-weapons policies in health facilities. They can also negotiate concessions that enable them to survive, such as by deferring to groups' cultural norms, especially regarding women. Armed groups' attitudes toward international law also affects their conduct. An oft-repeated truism holds that demanding adherence to the law and expecting results is naïve. Yet many armed groups have positive attitudes about international humanitarian law, and education and persuasion can influence conduct, especially if elements of the law are in harmony with the groups' own norms.[29] The ICRC has long trained armed groups in the law and appealed to local values that reinforce it. More recently, a Geneva-based NGO, Geneva Call, gained commitments from armed groups to comply with international law. It promotes what it calls a "deed of commitment" to abide by international norms and agree to training and monitoring of adherence. Fifty armed groups have signed a deed of commitment pledging not to use antipersonnel landmines, and twenty-six have signed a deed of commitment on child protection, including a prohibition on child soldiers.[30]

In late 2018, Geneva Call launched a deed of commitment on protection of health care and began soliciting signatories.[31] The deed's language generally tracked the Geneva Conventions and additional protocols and contained provisions that extended beyond legal obligations. It called on armed groups not to compel the disclosure of confidential patient information, whereas the Additional Protocols to the Geneva Conventions permit disclosure if national law allows. It also required signatories to respect "no weapons" policies for health facilities and transports, which the Geneva Conventions do not require. Incorporating norms from human rights law, the deed of commitment demanded that signatories ensure, maintain, and protect the local population's access to essential health facilities, goods, and services. Finally, it called on authorities within the armed groups to implement and enforce the commitments among its troops and demanded that commanders and supervisors be held accountable for subordinates' compliance. It is important to be realistic about the prospect that signing a deed of commitment will change behavior, yet also avoid the cynicism that armed groups cannot be influenced. Some groups embraced norms of humanity based on their own values. The *Ejército de Liberación Nacional* in Colombia, for example, had an ideology heavily influenced by Catholic teachings that supported "humanizing war."[32]

Finally, armed groups are not immune to outside pressure to conform to the law, especially where, as in the case of violence against noncombatants, they are seeking to dislodge the government and take over political control. These groups often want to be seen as legitimate, which amounts to a point of leverage for human rights monitors and others. In some circumstances, they are responsive to pressures from local communities, especially if from the same ethnic or religious group. As a result, generalizations about the conduct of armed groups toward health care are largely futile. Context, structure, objectives, recruitment approaches, ideology, and potential sources of restraint matter, and they may change over time.

## POLITICAL OBJECTIVES AND THE POSSIBILITY OF RESTRAINTS: THE TALIBAN IN AFGHANISTAN

Markus Geisser's career with the ICRC brought him to Darfur, Myanmar, the Democratic Republic of the Congo, Liberia, and Iraq. In 2009, Geisser was assigned to run ICRC operations in southern Afghanistan. How appropriate that seemed to me when I interviewed him, as he is a devotee of Sherlock Holmes. It was in Afghanistan, according to Arthur Conan Doyle's first Sherlock Holmes novel, *A Study in Scarlet*, that Dr. Watson had served with the British medical corps. The book tells us that

Dr. Watson experienced nothing there but "misfortune and disaster." Geisser, though, more resembles his hero than Dr. Watson. Like Holmes, his easy manner masked a shrewd mind and tough attitude, which proved useful in navigating complex relationships required for the security of health care services in Kandahar, where he remained for two years. The Taliban was strong in the region, the situation always volatile, and the fighting sometimes intense. The International Security Assistance Force (ISAF), the NATO-led military operation in Afghanistan, launched major operations there in 2010 and 2011, and the Taliban responded with a spring offensive, while also assassinating government officials, including the brother of Afghanistan's president. The region remained dangerous for Afghan and Western humanitarian aid workers despite the ICRC's constant efforts to affirm its neutral stance.

In four volatile provinces, Geisser oversaw ICRC's assistance to internally displaced people, supported local water board authorities, visited people in Afghan and ISAF detention facilities, established family links for detained Afghans, and offered health care. He also acted as liaison to all combatants to seek their compliance with the laws of war and to facilitate people's access to health care. When I interviewed him in London, where he was posted years later, he said he had felt like a "spider in the web of human contradictions," as he engaged with people who may have committed horrific acts. He said he tried to convince them to respect human life and health. Geisser loved the country and the work. Like many war zones, he said, southern Afghanistan was the perfect example of what Ryszard Kapuściński, a journalist and writer who covered political conflict in Central America and Africa for decades, called a "violent paradise."

As in all his previous assignments with the ICRC, Geisser sought to persuade all combatants to comply with the laws of war. It was hardly a straightforward task. He tried to figure out, as he told me, "What appeals to people who are portrayed as having no respect, no knowledge and don't care about the law." He relished the opportunity to "contribute positively, to maybe convince people who have done some pretty bad stuff that they have been responsible for directly or indirectly" not to engage in such acts again. He had encountered military forces like the Janjaweed militia in

Darfur, U.S. commanders in the Baghdad Green Zone, and rebel groups in the eastern Congo. "I haven't met too many combatants who simply didn't care," he told me. "They have interests—personal interests, political interests, economic interests. You can have rather sophisticated conversations" with them, especially "if they have some sort of political vision."

He described humanitarian negotiations as squaring a circle. He compared the challenge for humanitarians to a nonsmoker trying to convince a smoker to refrain from smoking in a designated smoking compartment of a train. Whether engaging with Afghan authorities, ISAF officers, or Taliban operatives, he said the first task was to develop personal contact and a relationship. That included showing patience and listening to their concerns. Geisser said you can anticipate a common response to appeals to adhere to the law: "You have to understand my situation." That situation could be unruly troops, demanding commanders, or pressure to achieve military objectives. Given that, he said it was important to be pragmatic and responsive but never forego discussion on why the rules of war are so important and must be respected. It was also essential, he said, to offer his interlocutors something. "You have to show you are useful one way or the other: provide humanitarian services to their communities; understand causes of violence as well as the potential restraints on committing violent acts; discuss frameworks familiar to them such as codes of conduct. This helps to start conversations about principles and what should change in commanding their troops." An ethnographic study of humanitarian workers seeking to persuade armed groups to adhere to the requirements of international law showed that they similarly relied on developing relationships with armed groups and devoted energy to understanding the often-shifting local context and the objectives and priorities of groups whose conduct they sought to influence.[33] At the same time, Geisser said, you do not refrain from making demands in these discussions, starting with guarantees for the security of your own staff. He offered another analogy, comparing gaining access for humanitarian action to negotiating a license to operate.

In Kandahar, meeting Taliban needs included increasing their access to health care. Filling that need also provided a point of leverage. The ICRC supported 70 percent of the funding for Mirwais Hospital, the second largest in Afghanistan and a referral hospital for all of the southern part of the country, covering thousands of square miles. With 620 beds, a surgical unit, and three operating theaters, it was capable of treating traumatic injuries from the heavy explosives used by all sides in the conflict. Its expatriate staff worked alongside health workers from the Kandahar Provincial Ministry of Health. It was open to all patients, regardless of affiliation or combatant status.

The huge territory the hospital covered in a mountainous area with ongoing armed conflict made travel to the hospital for wounded and sick people difficult. Roads were often too dangerous for official ambulances or ICRC vehicles to bring patients to Mirwais. In their place, the ICRC relied on local transport. In the early 2000s, with the agreement of all parties, the ICRC organized a network of about forty taxis in the four provinces around Kandahar and supplied identification cards to the drivers to help them get through checkpoints safely. Managing the program was challenging, requiring constant negotiations. These were complicated by the fact that the drivers were not ICRC staff. The system didn't eliminate all dangers of travel, well-illustrated by the killing of one driver in neighboring Helmand province. Still, the taxi system facilitated access to medical care for thousands of patients. In one case reported by Fiona Terry, Geisser's ICRC colleague, a taxi was stopped at a checkpoint as the driver and soldiers argued whether the patient should be sent to an interrogation center or a hospital. An ICRC representative spoke to soldiers at the checkpoint by phone and asked that the taxi be permitted to go to the hospital, explaining that the wounded man could be questioned later. The taxi was allowed to pass.[34]

Afghan authorities and the U.S. military often criticized the taxi network, calling it the "Taliban express," as it transported wounded Taliban soldiers as well as civilians to Mirwais Hospital. The wounded Taliban soldiers were of course entitled by the Geneva Conventions to medical care. But instead of merely citing the law in justifying the program, Geisser engaged with authorities including the governor of Kandahar province. He reminded them of the significant support ICRC "pumps into your hospitals" like Mirwais, a government-run facility, and its treatment of Afghan national police who, unlike Afghan army personnel, lacked access to ISAF medical services. To further aid and gain trust of the authorities, he said, "We started to assist the police with basic medical supplies and organized first aid trainings." Geisser commented that some may call this a carrot and stick approach, but he disagrees. He said, "Humanitarians have no sticks, just carrots. But they are not distributed without a purpose."

Geisser had no illusions that his work would guarantee compliance with the law. The point was shockingly illustrated on April 7, 2011, when Taliban operatives drove an ambulance loaded with explosives into a police and military training center outside Kandahar following an assault by fighters with suicide vests. Six people were killed. Dozens were wounded. Most of the casualties were Afghan national police. The Taliban claimed responsibility. ICRC condemned the use of a medical vehicle for an attack as a gross violation of international humanitarian law.[35] Geisser himself was incensed at the use of an ambulance as a weapon. He recognized, too, that attacks like this also could lead combatants to distrust ambulances, whether official or private ones like taxis, and massively hamper the delivery of medical assistance. As on similar occasions in the past, Geisser secured contact and discussed the attack with Taliban officials in charge of their operations in Kandahar. He reiterated the ICRC position and shared his fears about the impact of the attack on the transport of the wounded across frontlines and checkpoints.

The ICRC's pledge of confidentiality in conversations with parties to the conflict, which allows frank, candid discussions, prevented Geisser from sharing details of his exchange with the Taliban official with me, but he described it as "solid and robust." It is also difficult to know what influence the exchange had on the Taliban, but a few days later a Taliban spokesperson publicly stated that attacks like this one would not happen again.[36] Was the decision based on ICRC's demand to respect international humanitarian law, the potential restrictions on the taxi program and Taliban fighters' access to care as a result of the attack, or the Taliban's own code of conduct? Geisser says that only a combination of all of these factors "and probably many others" can lead to the restraint of violence by combatants and respect for international humanitarian law. Sometimes negotiation works. Often it does not. In this case, for years following the incident, the use of an ambulance to carry and detonate bombs remained a rarity in Afghanistan.

Engagement and tough negotiations with combatants to protect health care can make a huge difference, which is why they have become so central to the work of the ICRC, MSF, and some other humanitarian health organizations. The ICRC engages in discussions and negotiations on civilian protection with almost two hundred armed groups. MSF has published multiple books on the subject.[37] The importance of these negotiations skills is so high that ICRC, together with MSF, the Center for Humanitarian Dialogue, and UN agencies and international NGOs invested in a training center to study negotiation techniques, share best practices, teach humanitarians working in conflict zones, and advise organizations.[38] Local health providers, though, often lack the leverage, training, and resources those groups have, leaving their services far more vulnerable to violence. An extensive study by William Carter and Katherine Haver found that willingness and ability to negotiate with armed groups appears to depend more on the political positions of governments and donors than on the structure or conduct of armed groups. The study revealed that only about a third of the groups interviewed found it acceptable to negotiate with the Taliban. This finding was confirmed in my interviews with health managers in Afghanistan who said that the government looked askance on interactions with the Taliban. By contrast, the authors found that groups working in Somalia, South Sudan, and Syria were far more likely to think it appropriate to engage with armed groups.[39]

One of the potential sources of influence Geisser mentioned was the Taliban's code of conduct, the Layeha. First adopted in 2006, the code set out rules of conduct by its cadres and also elaborate investigative and disciplinary mechanisms for enforcement. Although skeptics have viewed the code as little more than propaganda, scholars and analysts have shown that the Taliban used it to advance both internal and external strategic objectives. It was initially adopted in part as a response to criminality, extortion, and banditry by fighters who had been recruited to the Taliban without a commitment to its ideology. Over time, the Taliban sought to strengthen control of operations, regulate the conduct of its soldiers, advance professionalism, and limit abuse of civilians in order to increase its legitimacy and better achieve its military objectives.[40] It received and responded to complaints made by the population regarding Taliban behavior and created a Commission for the Prevention of Civilian Casualties and Complaints that human rights monitors found took positive steps in some cases.[41]

During Geisser's time in Kandahar, the Taliban's attitude toward health care was evolving as the group sought legitimacy and competed with the Afghan government and ISAF for the support of the local population. The Taliban considered health care as a key means to advance that objective. Over time, Taliban leader Mullah Omar tightened rules against attacks on schools and hospitals. The shifting political objectives were reflected in 2010 revisions to the code.[42] The revisions included extensive guides to conduct in combat purportedly designed to protect civilians. The revisions also created a commission on health policy. Additionally, while the language was vague, the code suggested refraining from violence against local and international NGOs that provide health, education, and social services.

The restrictions on harm to civilians and health facilities, though, remained quite circumscribed to be in harmony with other dimensions of Taliban ideology, perceptions, strategy, and tactics. The Taliban often viewed Western aid groups as collaborators in the fight against it and often corrupt as well, though they tended to look more favorably on health groups.[43] The code excluded large categories of people from the definition of civilians: government officials, progovernment politicians and Afghans working for them, women's rights activists, and international civilians it considered aligned with the government. Under the Layeha, they could be subjected to targeted killings.[44] In May 2019, the Taliban took credit for an attack on a U.S. NGO, Counterpart International, that killed three people. It tweeted that Counterpart engaged in "harmful Western activities inside Afghanistan," and employed "foreign advisors" who acted with "brutality, oppression, terror, anti-Islamic ideology and promotion of Western culture."[45]

The code revisions also permitted improvised explosive devices to be employed for suicide bombings, subject to supposed but absurdly ineffectual safeguards to avoid civilian casualties. Likewise, it did not embrace the principles of proportionality and distinction, nor followed the requirements to take precautions to avoid harm to civilian objects, especially in cases where a hospital is near a military target.[46] As a result, the Taliban did not appear to try to avoid hitting a health facility if near a military objective or to forgo use of an ambulance to launch an attack. In January 2018 the Taliban placed a bomb in an ambulance in Kabul. It exploded on a busy street, killing more than a hundred people and injuring more than two hundred. When condemned for the attack, the Taliban responded with a statement saying the police were the target, as though that excused the attack.[47] In the first nine months of 2019, the Taliban carried out twenty-four suicide attacks with improvised explosive devices, causing more than 1,300 civilian casualties including almost 150 deaths.[48] The same year, a truck full of explosives detonated near a hospital in Zabul province, near Kandahar, whose governor said it was destroyed. The Taliban justified the attack as directed at a government intelligence office next door.[49] Similarly, when in its tactical interests, it would take over a health facility to gain a good firing position.[50]

Even with these major departures from international law, the Taliban's posture and conduct toward health care improved over time, albeit unevenly. In 2007, the ICRC and UNICEF acted as intermediaries between the government, the Taliban, and ISAF to permit house-to-house polio vaccinations to go forward safely in volatile areas. Mullah Omar, then the supreme leader of the Taliban (he died in 2013), signed a letter asking local Taliban commanders to cooperate and to allow the campaign to go forward without interference. Not all local commanders followed his directive, but many did, and vaccinators carried the letter with them. The immunization campaigns reached hundreds of thousands of children.[51] There was precedent for this kind of cooperation in vaccinations. Starting in the 1980s, armed groups and government forces in wars in Afghanistan, the Democratic Republic of the Congo, El Salvador, the Philippines, Sri Lanka, Tajikistan, and Peru reached agreements to permit vaccination campaigns. In El Salvador, the period when fighting ceased and vaccinations proceeded was dubbed "days of tranquility," and the name stuck. In the Democratic Republic of the Congo, in 2000, similar campaigns successfully vaccinated more than four million children, eliminating the polio virus, though periodic campaigns were required in later years as a result of importation of the virus into the country.[52]

The engagement of the Taliban with health providers continued, albeit with interruptions and complications, even after the CIA's fake vaccination campaign in Pakistan during its search for Osama bin Laden was revealed in 2011. The Pakistani Taliban and some other Islamic groups declared vaccinations a Western plot, forbade vaccinations, forced humanitarian groups out, and attacked and killed vaccinators. The Taliban in Afghanistan, by contrast, often continued to permit campaigns except in areas with active fighting—though on its own terms. The Taliban demanded and gained control of the hiring of vaccinators and determining when security conditions permitted campaigns to go forward. It also made money by brokering the use of vehicles for the campaign and providing "guides" for vaccinators. Its approach served multiple purposes: demonstrating its ability to provide essential health services to the population, controlling the work of NGOs, determining when vaccination campaigns met its conditions for security, and providing income through a "microenterprise."[53]

It used a similar approach with other health programs, valuing the services as a means of promoting its legitimacy by serving the population, but exercising power over them. Most of these services had been developed and operated by NGOs under contracts with the Ministry of Public Health as part of a plan to expand primary care, safe childbirth, and essential hospital services throughout the country. Except in the most insecure regions, health services operated in areas controlled by the Taliban as well as the government. The Taliban had no qualms about relying on government-financed services, but it sought to manipulate them. Ashley Jackson, one of the leading analysts of Taliban attitudes and conduct toward social services, explained that the Taliban's tactics gradually changed from attacking health clinics and other social services to coopting them.[54] The Taliban demanded that clinics meet its demands in their decisions on staffing, geographic reach, and operations, and that they forgo giving credit to the government for the services.[55]

Khalid Fahim of the Swedish Committee for Afghanistan told me about demands that the Taliban made regarding health-care management. The Taliban tried to control supervisors' decisions to visit health facilities in regions, move a particular clinic to another location, revise ambulance operations, and hire the medical staff. In each case, the organization pushed back and managed to negotiate a resolution. In other cases, the Taliban insisted on vetting administrators and doctors for their politics, both their real or presumed allegiances to the government, and their qualifications for the job. It sought to influence where health posts were located and what services were offered.[56] Fahim told me that during the COVID-19 crisis, the Taliban interfered in recruitment of health workers for the community-based health response, but also held community education activities concerning COVID-19. That activity, too, turned out to be double-edged, as the education sessions were held in health facilities, raising concerns by staff and patients that the facility would be targeted by others. The Taliban also distributed personal protective equipment and permitted health workers supported by the Ministry of Public Health to practice in areas it controlled.

At the same time, the Taliban often showed genuine interest in quality of care. Fahim told me that in Wardak, the intense interest of the Taliban in health services was sometimes helpful, as its representative offered feedback on shortages of medicine and monitored health services. In some provinces the Taliban appointed an official to act as focal point or liaison for health care. Some Taliban representatives even interacted and negotiated with local Ministry of Public Health officials and health provider organizations, though it had no contact with officials at the national level. The Taliban's interventions, however, could often be coercive. The director of a health agency (who asked not to be named for security reasons) explained to me that the Taliban frequently forced closure of clinics or abducted staff if it didn't get its way. In 2017, the Taliban forced the closure of twenty of his agency's health facilities for two or three months after he refused its demand to move facilities to places where populations loyal to the Taliban would have closer access to care.

Even large international NGOs like the Swedish Committee for Afghanistan, which had more negotiating leverage, were subjected to these pressures. Fahim told me that on one occasion the Taliban wanted to upgrade a comprehensive health center to a district hospital. When program officials explained that the upgrade was not appropriate under its standards, the Taliban forced the closure of dozens of facilities for two months. In the first ten months of 2019, the Taliban forced eighty-eight medical facilities in the volatile eastern region of the country to close for days or weeks and abducted and held three medical personnel for days before they were released.[57] During that period, the WHO reported 181 forced closures nationwide, with only 27 facilities reopened, though not all of them may have been the responsibility of the Taliban.[58] In many cases, health providers relied on community elders as interlocutors to keep services going or reopen them when closed. But elders, too, came under threat as a result of their interventions.[59]

The Taliban also used threats of closure to influence government policy. In 2017, the Taliban organized a campaign across fourteen provinces to pressure the government and NGOs to improve services in areas it controlled. Its demands included increased staffing, equipment, and facilities. Although in most cases changes were negotiated, in at least one province the Taliban forced closure of facilities for a month and a half.[60] After government security forces attacked a Swedish Committee for Afghanistan hospital in 2019 in Wardak province, near Kabul, the Taliban forced more than forty clinics in the province to briefly suspend operations. The same dynamic played out in Laghman province, near the city of Jalalabad in eastern Afghanistan, in 2017. Government security forces detained four private surgeons for treating the Taliban, and the Taliban responded by forcing closure of the facility for almost a week. The Taliban could also be mercurial in its threats. In 2018 it issued a statement saying it would no longer protect ICRC workers because it claimed that the organization was not doing enough to address poor conditions and lack of medical care for Taliban soldiers in a government prison in Kabul.[61] Despite its previous record of cooperation in polio vaccinations, in April 2019, the Taliban "banned" the World Health Organization and the ICRC from polio vaccination, which brought all of the campaigns in the country to a temporary halt during the second quarter of the year.[62] For the first half of 2018, the UN reported that the Taliban was responsible for the highest number of violations against health care.[63]

Despite its willingness to coerce, threaten, and force closure of clinics, the Taliban often refrained from direct violent attacks on them. One more factor was at play. Because of its political interests in governing the country, the Taliban was subject to external pressure from humanitarian organizations, community elders, and the human rights branch of the United Nations Mission in Afghanistan (UNAMA), operated in conjunction with the Office of the UN High Commissioner for Human Rights. UNAMA issued detailed, tough quarterly reports, and an annual review of civilian casualties, offering precise numbers and calling perpetrators to account. The Taliban's thinking, and to some extent, its tactics, appear to have been influenced by the reports.[64] Because of the Taliban's sensitivity to UNAMA's findings, it prepared lengthy written responses to them. It often contested facts and explained all the steps it took to prevent civilian casualties. In its answer to the 2018 UNAMA civilian casualty report, it claimed that "protection of civilians is a top priority," indeed a "religious obligation," and cited its investigation commissions as well as a special delegation to raise awareness of obligations, assess civilian casualties, identify causes, hold those responsible accountable, and explore better prevention strategies. It denied targeting civilians, using indiscriminate improvised explosive devices, or engaging in disproportionate attacks. It said that if one of its soldiers engaged in inappropriate conduct he would be disciplined. And it specifically claimed that it "does not target health workers, polio vaccinators, schools and education personnel, but rather provides them with security to the extent possible and tries its best not to interrupt their activities."[65]

Some of these responses amounted to a disingenuous public relations spin, but a review of the conduct of the Taliban over time reveals that the assumption that it was incorrigibly violent against health care is incorrect. True, it rationalized coercion and threats of closure against health facilities, inflicted violence on humanitarian groups it claimed to be allied with the government and its allies, and ignored rules designed to reduce civilian casualties. Yet it was restrained to some extent by its political objective to govern, its ideology and code, and by external pressures that capitalized on its quest for legitimacy. Its desire to be seen by communities as ensuring medical services, enabled communities, humanitarians, and human rights monitors some space and tools to pressure the Taliban to comply with norms. A nuanced analysis of the Taliban's values, military and political objectives, and perceptions of its environment informed negotiations like those Markus Geisser pursued and became the foundation for pressures on it to adhere to international norms.

In reviewing the evolution of the Taliban's logic on the protection of health care, and the pressures brought to bear on it, one potential player is missing. Ashley Jackson confirmed to me what directors of health organizations in Afghanistan told me: the Ministry of Public Health played no meaningful role in advancing protection. Doing so was seen as too political, as it risked accusations of support of or, as bad, complicity with the Taliban.[66] That stance can be a missed opportunity. There is another way.

## STRATEGIES TO END IDENTITY-BASED VIOLENCE: CENTRAL AFRICAN REPUBLIC

Gina Ngobe, a nurse at a Ministry of Health hospital in Bambari in the Central African Republic, told my colleague, Sarah Woznick, about a time where armed men accused her of killing one of their comrades after the medical staff could not prevent his dying from the wounds he received. She told Sarah, "You are scared to work. You're scared, maybe someone will shoot you." Her experience was all too common in a war that entered hospitals. Her colleague Marcelin Mentchechougo, a supervisory nurse at the hospital, said, "There are not only the threats . . . between the groups, but also by the companions. They want to blame the health care workers . . . because we are not from the other community." The "other community" was a reference to the fact that the war, which began in 2012 as a political conflict, had morphed into a sectarian one, as Muslim-dominated armed groups attacked Christians and Christian groups attacked Muslims. The violence became contagious, extending beyond both the political and sectarian to criminal gangs seeking lucre. Armed groups splintered and attacked others of their own kind. Mr. Mentchechougo pointed to the larger problem: "Health centers are the places that must be . . . respected by all." His experience was that they were not.

The violence and fear they experienced was replicated throughout the country. Armed groups invaded hospitals, killed patients, threatened and assaulted staff, often forcing health facilities to suspend their operations. The assaults exacerbated already extraordinary levels of disease and premature death in the country. The Central African Republic ranks 188th of 189 countries in the UN's Human Development Index, a measure of a long and healthy life, access to knowledge, and a decent standard of living. That dismal statistic is the result of a tragic history, dominated by organized cruelty. Over the course of at least two centuries, the country's people were subjected to exploitation, oppression, and violence, and incompetent, corrupt, and dysfunctional governance. In the precolonial era, the region was a major slave trading center. When France colonized what it called the Oubangui-Chari region of French Equatorial Africa in 1903, it did not invest in roads, a civil service, education, and health care, as it had in many other parts of its empire. Instead, France mimicked the practice of King Leopold of Belgium in neighboring Congo, ceding control of land to private companies seeking wealth from rubber, coffee, and minerals. As in the Congo, the companies engaged in terror against the population. To meet the need for three thousand porters a month to ferry supplies and products, companies imposed quotas on local chiefs to supply forced labor and enforced them by taking women and children prisoner, and by burning villages.[67] Many people who fled brutality in the Congo returned after experiencing worse under the French.[68] Scholars have characterized the French rule variously as a Cinderella story, a trashcan colony, or a dead-end street.[69] Between 1890 and 1940 the population declined by half. In 1950, only 8 percent of the colony's children attended school. At the time of independence in 1960, there was one hospital in a country the size of France itself.

Independence brought a succession of despotic, corrupt, and incompetent governments, punctuated by coups and violence. In 1979, France's frustration with its former colony led it to overthrow Jean-Bédel Bokassa, who had declared himself emperor, and for a time took back control of the country. The first free and fair election did not take place until 1993, and it proved to bring only mutiny and war. Scholar Stephen Smith has written that this "internecine violence amounted, in the long run, to ever more serious attempts at national suicide."[70] A series of conflicts, peace agreements, and peacekeeping forces did little to end the country's misery and maladministration. Another free election did take place in 2005, but again did not bring the rule of law, financial accountability, human rights protections, economic progress, or peace. Instead, the elected president, François Bozizé, continued arbitrary and oppressive governance and won a fraudulent election in 2011, which in turn led to another armed revolt. The insurgent group called itself Séléka, the word for alliance in the local language, Sango. Its grievances included the government's failing to protect people in the northeastern part of the country, ignoring a prior peace pact, and neglecting to investigate atrocities its forces committed.[71] In late 2012, the groups were joined by combatants from Chad and Darfur who hoped to profit from overthrowing the government. The Séléka quickly captured towns and marched toward Bangui, the capital.

Neighboring states negotiated a peace agreement, but President Bozizé reneged on it. By March 2013, the Séléka, carrying machetes and arms funneled through the country's neighbors, captured Bangui. President Bozizé fled, and the Séléka's leader, Michel Djotodia, took power. As a show of purported national unity and in light of the atrocities the Séléka had committed against civilians during its campaign, in September 2013 Djotodia dissolved the group. But the fighting soon resumed as disparate locally led self-defense groups, former soldiers, and others, organized militias, called anti-Balaka, to attack former Séléka members. The latter responded by reconstituting, now calling themselves ex-Séléka. Violence quickly escalated, with new atrocities committed by both sides. By December 2013, thousands of people were dead.

Though the Séléka had been dominated by Muslims, an oppressed minority in the Central African Republic, its campaign and takeover did not originate in sectarian hostility.[72] Soon, however, each side began to exploit religious differences to mobilize and incite hatred. Each side targeted civilians of a different religion for abduction or killing.[73] The ex-Séléka committed atrocities against Christians, and the Christian and Animist anti-Balaka forces attacked Muslims. By early 2014, more than eighty thousand Muslims had fled the country.[74] Over time, splits in the main factions led to more than a dozen armed groups competing over resources, including diamonds, and power, and groups of the same religion fought each other, often over local grievances. Some of the groups originally formed to protect their own communities preyed on them.[75] In the chaos, criminal violence by rogue members of armed groups and ordinary criminals proliferated against civilians and humanitarian organizations.

In October 2013, the UN Security Council found "a total breakdown in law and order, the absence of the rule of law, inter-sectarian tensions" and armed groups' engagement in "extrajudicial killings, enforced disappearances, arbitrary arrests and detention, torture, sexual violence against women and children, rape, recruitment and use of children and attacks against civilians." It warned of a potential "spiral into an uncontrollable situation."[76] It authorized an African Union-sponsored peacekeeping force that included French troops. Djotodia resigned in January 2014, replaced by the country's first woman president, Catherine Samba-Panza, who vowed to end corruption, protect Muslims and Christians, and reorganize the military. Later that year, with the fighting and displacement still raging, the Security Council voted to send a contingent of UN peacekeepers, under the name UN Multidimensional Integrated Stabilization Mission in the Central African Republic (MINUSCA), that over time grew to almost eleven thousand troops and more than two thousand police. The council empowered MINUSCA with a strong mandate to protect civilians and neutralize armed groups, but it was too small a force to change the dynamic of the war, and had gaps in its capacity.[77] By mid-2018, armed groups controlled 80 percent of the country. More than six hundred and fifty thousand people had been displaced, and another half a million people had fled the country. In 2019, fourteen of the armed groups entered into a peace agreement to integrate their representatives into the government and to establish joint military units, but implementation lagged. In the run-up to a presidential election in December 2020, the Constitutional Court disqualified former president Bozizé from running. Armed groups violently tried to disrupt the election, and turnout was low. The Constitutional Court certification of the reelection of President Touadéra did not end the violence, including a siege in Bangui, when more than two hundred thousand people were displaced.

Bambari, a market town in the middle of the Central African Republic, with a population of about forty thousand people, has the distinction, unfortunate in war, of being at a crossroads for travel from the capital to the eastern parts of the country, which included the country's diamond mines. As a result, it became a strategic point for a slew of armed groups that fought the government, each other, peacekeepers, and civilians from other ethnic or religious groups. The war periodically brought clashes that intruded into Bambari's hospital, whose surgery, pediatric, and malnutrition programs were operated by MSF, and whose maternity ward was run by the International Medical Corps, both in collaboration with the Ministry of Health. Both NGOs had a no-weapons policy in their health facilities, but armed groups often defied it to search out their perceived enemies, whether fighters or civilians.

In the spring of 2014, fighting displaced more than ten thousand people in Bambari in the midst of the rainy season, which led to shortages of shelter, water, sanitation, and food. Patients in its hospital were attacked by forces associated with rival ethnic and religious groups. In 2016, twenty-five people were killed in clashes between ex-Séléka and anti-Balaka groups there. The intervention of MINUSCA helped stabilize the town and disarm fighters in 2017, but violence flared up again in 2018. In mid-May, armed groups returned to Bambari, where forty thousand displaced people were living in the town and its outskirts. Their makeshift shelters offered little protection from rain and lacked access to clean water and electricity. Two armed groups each took control of a part of the city, looting government buildings and facilities in the process. Nine civilians were killed, and more than seven thousand more people were displaced. MSF treated seventy people wounded with gunshot or machete injuries at the hospital.[78]

Two weeks later, an ex-Séléka faction, the Union for Peace in Central African Republic (UPC), fought with local police and anti-Balaka groups. Twenty more civilians and police were killed. The hospital, located between contending groups, treated dozens more wounded people, mostly from gunshot wounds, while three hundred displaced persons initially sought refuge in the hospital before fleeing the city. The following week, dozens of UPC fighters entered and began shooting inside the hospital to extract one of their fellow soldiers. Muslim patients hid or fled, fearing retaliation from anti-Balaka forces. They were right. Anti-Balaka forces came to the hospital seeking out UPC fighters and terrorizing patients and staff.[79]

Marcelin Mentchechougo, who had been working at the hospital with MSF for four years, was on duty as armed men with machetes entered the intensive care unit while others shot their way into the operating theater, in search of Muslim patients. They seemed "pushed by anger," he recalled, "pushed by violence, blinded by violence." He and his colleagues wanted to reach the safety of the hospital's residential staff compound but "every time we tried to get out, we were forced to take cover." As the armed men searched for Muslim patients, his most vivid memory was of a woman belonging to the predominantly Muslim Puehl ethnic group. "People coming into the hospital were demanding, 'Where are they . . . bring out the Puehls!' So, this woman, I hid her behind, with a mattress. . . . She was petrified with fear. And I thought, if she had died that day, perhaps I would be responsible for her death. So, it was a moment, an image I have never forgotten." He felt helpless. "I was there but I could not do very much. Because yes, I could provide care, but I couldn't do anything else. So, for me, I was powerless. . . . People think that you can bring a solution, but unfortunately, you can't." And yet he took a modicum of hope in the fact that during this crisis "the patients trusted us so much because, wherever we go, they think that is where there is safety."

The patient remained hidden and escaped death. Not everyone was so fortunate. A veteran nurse who asked to remain anonymous told Sarah, "There was a little child here, from the other community. When things exploded on May 14, they came in with their weapons. We told the children, 'Little ones, go home. Don't stay here.' They refused. Then, a bullet was fired into the hospital and pierced the child's abdomen. The medical staff took him to the operating room for an exploratory operation." He added, "We made an effort to find blood for the patient. Unfortunately, the next day at 2 p.m., the child died."

After the second incursion and armed robbery at its compound later in May, MSF evacuated some of its staff until mid-June and had to suspend a malnutrition program and treatment programs in one of its community-based clinics. It set up mobile clinics in the countryside to treat displaced people. Mentchechougo said, "All of those who left went back home with their malnourished children." Many may have died. Although the hospital remained open, many patients and families, even those suffering malnutrition or tuberculosis, feared assault within the walls and stayed away. Mentchechougo explained that "those who didn't return, we do not know their fate." He said, "People no longer trust that health structures will remain protected." The data bear him out. In April the hospital admitted 230 patients. In June, only 70 came. Although patients gradually returned, many of them had delayed care until their condition was more critical and difficult to treat. Some whose conditions would have been treatable if they had come earlier died.[80]

As in Bambari, many of the attacks on health care during the war were perpetrated against patients in hospitals, whether fighters or noncombatants, in the midst of care. In one of the most horrifying events of 2017, during fighting in the town of Zemio, in the east of the country, two armed men entered the hospital and killed an infant in the arms of her mother as the family sought to take cover. Armed men again attacked the hospital the following month, this time killing eleven civilians from among thousands who had gone to the hospital seeking shelter.[81] The hospital closed. As a result of the violence in Zemio, twenty thousand people, almost the town's entire population, fled across the river into the Democratic Republic of the Congo, or to the surrounding bush. Four months later Zemio remained a ghost town. The region where Zemio is located has triple the prevalence of HIV/AIDS as other parts of the country, and at the time of the attack, sixteen hundred patients were receiving antiretroviral medications. Many of them lost access to the drugs, putting their lives at risk.

In the absence of security, it was largely left to health providers to fend for themselves in dealing with security threats to their facilities, staff, and patients. Their most common strategy, as elsewhere, was to show strict impartiality, including treating wounded combatants, as a means to gaining acceptance by all communities and armed groups. They also cultivated relationships with local leaders who might influence, or at least intercede with, armed groups.[82] MSF, like ICRC, but unlike some other health providers, invested heavily in outreach, dedicating staff and resources to developing and sustaining relationships with communities and with leaders of armed groups.[83] It communicated frequently with them, was transparent about hiring decisions, and met the medical needs of members of armed groups. It also took advantage of the leverage it had owing to needs of fighters and their families for health care. At the same time, it made demands of the groups. It insisted that no weapons be brought into health facilities and that the groups not interfere with health care activities. It openly condemned groups when they breached their obligations. Security was never assured, but over time MSF's investment in relationships managed to head off attacks, and in some cases avoid potential catastrophes in frightening circumstances.

A major incident in the northern town of Batangafo, two hundred miles north of Bangui and home to thirty thousand people, in 2018, provides a telling example of the threats MSF faced and how it responded. The town lacked any police or security forces. During that year, MSF already experienced more than two hundred security incidents, about a third involving civilians against other civilians. The line between criminal and political violence, between civilians and combatants, and between protectors and aggressors, had blurred.[84] That fall, tension and incidents of violence were growing. In October, assailants, later determined by MINUSCA to be ex-Séléka, set fire to an internally displaced persons' camp that was home to twenty thousand people, burning and looting houses and its market. Fifteen people were killed and another twenty-nine wounded. More than ten thousand people sought refuge in MSF's large hospital compound. Many of MSF's own hospital staff and many local staff of other NGOs joined them. It was the fourth instance since 2013 when people displaced in the town had sought shelter on the hospital grounds. In the aftermath of the attack on the camp, ex-Séléka and anti-Balaka forces each brought reinforcements to the town, while MINUSCA troops were sent to try to avoid a conflagration.[85]

The presence of so large a group of people in the hospital compound created major management, operational, and security challenges, including the possibility of violent reprisals on the hospital grounds. Ex-Séléka commanders accused MSF of lacking neutrality and hiding anti-Balaka forces in the hospital. They demanded that MSF expel the thousands of frightened and traumatized people from the compound. As the displaced people needed food, shelter, and water, MSF refused the demand, instead providing what necessities it could to them and built latrines, while it sought to control weapons entry onto the premises. Meanwhile, anti-Balaka troops blocked access to the hospital. Ex-Séléka commanders responded by demanding access and threatened further violence if the blockage continued. MSF, supported by the UN humanitarian coordinator, and to a much lesser extent, MINUSCA, managed to diffuse the situation and avoid further violence. It temporarily suspended outpatient services so it could focus on care of people with severe injuries. Additionally, MSF conducted more than two hundred medical visits in the Lakouanga neighborhood of the town, where access to the hospital was severely impeded. It continued to enforce, as best as it could, its no-weapons policy in the hospital. It sent staff to treat ex-Séléka fighters who could not enter the compound.

The situation remained volatile. Two weeks later an ex-Séléka commander threatened to burn down the hospital if MSF did not expel the displaced people and move an ad hoc market they had created within the compound after their market was destroyed. MSF again refused and also continued medical activities. The perception of the hospital as a safe place, and despite accusations to the contrary, of MSF as impartial, remained. The crisis finally diffused after more than two weeks. In a report on the event, MSF condemned the violence and threats of violence the armed groups inflicted on displaced people and medical care as "a deliberate action to inflict collective punishment to thousands of civilians in an environment of impunity."[86] What is remarkable, though, is how much worse the outcome could have been. MSF's credibility with communities and armed groups, reputation for impartiality despite accusations of favoritism, provision of medical services to people including combatants who could not reach the hospital, and refusal to yield to demands to harm displaced people, all contributed to diffusing a potential catastrophe. As in Bambari, though, the events had serious and continuing consequences for access to health care. For two months after services were fully restored, patients remained fearful of traveling to the hospital, resulting in a major decline in the number of people who came for care.

In 2017, health care providers gained a new ally in their efforts to protect the security of health care. After a free election in 2016, the new president, Faustin-Archange Touadéra, a former mathematics professor, appointed Dr. Pierre Somse to be minister of health. Dr. Somse left a comfortable job with the UN's HIV/AIDS agency to return to take on the stunning challenge. Even before the war, more mothers died in childbirth in the Central African Republic than in all but a handful of countries. Infant mortality and chronic childhood malnutrition were also among the highest in the world. During the war, more than 70 percent of health facilities had been damaged or destroyed by violence and looting.[87] A few months before he took the job, the UN reported that two-thirds of the population lacked access to health care.[88] Displaced people were especially vulnerable to malaria, the country's most severe health problem, as they often had to sleep outside, unprotected by bed nets that shielded them from mosquitos.[89] The health workforce was severely depleted. The basic components of a health system, such as human resource management, health information systems, and planning, were nonexistent or extremely weak. The country's health system was so broken that MSF, which receives no funding from governments, financed more the 30 percent of the country's health care, employing more than two thousand local staff along with more than two hundred expatriates.[90] And, of course, health care was itself caught up in the violence of the war, which jeopardized treatment for malaria and chronic malnutrition among children. The violence also made it ever more difficult to recruit qualified medical staff to work in vulnerable clinics and hospitals. More than half of health facilities were being run by individuals with only the most minimal training, and many lacked doctors or nurses. International donors committed to developing health systems in poor countries largely ignored the Central African Republic until 2019, restricting their aid to humanitarian relief that did not build local capacity.

Dr. Somse's decision to take the position in these circumstances, though, was in character. Growing up, Dr. Somse's mother, a midwife, allowed him to accompany her to births, inspiring his interest in health care. He told Sarah Woznick during an interview in Bangui in 2018 that as a preadolescent, after he met a French doctor, he thought, "I want to be like him." But he was also religious and attracted to the priesthood. He hoped to pursue both careers, but soon abandoned the idea as impractical and chose medical school. He brought his religious calling to medicine and infused his work with a sense of responsibility that surpassed the Hippocratic devotion to patients. When offered the position of minister of health, Dr. Somse had few illusions about the task. He had been trained in public health and well knew what the country lacked. But he said, "I could not afford to be away when the country was in trouble."

Once in the job, Dr. Somse quickly realized that building a functioning health system, essential as that was, would not suffice. He felt he had to address violence against health care. Outside the security apparatus and lacking political clout, health ministers are typically reluctant to address major security issues, much less engage with UN peacekeepers, government security forces, or armed groups. Health ministries' contributions to protection of patients and health workers is so rare that in fifteen essays commissioned by a respected British think tank on the crisis of civilian protection in the Central African Republic, none of the authors mentioned a role for the Ministry of Health. The gap is evident in discussions of humanitarian security.[91] A rare exception has been Colombia, where the Ministry of Health initiated a campaign called *Misión Médica* that promoted the protection of health care, established an emblem for all medical facilities and staff, issued a manual on the protection of health care, distributed posters, collected data, and ran radio spots urging respect for health care. Others are beginning to follow. The Ministry of Health in Burkina Faso, which has experienced extensive violence against health care, has collaborated with defense officials and the ICRC toward legislation that could offer greater protection of health care. The Doctors Union in South Sudan developed a proposed policy prohibiting weapons in health facilities along with other protections, and presented it to the government.

Early on in his tenure, a seemingly small incident at the hospital in Bambari convinced Dr. Somse of the need to act. A Muslim woman fell down a well and suffered an open fracture in her foot. By the time she was rescued four hours later, she had developed sepsis. Despite surgery, she died in the hospital. Her family accused a Christian nurse of poisoning the woman. A community health director informed Dr. Somse about the incident but treated it as a minor concern. But Dr. Somse realized that the nurse was vulnerable to retaliatory ethnic violence. He asked his government to open an investigation into the death, which revealed that the woman had not been poisoned. The family accepted its conclusion.

His commitment to speedy intervention in order to diffuse the potential for violence helped shape his response to an even more frightening incident in Bangui. On May 1, 2018, members of an ex-Séléka group attacked the Notre-Dame de Fatima Catholic Church in Bangui, where thousands of people were attending a service, killing at least sixteen worshippers. An angry crowd, including Christian youths with machetes, headed to the hospital to retaliate, killing a Muslim man who was accompanying a patient along the way. After learning of the incident, Minister Somse realized that Muslim patients in the hospital were at grave risk of a massacre. "Knowing the context, I knew I had to go there very quickly," he said. The "country could have exploded." Placing himself in the midst of an angry and unpredictable crowd put his own life at risk, but he didn't hesitate: "I told them to close the entrances to the hospital and hide the Muslims as the young people with machetes were preparing to attack." He also worked with the Red Cross and MINUSCA to evacuate the wounded to another hospital.

When I listened to the recording of Sarah's interview with Dr. Somse, I was intrigued. In March 2019, when he was invited to address the UN Security Council about violence against health care, we met for dinner. We went to an Italian restaurant on 42nd street in Manhattan, an incongruous setting to discuss the problems he faced in his home country. In a quiet but compelling way, he laid out the foundation of his strategy and his sources of hope. Dr. Somse said he discovered that despite its weaknesses, "the health system remains the only trusted place amid this epidemic of violence, and where hospitals or humanitarians are attacked they retain the bond with communities." He noticed, too, that despite all the violence against Muslims in certain communities, "We always see Muslims coming to hospitals, because they trust the health professional; they trust the space. For me, medical space is a safe haven for peace." He also saw the hospitals as a vehicle to advance a modicum of social cohesion in a society that is being ripped to pieces. He came to believe that the function of the hospital is "more than just giving care. It is really securing a space where people start living together again." His attitude echoed Marcelin Mentchechougo's view after practicing nursing during the entire war, when he said, "These same people maybe have done wrong against health structures. When they are hospitalized, it is at this moment that they know the greatness of the health care staff. They see, for example, the gentleness, the patience with which we transport them, we clean their wounds. I think that often after healing, it changes them a little."

I asked Dr. Somse about his relations with the armed groups who inflicted the devastation on the country. He told me that it was essential to establish and maintain regular contact with their leaders. He found many of them open to discussions with him because "they are honored to be taken seriously." His goal was to "convince them that this a sacred medical space." For his part, Dr. Somse was transparent with them about the hospital's activities and the communities that were being served. He added that he didn't pull punches: "I praise them if they behave and call them out if they don't." This sometimes included publicly condemning their acts of violence against hospitals, staff, and patients, and demanding their adherence to humanitarian law. He was realistic, though, about the uncertain success of his efforts: "To a certain extent they listen."

As we lingered over the remains of our pasta, he shared a vision of the role health ministries can play in ameliorating violence. He said that they have to go beyond ruing the violence and viewing it as utterly beyond their control. Wherever possible they need to actively devise strategies for protection of health care and supporting the staff and patients. He believed, too, that humanitarian organizations and ministries had to address the often-wide gulf between them. There were often suspicions on both sides about commitments, values, and relationships with communities that had to be addressed. In some circumstances, he said, because of its local knowledge and relationships, the Ministry of Health was likely in a better position to navigate community tensions than humanitarian organizations. The next day, Dr. Somse told the Security Council that his dialogue with the groups was productive. "When they have problems on the ground they call me because the government has the responsibility to protect them. Now when MSF has a problem, they contact me, and I get in touch with Ministry of Security and Defense" to try to solve the problem. "We are working toward the same end."[92] Inevitably, tensions, sometimes major ones, could arise in the relationship, especially when his own government's military and security forces breach their obligation not to interfere with health care. In December 2019, police detained four MSF staff in Bangui in the apparent belief that they had helped a member of an armed group avoid capture. It wasn't the first time security forces have accused medical groups of supporting rebels. The detentions severely disrupted the operations of its hospital, and MSF expressed outrage at the infringement.

I spoke to Dr. Somse again when Sarah and I, along with our Johns Hopkins colleague Natalya Kostandova, traveled to Bangui in early 2020 for a research project there on the long-term impacts of violence against health care. He elaborated on his approach to helping health services survive the conflict, especially as communal violence was expressed in hospitals. At the simplest level, he arranged for fences to be built around some hospitals. He developed procedures for the staff in each hospital to stay in touch with him in volatile situations. He insisted that incidents of violence be reported. He reassured staff at risk of violence of his support. He collaborated with the ICRC on a public education campaign that reached out to community leaders and organizations, religious leaders, neighborhood representatives in Bangui, youths who had blocked hospital access, and armed groups. The campaign distributed posters, briefed journalists, and ran radio spots.[93] He began to create a working relationship with peacekeepers to help them support health facilities and resolve rather than inflame volatile situations. He said that in cases where Christian groups distrusted peacekeepers from Muslim countries, he asked MINUSCA to back off. Even though the state was weak, it should not be surprising that his outreach to the armed groups did, at times, succeed. As political scientist Rachel Sweet's research in the Democratic Republic of the Congo showed, even in the most fragile states, bureaucracies can have significant influence over armed groups, including the ability to negotiate with them. Their engagement can both rely on and increase state legitimacy in volatile regions.[94]

The work of ICRC, MSF, the Ministry of Health, and other NGOs in seeking to reduce violence against health care by armed groups appeared to have made a difference in the Central African Republic, especially those with clear political agendas. The violence hadn't ended, but incursions into hospitals for sectarian reasons seemed to be decreasing. Vaccination coverage was also up, especially in areas controlled by armed groups. When my colleagues and I visited Bangui in early 2020, Dr. Somse, health providers, and representatives from UN agencies all told us that criminals, rogue elements of armed groups, and family members unhappy with the care their loved ones received were now responsible for most of the violence against health care, with fewer incidents generated by political or sectarian motives. Their major concerns were robbery of and sexual violence against patients walking to a clinic or hospital, attacks on vehicles on roads, and looting of facilities. In 2018, the last year for which there is good data, almost half of the recorded incidents of assaults on health care involved looting of medical supplies in facilities, compared to four involving armed entry.[95] The data are consistent with the UN's humanitarian agency reports of security incidents against humanitarian groups through October 2019, where more than half of them involving opportunistic crimes. One NGO leader told us that the amounts at stake are often trivial, but the consequences could be draconian. The robberies could lead to suspension of medical activities for days or more, leading to the departure of health staff, severe disruption of vaccination campaigns, and deterrence of patients from coming to the hospital.

Aside from efforts at prevention, ending impunity for acts of violence was also broadly recognized as essential, for the shortage of police, courts, judges, and prisons reinforced impunity.[96] In 2015, with UN financial and staffing support, the Central African Republic established a special criminal court, with primacy over regular national courts, to investigate and prosecute serious crimes committed during the conflict. In late 2018 the court held its inaugural session. It faced enormous challenges in funding, security, and protection of witnesses and victims.[97] Nevertheless, more than thirty cases had been referred to the court for investigation, and ten transferred to the investigating judge. With support, the court has the potential to bring some level of accountability for the perpetrators of violence against civilians.

Dr. Somse came to believe that dealing with violence should become a discipline within health care management, toward developing a systematic approach to the problem of violence against health care. For the moment, though, he had to cope with postelection violence, which included new assaults on health care.

# HEALTH CARE IN A CALIPHATE:
# ISIS IN IRAQ AND SYRIA

In 2013, Abu Bakr al-Baghdadi, the leader of the Islamic State in Iraq, moved into Syria and declared an Islamic State of Iraq and the Levant (known mostly in the West as ISIS) and declared himself Caliph. In Syria, the group was originally affiliated with Jabhat Al Nusra, an armed group associated with al-Qaeda that competed for hegemony with prodemocratic groups such as the Free Syrian Army. The affiliation between al-Baghdadi and Jabhat al Nusra didn't last, as the latter was more focused on overthrowing the Assad regime than in establishing a caliphate. With the help of the foreign fighters it recruited, in 2014 ISIS rapidly captured large portions of eastern Syria, taking Raqqa in January 2014 and, later that year, large swaths of Iraq, including the cities of Mosul, Tikrit, Fallujah, and Ramadi. Raqqa became the caliphate's capital.

ISIS's brand of Islam is based on a fundamentalist, millennial conception of religion that views violent jihad as a religious duty to achieve cultural cleansing and to impose God's law. It does not distinguish between civilians and combatants, only between Muslims and non-Muslims. Additionally, Muslims who resist its theology may be killed as well.[98] It approves suicide attacks and beheadings to strengthen Muslim resolve and terrorize apostates.[99] After public beheadings, ISIS often displayed the mutilated bodies of the victims for days at a time.[100] When it captured parts of Syria and Iraq, ISIS's civilian administration imposed its version of Sharia law, enforced by a morality police. It banned music, enacted severe restrictions on how women dress and move around, and punished offenders for crimes such as smoking or theft by flogging and amputation. It kidnapped and killed journalists and humanitarian workers. It considered ethnic Yazidis living in these areas to be infidels and raped and enslaved its women. ISIS, like many radical groups, expresses particular contempt for the West and its law. A 2007 al-Qaeda propaganda video said, "The amount of respect we hold for your international law is even less than you show for our defined Islamic Shariah," and cited "international infidel law."[101]

Because of the dangers to human rights organizations and journalists in ISIS-controlled areas and with local health workers reluctant to speak about their experiences for fear of reprisals, the record of ISIS's conduct toward health care is sparse. The available evidence shows, though, that ISIS fighters consistently abused and threatened doctors and nurses seeking to care for their patients in accordance with professional standards. Some who objected were kidnapped, others executed. In 2013 and 2014 it abducted five foreign MSF doctors, six staff of the International Committee of the Red Cross, and one from the Syrian Arab Red Crescent.[102] It issued instructions for its sympathizers to attack hospitals in the United States.[103] During military campaigns, ISIS used hospitals as staging areas for operations, military headquarters, and weapons depots.

As ISIS rapidly gained territory in northwestern Iraq and eastern Syria, it faced two problems regarding health care services. First, it had no medical corps or facilities for its wounded fighters; second, because it purported to operate a state, it needed to provide health services for the population under its control. Addressing the first problem was its priority. It used slick videos to recruit foreign doctors, including from Europe.[104] ISIS also demanded that health workers in areas it controlled give medical priority to its fighters. The fighters also received free care, while civilian patients had to pay sometimes exorbitant fees, unaffordable to many, especially given the widespread impoverishment that followed ISIS's takeover. It frequently commandeered civilian hospitals in captured cities, sometimes emptying them of patients to make room for its own wounded combatants.[105] It often compelled the medical staff working in the facility to abandon civilian patients and treat its cadres, and to leave their own clinics and practices to treat fighters in hospitals or the battlefront. Dr. Omar Amouri, an orthopedic surgeon, was forced to work in an ISIS hospital for two and a half years before he escaped to Kurdistan.[106] When ISIS captured Mosul in 2014, a doctor told a reporter from the *Guardian*, "As a doctor, I am supposed to treat all people equally, but they would force us to treat their own patients only. I felt disgusted with myself."[107] ISIS also took blood from blood banks for its fighters, forcing civilians needing blood to supply their own.[108] As a result, many doctors fled even as they were threatened with confiscation of their property.

To compel health workers to bend to its priority, ISIS resorted to executing doctors who refused to travel to the front or hospitals in other locations to treat its wounded.[109] ISIS also took health workers' medical instruments for use in military hospitals, leading some health workers to hide them. Once the military assault on ISIS began, the distortions of medical care worsened. In West Mosul, residents told Amnesty International investigators that ISIS regularly denied civilians both routine medical care and emergency treatment for wounds suffered during the battle. A man injured from a mortar attack told the investigators that when they came to al-Jamhuri hospital in West Mosul, he was turned away as doctors told him the hospital was only for ISIS fighters.[110]

The second problem, health care for people in the areas it controlled, was serious as well, as ISIS aspired to be a state with a full administrative apparatus to provide services and establish its bona fides with the population. Health-care bureaucrats from the previous governments remained in their positions. ISIS appropriated the British National Health Service logo as a marketing strategy to demonstrate its commitment to population health. Services deteriorated and some had to be curtailed, however, as supplies and staff dwindled. Primary care and maternal, newborn, and child care in local clinics especially suffered.[111] Unlike some radical groups, most notably the Pakistani Taliban and Boko Haram in Nigeria, ISIS permitted polio vaccination campaigns to go forward, though it initially refused to allow the vaccinators to go door-to-door, instead requiring people to bring children to medical centers.[112] It imposed other severe restrictions on medical services. It forced closure of private clinics and banned medical providers from bringing in medication to areas under its control. The medications it allowed were of dubious quality or past their usage date.

ISIS ran health services to reflect its ideology, particularly regarding women. Female health providers were often segregated from their male colleagues and forced to obey a strict dress code including full facial veils, even while seeing patients. They were also forbidden to work at night.

Women in labor were often denied medication and entrance to the hospital if they were not wearing a veil. In Mosul, some of the women health workers went on a strike that resulted in the relaxation of rules on men and women working together.[113] After ISIS's defeat in Mosul in 2017, colleagues of mine at Johns Hopkins and Iraqi researchers interviewed twenty health care professionals there, most of them female, who had worked in clinics and hospitals under ISIS control. They described how they were constantly watched at the hospital by the morality police, known as Al-Hesba, to check for deviations from strict rules on clothing, gender separation, and other edicts. They reported that the police were frightening, violent, and unpredictable. Women were censured for wearing the wrong color clothes and men for having trousers that were too long, or beards that were too thin. One female health worker was forced to marry a man she was alone with to avoid his execution. If the health workers refused to work, they could be killed. One said, "We pray to God daily to complete the day without trouble." Even coming to work could present challenges for women as they were prohibited from riding in a car with others unless a male escort was present; if they did not come to work, though, they would be punished.[114] Patients often feared going to public health clinics, instead seeking care at clinicians' homes.[115]

Humanitarian groups that tried to work in ISIS-controlled areas faced huge risks and could not sustain a presence. In May 2013, before ISIS arrived, MSF France opened a hospital in Qabasin, Syria, near another town, Al-Bab, that had been repeatedly bombed by the Assad regime. Qabasin was home to about twenty thousand people, a mix of Kurds and Arabs, and included supporters and opponents of the Assad regime. Before coming to the town, MSF reached out to all communities, local council officials, and armed groups to gain feedback and acceptance. "I drank a lot of tea during this period," the project coordinator commented, referring to all the outreach meetings he had.[116] Some people in the town were not pleased with having a hospital in the town, as they worried that it would become more susceptible to regime bombing. MSF gained enough local support, however, to open a hospital. It did not only offer trauma surgery, which was its primary work in Syria: in response to community needs and preferences, it also offered general medical care. Administrators also thought offering services beyond trauma surgery might lower the risk of the regime bombing the hospital on account of treating armed group fighters.[117]

Three months after MSF arrived, ISIS took the town. ISIS permitted the local governing council to remain in place and didn't introduce the kind of radical measures it imposed on many other towns it controlled. It gave assurances that MSF could stay, allowed women and men to work together, and provided written guarantees of security. Even so, MSF gave its fourteen international staff the option of leaving; nine accepted. Gradually, international staff began to return. Nevertheless, ominous signs began to appear: an MSF surgeon was kidnapped and murdered in the Syrian town of Bab al-Salama; some Twitter chat suggested that MSF staff were spies; and the French Ministry of Foreign Affairs warned MSF of threats to kidnap two of its doctors. In November, the president of MSF France visited Qabasin. ISIS reassured him that security guarantees would remain in place, but the commitment proved worthless. In January 2014, five MSF staff were kidnapped in Idlib and held for five months, apparently in connection with an offensive by other armed groups against ISIS. In response, MSF again evacuated international staff from Qabasin but kept the hospital open with national staff. Threats against them persisted. When the five hostages were finally released, ISIS asked MSF to stay in Qabasin, but the organization wanted higher level guarantees of its safety. It received none. In August 2014, after a year in Qabasin, MSF left the town and all ISIS-controlled areas in Syria.[118] Health care, such as it was, was left in the exclusive hands of ISIS.

The MSF experience showed the enormous challenges of negotiating with ISIS for security. Despite its propaganda, ISIS's commitment to the health of the population was weak, which limited MSF's ability to offer incentives to respect health care. Sources of external pressures available to compel it to respect health care were lacking. In their place was a campaign by the U.S. and its British, Iraqi, and Kurdish allies to dislodge ISIS from the territory it held by military means. It was one that brought yet more violence to hospitals. The fighting included fierce, prolonged, and difficult battles to wrest control of Raqqa, Mosul, and other ISIS-controlled territory. The U.S.-led campaign launched more than thirty-four thousand air and artillery strikes.

Lt. General Stephen Townsend, commander of the campaign against ISIS, claimed that its "extraordinary efforts" and "rigorous standards in our targeting process" ensured compliance with principles of "military necessity, humanity, proportionality, and distinction."[119] The U.S. said it relied on informants, advanced electronic surveillance and drone footage, and bureaucratic approvals to avoid significant civilian harm. General Townsend claimed that the coalition's meticulousness reduced civilian casualties to a tiny number, with only a third of one percent of engagements resulting in any of them.[120] Monitoring groups including Airwars and Amnesty International, by contrast, reported thousands of casualties.[121] General Townsend dismissed their reporting as based on allegations not facts, and claimed they were not credible based primarily on the lack of correspondence between the locations and dates of strikes reported by the monitoring groups and the coordinates recorded in U.S. logs.

It turned out that the U.S.'s methods of determining numbers of civilian casualties were faulty and its logs were flawed. An eighteen-month-long investigation by the *New York Times* inspected more than one hundred sites of air and artillery strikes, interviewed hundreds of witnesses, examined remains of ordnance, reviewed satellite imagery, and held discussions with officers in Qatar, where the airstrikes were controlled. ISIS's use of hospitals, apartment blocks, and other civilian structures as barracks, command centers, and weapons sites exacerbated the military challenges coalition forces confronted in dislodging it. Yet the ISIS tactics were not responsible for many of the casualties. The *Times* investigation found instances where there were no ISIS fighters or likely targets in the areas struck; rather, too often, strike planners conflated civilians with fighters. Target planners often relied on faulty intelligence. Determinations of casualties were made without any site visits. The flight logs, the principal source of evidence to discredit the reports of human rights monitors, were often inaccurate. As a result, the investigators found that airstrikes resulted in civilian casualties not one third of one percent of the time, as the coalition reported, but in 20 percent of airstrikes, a rate thirty-one times higher.[122] In the battle for Mosul, the WHO reported that as of mid-May 2017, more than 70 percent of the injured were civilians, more than a quarter of them children (it did not attribute responsibility for them).[123]

Another factor may have been at play in the high number of civilian casualties. In 2017, four months into the new Trump administration, and on the eve of the battle for Raqqa, newly appointed Secretary of Defense James Mattis announced the coalition was employing a new strategy against ISIS. The plan was to move from what he described as attrition, by which he meant forcing ISIS troops away from military objectives, to "annihilation," that is, surrounding and killing the fighters. General Mattis said, "Our intention is that the foreign fighters do not survive the fight to return home."[124] He acknowledged that there was a prospect of civilian casualties as a result of the strategy, but said, "Civilian casualties are a fact of life in this sort of situation. We do everything humanly possible consistent with military necessity, taking many chances to avoid civilian casualties at all costs."[125]

General Mattis's invocation of military necessity as a justification for civilian casualties was right out of Francis Lieber's philosophy. Notwithstanding his expressed desire to "protect the innocent" and avoid civilian casualties, and claims of having "taken chances to do so," the policy amounted to using tactics in the battle deemed necessary to win a just war, notwithstanding the civilian casualties inflicted. The Pentagon had long since embraced duties of precaution, distinction, and proportionality that rejected invoking military necessity to permit civilian harm. However, as Anand Gopal, one of the authors of the *New York Times* investigation explained, in the battle against ISIS, the U.S. military used a very elastic approach to the obligation of proportionality in attacks, resulting in increased risks to civilians in order to avoid harm to its own troops.[126]

Under the new strategy, airstrikes against ISIS after Trump assumed the presidency increased by 50 percent, and Airwars assessed that civilian casualties from them doubled from the last year of the Obama administration, most of them in Raqqa.[127] Frances Brown, who observed the change in approach, serving as a member of the National Security Council staff under both Obama and in the first six months of the Trump administration, put it more bluntly, that "when the new [Trump] team came in, human rights concerns were relegated to a way-back-seat compared with the new commander-in-chief's declared preference to 'bomb the shit' out of ISIS.'"[128]

During the four-month-long battle for Raqqa that began in June 2019, begun just after Mattis's remarks, Kurdish commanders used iPads containing satellite maps and GPS coordinators, identified targets for shelling and airstrikes, and forwarded them to American soldiers, who called in airstrikes.[129] Luke Mogelson, a correspondent for the *New Yorker* who was in Raqqa during the battle, reported that many of these strikes seemed "incongruous," as there did not seem to be ISIS fighters in the area. When he questioned a Kurdish commander who the target was, he said that it was for snipers.[130] The U.S.-led coalition used missile attacks, airstrikes, and more than thirty thousand shells to pummel the city. The assault was so intense and so constant—"every minute of every hour," an advisor to the chair of the joint chiefs of staff said—that the barrels of two nine-thousand-pound artillery pieces burned out, a result of the constancy of their use.[131]

Returning to Raqqa two years later, Mogelson wrote, "When the last *ISIS* holdouts surrendered, the layout of the city was unrecognizable. Months of labor were required just to uncover the streets."[132] He continued that the scene was "visually disorienting," with roofs at strange angles, concrete staircases dangling, and slabs of concrete that seemed to be undulating. "It's as if the cumulative energy of the American bombardment had scrambled the normal order of things, leaving behind an Escher-like reality to which the mind needs time to adjust."[133] The U.S. military has denied that its campaign led to significant numbers of civilian casualties in Raqqa, but independent investigations revealed that of the eighteen to twenty-five thousand civilians trapped in the city by ISIS, sixteen hundred were killed.[134]

The tactics brought destruction of major hospitals. During the battles for Fallujah and Mosul, before the Raqqa assault, ISIS had established military positions in hospitals. As a result, they became legitimate targets, but the law requires that a warning be given before an attack and steps be taken to minimize harms to civilians. There is evidence that in Hamam al-Alil, outside Mosul, and in Fallujah, warnings required by the Geneva Conventions before the attacks were not given.[135] In Mosul, the coalition bombed hospitals as its forces closed in on the city, apparently without warning; ISIS looted and destroyed others. Only four of the thirteen hospitals survived the battle, resulting in a 70 percent reduction in beds.[136] During the battle for Raqqa, ISIS fortified the city's large main hospital and used it as a command post.[137] Mogelson told me that he saw gunners' nests at windows on the top floor of the hospital. ISIS built berms around the hospital to protect it from shelling. The building remained functioning as a hospital, though, both for ISIS fighters and for the estimated eighteen to twenty-five thousand civilians trapped in the city, and used as human shields by ISIS.[138] The coalition attacked the hospital, apparently without warning and certainly without precautions to minimize civilian harm. The assault brought down pipes and ceilings, destroyed examination tables, X-Ray machines, CT scanners, and MRI machines. The hospital's walls were scorched by fire.[139] The closest well-functioning trauma hospital was ninety miles away, in the town of Kobane. Aid convoys with medical supplies could not reach the city. Racha Mouawieh, a Physicians for Human Rights researcher, reported that "the stories coming out of Raqqa right now are truly nightmarish. The city has been under nearly continuous bombardment since June, demolishing hospitals and clinics. Raqqa is a deathtrap where civilians who have already suffered for years under ISIS rule now also suffer the deadly consequences of the fight against ISIS.'"[140]

There are at least sixty-seven Salafi-jihadist groups in the world, most of them operating in the Middle East, North and sub-Saharan Africa, and Central and South Asia.[141] ISIS, al-Qaeda, and affiliated groups were involved in twenty-eight civil wars in the world in 2019.[142] Not all of them undermine and manipulate health care as thoroughly as ISIS. They pose enormous, but not always insurmountable challenges to local health providers. In Syria, for example, Hay'at Tahrir al-Sham (usually referred to as HTS), a merger of Jabhat al-Nusra and three other groups, which largely controlled Idlib, dominated the provision of services. Its civil governing arm sought to impose Sharia law inside hospitals, including dress codes and separating patients and doctors by gender. Some visitors were arrested. Local doctors and medical managers, however, pushed back, temporarily suspending their work and issuing a statement of protest.[143] They protested, too, when HTS fighters kidnapped doctors. Combatants stormed into hospitals looking for enemies and in one case arrested a nurse. Some doctors and nurses refused to work in HTS-controlled areas at all. The doctors and nurses used the leverage they had, the threat of suspending or ceasing services, in countering HTS's efforts to divert aid or control the facilities. With support of the local population, and the need for health care, the local Health Directorate persevered and maintained health services with integrity and professionalism, acted as a buffer between medical groups and armed groups, and prevented HTS from taking over the health sector.[144]

Of all the quandaries posed in securing protection of health care in conflict, the most difficult may be in dealing with radical groups. Traditional strategies of engagement and negotiation are of limited use, though some leverage exists because of the need for population health. At the same time, the grave violations by those groups cannot justify bombing and shelling of health facilities under the guise of military necessity that grossly depart from obligations militaries have under the Geneva Conventions to respect and protect health care, warn before attacks on health facilities, and minimize harm to civilians. Compounding the violence just brings more disproportionate death and suffering.

## VIOLENCE AND THE FAILURE OF GOVERNANCE: DEMOCRATIC REPUBLIC OF THE CONGO

In March 2019, Dr. Richard Valery Mouzoko Kiboung, an epidemiologist from Cameroon, came to the city of Butembo in the Democratic Republic of the Congo (DRC) to support a global response to an Ebola outbreak that began in August 2018. A father of four, well-liked by his colleagues, Dr. Mouzoko was part of a team in a hospital in Butembo that helped serve a population of about a hundred and fifty thousand people. About four weeks after he arrived, on April 19, armed men burst into a staff meeting and, according to witnesses, demanded that all expatriates leave and shouted that Ebola did not exist in the Congo. The armed men shot and killed Dr. Mouzoko and wounded others.[145] Health workers and officials were shaken by his murder, the latest in a plague of attacks on Ebola responders and health facilities in the eastern Congo that numbered three hundred in 2018 and 2019. They represented the most sustained and dramatic instance in memory of violence directed against well-funded and globally coordinated efforts to control a major outbreak of a deadly infectious disease.

The director general of the World Health Organization, Dr. Tedros Adhanom Ghebreyesus, paid tribute to Dr. Mouzoko and spoke of the terrible implications of his murder: "The death of Dr. Mouzoko also underscores that when health workers are targeted and attacked, it has huge ripple effects that are felt by the people they served, the communities in need, and of course their loved ones, friends and co-workers. It's a loss for everyone, everywhere."[146] Those ripple effects were felt immediately, as the WHO suspended the Ebola program in the hospital. Equally disturbing, responsibility for his murder was unclear. In the months after the attack, police arrested more than fifty individuals in connection with the attack. About half of them were affiliated with the Mai-Mai, an assortment of so-called community self-defense groups in the region. The mass arrests renewed questions not only about who had organized and committed the attacks, but the legitimacy of DRC's security and other agencies, and their competence to stop the attacks and achieve justice.

The disease struck two provinces, North Kivu and Ituri, along DRC's eastern borders with Uganda and Rwanda, and home to more than eight million people. Ebola is a terrible viral disease that causes internal bleeding, tissue inflammation, and hemorrhaging. After symptoms develop, it can be transmitted to others through any contact with bodily fluids, including sweat, blood, mucus, and vomit, and through clothes, bedding, and other objects exposed to these fluids. Globally, half the people who are infected die, but in the DRC epidemic, the death rate was even worse: two-thirds of infected people did not survive. Through experience of prior outbreaks, including one in West Africa a few years before, it was known that the key to stopping an Ebola epidemic is an intense and rapid public health response consisting of disease surveillance, isolation of victims so they do not spread it to their families, the tracing of victims' contacts so they could take precautions to limit further spread, infection control, treatment, safe burials, and—newly available in the DRC outbreak—vaccinations. Large numbers of health workers and support personnel must be enlisted to carry out all these activities and the community engagement that underpins them. The nature of the disease, though, including its lethality and transmission through mere touch, also explains the profound challenges communities and families face in dealing with a disease. Apart from anxiety about a frightful disease, families often have to forgo deeply meaningful forms of support for the sick and cultural rituals in preparing the dead for burial. Isolation separates loved ones from one another at a time of dire need. Contact tracing requires buy-in and cooperation from communities. As Jeremy Konyndyk, who helped lead the U.S. response to the Ebola outbreak in West Africa, said, "This is one of the really pernicious things about Ebola, it is a disease that preys on very basic human instincts and human emotions."[147]

Having learned lessons from its initially lackadaisical response to an Ebola outbreak in West Africa in 2014, the WHO responded with alacrity and coordinated closely with the DRC's Ministry of Health. With financial support from the World Bank, more than a thousand health workers, including Dr. Mouzoko, the majority of them from other countries, descended on the region to mobilize a response. Money poured in to hire local support staff, rent vehicles, and procure supplies. Hazmat-suited staff opened treatment centers and health workers fanned out to remote areas to contact trace, engage in community education, and vaccinate people. It was a massive public health response, staffed by competent professionals. Because of the demands made on individuals, families, and communities, though, a successful Ebola response requires that epidemiological approaches to control be implemented in true and effective partnerships with communities. The communities need to have confidence that the control plans respect their values and traditions and affirm their agency.[148] That means not just sending educational messages about the disease and how people should respond but also ensuring active community participation in the development of virus control plans and in their execution.

The recent history and politics of the eastern DRC conspired against fulfillment of these requirements. The outbreak took place after two decades of armed conflict in eastern DRC, involving more than seventy armed groups, including well-financed entities like the Allied Democratic Forces and many local self-defense groups including the Mai-Mai. Large urban areas including the epicenters of the outbreak, the cities of Beni and Butembo, mostly escaped the violence, but about twenty armed groups nevertheless operated in the area. People in rural communities were especially prey. The Allied Democratic Forces and other groups committed massive human rights violations, including massacres of civilians. Only one major armed group active in the region, the Alliance of Patriots for a Free and Sovereign Congo, signed the Geneva Call's deed of commitment pledging to respect health care. In the two years starting before and lasting after the outbreak began, almost two thousand people were killed in eastern DRC and another three thousand were abducted.[149] Almost two million people had been newly displaced by the fighting.[150] There was little response from the international community. In June 2018 alone, on the eve of the Ebola outbreak, there were sixty-two clashes among armed groups, fifty-nine abductions, and fifty-eight kidnappings.[151]

Government military forces, supplemented by a UN peacekeeping force of eighteen thousand troops, were supposed to protect civilians. The Congolese armed forces' leadership, however, was often corrupt, inept and, worse, engaged in alliances with and transferred arms, intelligence, and Congolese military uniforms to armed groups.[152] Some units also collaborated with armed groups in trafficking of timber and minerals.[153] In 2015, there was extensive evidence of complicity by some members of the army in a gruesome massacre of twelve hundred civilians. In 2019, the UN High Commissioner for Human Rights found that government as well as UN peacekeeping forces had failed to protect communities against armed groups and indeed had committed 20 percent of the violations.[154]

In the years before the outbreak, the abdication of the government's security responsibilities also contributed to the deterioration of access to health care. Rachel Sweet, a scholar and analyst who spent a decade in the eastern DRC, told me that insecurity forced the closure of many health clinics, thereby weakening an already dysfunctional health system. The system was fragmented, underfunded, and inefficient.[155] A World Health Organization report described it in 2015 as the product of "three decades of non-governance," resulting in the "alarming" health status of the population.[156] Health spending was twelve to thirteen dollars per capita in 2012, and the leading source of financing for health was user fees, representing 40 percent of total spending.[157] Quality of care was low. In the east, access and quality were even worse, a product of the neglect of the region by the central government, based in the country's capital, Kinshasa, fifteen hundred miles away. Global health analyst Stephen Morrison wrote that, for DRC's "crisis-prone, fractured, repressive form of governance, what happens in the distant, remote east has been and remains a residual concern."[158] Even at the height of the Ebola epidemic, two to three times more people in eastern DRC died from a measles outbreak than from Ebola, with more than six thousand, mostly children under five, dying in 2019 alone.[159] Clean water was scarce. To make matters worse, at the time Ebola broke out, the minister of health, Dr. Oly Ilunga Kalenga, was engaged in a power struggle within the government in the run-up to national elections.

It was against this stew of insecurity, indifferent and sometimes predatory governance, and neglect of health needs, that the World Health Organization and DRC's Ministry of Health mobilized in the summer of 2018 to try to bring the outbreak under control. Many communities deeply distrusted the government, reasonably believing that it had utterly failed either to serve or protect them, and that the Ministry of Health was consistently unresponsive and uncaring about their needs. A randomized survey of almost a thousand people in the region taken a month after the outbreak began revealed that fewer than a third of people interviewed trusted government officials to act in their interest.[160]

The initial Ebola response reinforced the distrust. Few of the health workers who came to help spoke local languages. Community education and engagement programs were fragmented, ill-coordinated, bereft of local leadership and NGO participation, and were essentially a one-way street. Experts came to towns and villages to offer information and set out requirements for behavior, including safe burials, and sought to overcome "resistance" to response efforts. They did not generally solicit the views and concerns of community members, much less invite them to help fashion the response and ensure accountability to them.[161] The work of organizations that prioritized engagement of communities was sometimes undermined by other groups that arrived in the same place, uninvited, with armed escorts.[162] Communities even lacked a coherent account of how the outbreak suddenly appeared, as it seemed to come out of nowhere. The infusion of large amounts of cash to finance the interventions amplified the distrust, as it enriched, often corruptly, well-connected entrepreneurs, operators, politicians, and aid workers, in what became known as the "Ebola business."[163] Congolese left out of the bonanza witnessed the vast sums of money distributed with understandable suspicion and anger. The large sums distributed may also have had the perverse effect of incentivizing some people to sabotage prevention and treatment programs in order to keep the funds flowing to them.

The distrust undermined whatever modicum of confidence and trust communities had in Ebola responders and impeded people's willingness to make the radical changes in behavior demanded of them.[164] Many people also questioned why such an enormous international effort was focused on a single disease that wasn't close to being the largest killer in the area, especially as their basic health needs had so long been, and continued to be, ignored. Despite WHO plans to link the Ebola response to improvements in primary care, including enhancing measles prevention and treatment, the initiative didn't come to fruition, leading to even more community skepticism. Poor governance also provided an atmosphere ripe for disinformation, which local politicians and others exploited in order to advance their own agendas.[165] Social media was replete with claims either denying the existence of Ebola, or peddling conspiracy theories about the cause of and responsibility for the outbreak. Rumors circulated of people being killed when they arrived at a treatment center, and safe burials used to harvest organs. Security, too, remained poor. In the first three months after the outbreak, attacks attributed to the Allied Democratic Forces targeted government forces three times, killing more than thirty Congolese soldiers.[166]

As the backlash intensified, health officials and some community leaders pushed for more positive messages about the outbreak response, including better explanations of why isolation and restrictions on movement were so important, why contacts had to be traced, and why everyone should cooperate to save lives. These were reinforced by radio spots.[167] The messages, though, were overwhelmed by another event four months into the response. As if to reinforce the conspiracy theories, the government cited the Ebola outbreak as a basis to suspend voting in North Kivu in a presidential election in December 2018. The region's people, who largely favored the opposition to the current government, were left without an electoral voice. David Gressly, who later became the UN's coordinator for the Ebola response, said that the election suspension exacerbated local suspicions that the Ebola crisis was manufactured and led to even more mistrust and anger at the government.[168] The WHO's oversight and advisory committee's extensive review of the Ebola response found that "at a stroke, this [election decision] tainted the response by association with a narrative of political disenfranchisement" just when a new strategy was being rolled out to address the growing medical crisis. The postponement, it found, caused "huge damage to the response."[169] The election suspension also gave groups with a political interest in manipulating the crisis a hospitable environment to spread disinformation and encourage violence.[170]

After the suspended election, violence against responders, mostly by local, so-called self-defense groups, escalated.[171] In mid-February of 2019, civil society members in Butembo wrote an open letter to responders claiming that the Ebola response was linked to political parties and that health workers were "complicit with these political actors." The letter said, too, that a Congolese physician who was in the leadership of the local response (and coauthored articles on the outbreak for international journals) was also campaigning for the handpicked successor to DRC's president and assisting other candidates, often during work hours. In the writers' view, the politicization explained why "some population members began resisting the response teams."[172] Statements on social media and other channels alleged that Ebola was a weapon of war, a means for political exclusion, or a talking point in the run-up to local elections in March.[173] Ten days later, unknown attackers burned an Ebola treatment center run by MSF in the town of Katwa, outside Butembo, despite its decades-long presence and good relationships with the community.

A flyer circulated after the attack accused the Ebola responders of conspiring to experiment on local people and being in league with the despised Ministry of Health.[174] Soon afterward, a leaflet demanded "justice at the polls" from "thieves [who] steal the elections." The authors claimed that they did not oppose the police or army "so long as they build our homeland," but warned that after the attack on the Katwa treatment center, "we will carry out even larger plans than what you have seen today. Citizens, let us rise up!!!"[175] Posters appeared demanding that Ebola treatment center workers leave, and that people not seek care in them.[176] A few days after the Katwa attack, another MSF treatment center was attacked in Butembo. Flyers circulated there containing explicit threats, including one on April 20 that claimed that Ebola does not exist, and that "we are informing the Ebola response teams that we will eliminate them by force" and that "we warn that hospital and treatment centers will face destruction here in Butembo and elsewhere."[177] Whether Dr. Mouzoko's killing was related to these and other threats, the result of power struggles among armed groups, or some other reason, could not be established.

Grievances were so widespread that it was often difficult to learn who was responsible for each attack. Suspected perpetrators included youth groups encouraged to commit violence by politicians to advance their own agendas, groups angry at being left out of the financial windfall of the Ebola economy, and even security forces. Meanwhile, the effort to control the epidemic faltered. After attacks, treatment centers temporarily closed, case finding and contact tracing fell off, and targeted vaccination programs were suspended. People feared coming to Ebola treatment centers. Ebola transmission rates increased following an attack and were sustained for many more weeks afterward.[178] Ten months into the response, despite exhausting and dedicated work by responders, cases were increasing faster than at any time since the outbreak began and indicators of success in contact tracing were declining.[179] The virus spread further geographically and more people died.[180] Subsequent research confirmed that violence directed at the Ebola response had a larger impact on the spread of the disease than the overall violence in the region.[181]

After the attack on MSF and other treatment centers, the minister of health and WHO announced a new plan for greater coordination of protection for Ebola responders that brought accompaniment by fully armed military, police, and UN peacekeeping forces. But the enhanced security did little more than increase communities' antagonism and limit their cooperation. Security forces sometimes used coercion to bring people in for testing and treatment and used disproportionate force against demonstrators and alleged attackers.[182] After the two attacks on its treatment centers, MSF severely criticized the militarization of the response as both unethical and counterproductive.[183] A vicious cycle had ensued. Violence led to militarization, which in turn exacerbated fear and suspicions, which led to further violence and increased transmission. At the same time, the continued threats and volatility led health workers to become even more vulnerable and terrified. After the killing of Dr. Mouzoko in April, health workers demonstrated in the streets and threatened to go on strike if they were not protected. In June 2019, Aruna Abedi, the DRC's regional coordinator for the Ebola response, announced that security entities would enforce rules on prevention behavior, including hand washing and temperature taking. He supported the use of force if people resisted burial protocols. He was quoted in a meeting as saying, "We tried community engagement. It doesn't work. We need to use force."[184]

To address the crisis, the UN secretary-general appointed a coordinator to oversee all dimensions of the UN's Ebola response in the DRC, including health, security, humanitarian activities, and financing. The Ministry of Health adopted a new strategic plan that emphasized far greater consultation with all segments of communities, engagement of chiefs and religious leaders, promotion of local ownership of the response, and avoidance of the appearance of financial or political favoritism. Transparency increased. These initiatives brought greater positive messages about the response.[185] Efforts were also made to increase the use of "area patrols" instead of armed escorts in order to dissociate the Ebola response from the military and police. It proved difficult to move away from direct armed security, however, as many Ebola responders valued it and were fearful of losing it. Increased coordination between MONUSCO and Ebola responders was also piloted to dissociate security from the Congolese military and police, but years of mistrust, along with budget problems, inhibited cooperation. The UN also launched a new and ambitious strategy to complement the Ministry of Health's plan and ensure political engagement, security coordination, humanitarian assistance, and financial accountability.

Still, violence continued. In the fall of 2019, the Congolese military launched an offensive against the Alliance of Democratic Forces, which led it to renew attacks on civilians and worsened security still further. In November, health workers were warned to leave or face "the worst."[186] A few days later, a Mai Mai group killed four people in the mining area of Biakato, the worst attack on responders since the beginning of the outbreak. The same day a police officer at a health office in a small town was killed. Will Cragin, then a UN coordination official based in Biakato, told me that the reasons for the attack were not clear, but that the "Ebola business," the death of a family member of a prominent Mai-Mai in the nearby town of Lwemba, anti-MONUSCO sentiment, and broader political and security tensions were likely contributing factors. No perpetrators were identified. Michael Ryan, WHO's executive director for health emergencies, explained the two mutually reinforcing consequences of the attacks: an interruption in efforts to control Ebola and more distrust of authorities, and "a small but worrying increase in cases and maybe losing some of the gains."[187]

With the new initiatives and leadership, the courageous and dedicated work of health workers, and the decision to ground the response in respect for and relationships with communities, the spread of Ebola finally waned. In late June 2020, almost two years after an outbreak that was supposed to be controlled in a matter of months, the Ministry of Health declared the outbreak at an end. By then, more than twenty-three hundred people had died.

Assessments of the Ebola control effort in DRC blamed the persistence of the epidemic on the World Health Organization, foreign governments, UN peacekeeping forces, and the Congolese government and its military. They also pointed to inadequate coordination among the many players involved in outreach to communities, insufficient financing, and especially the clumsy approach to community outreach and trust building.[188] Underlying all these was the "driving force," as a WHO oversight and advisory committee put it, of "shattered health systems, conflict, and traumatized and deprived communities."[189] Fashioning a response in the DRC would have been enormously challenging under any circumstance. Armed groups such as the ADF would likely have sought to exploit the disease for their own purposes, as would opportunistic and corrupt politicians. Yet the combination of the failure to meet people's health needs for prior decades and during the response, predatory security forces, and poor governance, bear a heavy responsibility for the length and lethality of the outbreak. A government that sought to protect the health needs of its people and whose armed forces were competent, professional, and acted with financial integrity, would almost certainly have avoided much of the persistent violence against the Ebola response and brought the outbreak under control more quickly.

It is useful to compare the response to the outbreak in eastern DRC with the large Ebola epidemic in Sierra Leone, Liberia, and Guinea in 2014. In West Africa, the countries' health systems were too weak to bring the initial outbreak under control, the WHO reacted too slowly, community engagement at the start was inadequate, and security forces at first reacted with coercion and sometimes violence. Governments in those countries, however, were mostly seen as legitimate and the mistakes at the start were addressed. In Liberia, after initial missteps in the response, a new management structure, led by an assistant minister of health, was put into place that relied heavily on community actors to lead the response, and which empowered local leaders.[190] After security forces in Liberia shot a civilian during a quarantine of an entire community, they retreated from an active role in the response.[191] The circumstances of the outbreak in eastern DRC, by contrast, including the lack of minimally effective governance and population health, manipulation of elections, mistreatment of communities, and the use of armed security that inspired fear rather than trust, created an environment for incubating suspicion and hostility and provoking violence. There was no trust because there was no basis for trust.

These governance considerations, however, are rarely discussed among strategies to protect health care from violence in armed conflict. For example, the many recommendations by the ICRC to protect health care from violence do not address good governance and the conduct of security forces.[192] In some contexts, these are the most important factors in preventing the violence. Fear of a potentially fatal disease, distrust in governance, disinformation and conspiracy theories, abusive security forces, and political agendas all contributed to violence against health workers in the COVID-19 pandemic.[193] In Colombia, for example, a wave of violence against health care during the COVID response was preceded by years of war and distrust in a fragmented health system.

At the time the outbreak in DRC began, of course, the history of poor governance and consequent lack of trust could not be undone. As was finally demonstrated late in the response, however, there were ways of ameliorating the risks without a heavily militarized response. The key was community engagement and leadership based on recognition of people's knowledge and respect for their ideas. In one of those frequent "what to do" panel discussions about vexing challenges in global health that take place in Washington, Ella Watson-Stryker, a humanitarian adviser to MSF with long experience in outbreak response, shared a strategy. She said that despite—even because of—the history of marginalization and resulting lack of trust in DRC, the response priority should be respecting the people being served, supporting their agency, and deferring to communities' decisions even when they seemed against their health interests. That approach is both consistent with humanitarian values and promotes public health:

So that you know that when you go to the village, and they say we don't want you here, and you say 'ok, I'm going to back off; can I come back tomorrow.' And you know that some people in that village are going to die from Ebola. But if you wait and go back the next day and you ask permission again and the community knows that you're not going to force them to do something, but that in the end it is their choice. In the end you will save more lives and prevent the spread of the virus.[194]

Hers was thus a principled but also pragmatic position, that the careful and respectful engagement of communities would likely pay off in greater security. But for policy types sitting in the room, it must have given pause, as it would come at a short-term cost that would no doubt be difficult for global public health officials to swallow. That approach could provide an opening for skeptics, worried donors, and others to criticize the loss of valuable time and paying for the time to build trust through more deaths in the short term. But such a decision would not only be principled, but possibly the most effective means to gain essential trust and avoid forced suspension of services. Its success is not guaranteed. Prevention of violence sometimes requires risks.

# 8

## CHALLENGES IN MAKING NORMS MATTER

R ONY BRAUMAN, A physician who joined MSF in its earliest days and was its president for a dozen years, noted that while Henri Dunant sought to enable health care settings to be "oases of humanity" in the midst of war, those oases "don't change the horrifying reality of war, which is a wrecking ball." Even so, he said, "I think we should take him up on that."[1] The oases are needed more than ever. Since Dunant's time, ever more lethal weapons have become more easily available, wars are often fought in dense urban areas, and they go on for years. Millions of people are subjected to displacement, deprivation, and disease. And there is hardly an armed conflict where health care is an oasis; instead, it is greeted with violence.

### THE NEW NORMAL?

The assaults occur with such regularity and without consequence that Margaret Chan, former director general of the World Health Organization, declared, "The sense of outrage has been muted. The fact that these attacks have become so widespread must not be tolerated as the new normal."[2] That phrase, "new normal," is now regularly heard in debates in international forums on the vulnerability of health care, suggesting that attacks on health care are increasing. David Miliband, the former British foreign secretary, and president of the International Rescue Committee, offered another take on the "new normal." He called this "the age of impunity." It is a time, he said, where "anything goes. War crimes go unpunished and the laws of war become optional." Combatants, he said, "believe they can get away with everything because they can get away with anything."[3] An entire book of essays is devoted to the question, *Do the Geneva Conventions Matter?*[4] In 2019, celebrations of the seventieth anniversary of the Geneva Conventions were tempered by the knowledge that their proscriptions were so often ignored, even scoffed at. Proponents were on the defensive, reflected in a speech by ICRC's president, Peter Maurer, who felt compelled to address the question of whether the conventions were "useless."[5] Meanwhile, authoritarian governments are on the rise, suppressing dissent and showing little compunction about punishing protesters and medics who treat their injuries.

Historically, though, violence against health care is not a *new* normal. As chapter 1 showed, since the adoption of the original Geneva Conventions, there has never been a golden age of protection of the wounded, the sick, and their caregivers from violence. From the siege of Paris during the Franco-Prussian War just a few years after the original convention; through World War I; Mussolini's war in Ethiopia; strategic, incendiary bombing in World War II, and Korea, Vietnam; and insurgency campaigns in the 1980s, hospitals were brought to ruin and health workers punished as enemies or subversives. One major difference now is that the attacks are more visible and widely reported than in the past, and that very reporting leads to the belief that the problem is worsening. This phenomenon is analogous to criticisms that violations of human rights have gotten more pervasive since the major international human rights treaties were ratified. Kathryn Sikkink, a political scientist who studies human rights, pointed out the flaw in the argument, that as the business of human rights organizations includes reporting violations, documentation of abuses has risen as the field has expanded, thus creating the illusion of increasing violations.[6] In the past decade, violence against health care has been tracked as never before, though it is still incomplete and unsystematic. Investigations at the behest of UN human rights bodies offer detailed analysis.

There is evidence, too, that during the last half century, commitments to and the strengthening of norms, along with public opinion and political pressures, have led combatants to refrain from violence against civilians. A wide-ranging statistical study by Jessica Stanton found that in civil wars between 1989 and 2010 more than 40 percent of conventional militaries and armed groups did not engage in severe violence against civilians.[7] As the case studies showed, internal and external demands have led to greater efforts at compliance with the law. Israeli reforms during the second Intifada and the modest changes in the Taliban code of conduct toward health facilities, limited as they were, likely saved lives. More profoundly, revulsion at the moral acceptability of indiscriminate bombing led to a major decline in its use by Western militaries.[8] The result is that civilian casualties from bombing by Western air forces are mostly measured in the hundreds, not in the tens or hundreds of thousands. The U.S. airstrike against an MSF hospital in Kunduz, Afghanistan in 2015 was viewed not just as unlawful and inexcusable but scandalous. The attack made the front page of the *New York Times* for a week running and elicited an apology from President Obama. To be sure, Western militaries sometimes bend or break the rules, as in the bombing of Raqqa and elsewhere in the war against ISIS, and other armed forces regularly breach them, as the case studies show. That is an unfinished business, not an indication of the hopelessness of compliance with the law.

The proper question to ask is not whether a new normal has come into being, but what the obstacles are to strengthening adherence to the norms and how they can be overcome. The major obstacles have become quite evident. Domestic and international incentives toward compliance remain too weak and recalcitrance, resistance, and stonewalling pay off. War crimes go unaddressed. UN mechanisms to promote accountability are undermined by narrow but powerful interests. Temptations to resort to military necessity as a justification for wrongdoing remain strong. To change direction toward greater protection of health care in war and times of political strife, four key steps are essential. First, we need to understand the drivers of the attacks, as I have tried to do in this book. Second, we need to reinforce norms that protect health care that have been chipped away, often without acknowledgment. Third, governments, state militaries, and armed groups have to follow through on commitments they have made to undertake the actions needed to prevent attacks on health care and end impunity. Fourth, new sources of leadership and solidarity must demand action and support those dedicated to protecting health care in war and in circumstances of political violence.

## THE LOGICS OF VIOLENCE
## AGAINST HEALTH CARE

Much of the violence by both state militaries and armed groups against health has a logic Francis Lieber would understand and appreciate, to advance their military objectives by harming the enemy and conceivably ending the war more quickly. The case studies suggest five dimensions of this logic, each with variations, summarized in table 8.1. These forms of logic, which may overlap in particular cases, are a form of the "ruthless pragmatism" Hugo Slim described in the context of violence inflicted on civilians to advance military aims in war.[9] The logic may be accompanied by attitudes, emotions, motives, and beliefs about enemies, including hatred, dehumanization, genocidal thinking, and revenge, that lead to disrespect for the wounded and the sick, as well as health services. These factors, often a product of history or contemporary propaganda, were likely present in wars in Chechnya, Kosovo, Myanmar, Syria, the Central African Republic, and the Israel-Palestinian conflict. It is often difficult to disentangle the motives and attitudes from the military logic, but it is worthwhile nevertheless to try to identify those logics. The case studies also suggest that multiple logics can be present or overlap. The first four logics can be rationalized as a form of military necessity.

The first dimension is denying health care to the wounded and the sick because they are enemies (or deemed to be, such as political protestors), or claimed to be affiliated with terrorism, and punishing health workers and facilities who provide care. This logic can also lead to violent entry into hospitals to make arrests, the killing of enemies in hospitals, or retaliation for perceived use of health facilities as a refuge. This logic may be employed to reduce the military effectiveness of enemies, prevent troops from coming back into the fight, advance counterterrorism objectives, discourage or end protests, or simply get rid of enemies.

The second logic is strategically destroying or manipulating access to health care to entire populations or subpopulations through violence against, threats to, or interference with health assets, health workers, and health services. The use of this logic is often tied to attacks on civilians and civilian infrastructure generally, to demonstrate the futility of support for an opponent through collective punishment, or advance territorial aims by forcing population movement. The strategy can also focus more directly on health care, employed to deplete essential health services needed to sustain the opposition, and the population allied with it, or undermine the authority of health workers to the extent that they are community leaders or elites. Of the case studies, Syria is the clearest example of these strategic attacks on health care. Strategic violence or threats can also serve ideological or political purposes, for example ISIS's killing of Westerners, the killing of vaccinators by some radical groups, and the Taliban's intimidation of health providers to show that it can ensure health care for the population and control entities that offer it.

The third logic is gaining tactical advantage through interference with health care. The conduct includes using health facilities and transports to store or transport weapons, launching attacks from hospitals or ambulances, demanding treatment priority for fighters, looting health supplies to help finance operations or to meet the medical needs of troops, abducting health workers to serve the group's own combatants, and misuse of the Red Cross/Red Crescent protective emblem to disguise military operations.

The fourth dimension is elevating the logic of convenience and efficiency, often masquerading as military necessity, over responsibility to protect and respect health care in war. It is reflected in not bothering to take precautions to avoid harm to the wounded and the sick or their caregivers required by principles of distinction and proportionality in attacks, and denying or obstructing safe medical evacuation in combat and expeditious passage through checkpoints. It is also evidenced in violent intrusions into hospitals for searches, arrests, and interrogation. In some cases, particularly obstructions at checkpoints, shooting at medical transports, and hospital intrusions, the decision may elevate force protection over respect for the wounded and sick. Finally, abdication of responsibility is evident in cases where a health facility is employed for military purposes, and thus loses protection, but the attacker does not provide a warning before an attack, and fails to take precautions to minimize harm to patients and staff.

For purveyors of arms or military assistance, the failure to take responsibility includes supporting parties, allies, or proxies that violate the law without the assessments required by the duty to ensure respect for health care, as well as domestic arms transfer laws. This logic has a political as well as an inconvenience dimension. These supporters rationalize their conduct through the primacy of political and diplomatic considerations when making decisions about support for partners or proxies, but in fact they are casting aside their legal obligations. They either deny responsibility for the conduct of the other party or avoid any serious effort to assess the violations committed by short-circuiting requirements to examine it. The support by the United States and United Kingdom for Saudi Arabia's war in Yemen, and the rationalizations offered for it, is the quintessential example of this conduct.

The fifth logic aims to express dissatisfaction with either the quality or organization of health care or governance generally, and to undermine it. When planned and executed by an armed group or political organization, it can have a strategic dimension, including manipulations and exploitation of dissatisfaction to undermine government, including spreading

**TABLE 8.1** THE LOGIC OF VIOLENCE DIRECTED
AGAINST HEALTH CARE

| ACTS | POTENTIAL OBJECTIVES/LOGIC | EXAMPLES |
|---|---|---|
| Deny health care to enemy fighters or political protesters; punish health workers for providing it, including criminalization of health care | Reduces military effectiveness of enemies<br><br>Prevents troops from coming back into the fight<br><br>Advances counterterrorism objectives<br><br>Discourages protests | Afghanistan, Central African Republic, Myanmar, Russia, Serbia, Syria, Turkey, new counterterrorism laws |
| Strategically target health care: bombing, burning, and shelling hospitals, arresting and killing health workers, threatening health providers to change their services or practices, killing Westerners | Demonstrates futility of support for an opponent through collective punishment<br><br>Advances territorial aims by forcing population movement<br><br>Depletes health services needed to sustain population<br><br>Controls health services<br><br>Advances ideological or political agendas<br><br>Disempowers medical elites<br><br>Undermines government | Central African Republic, Democratic Republic of the Congo, Myanmar, Kosovo, Syria, Russia (in Syria), the Taliban's violent manipulations of health services, ISIS killing of Westerners |
| Tactical interference with health care: storing weapons in health facilities; taking over a hospital or clinic; launching attacks from hospitals; requiring treatment priority for | Increases immediate tactical military advantage<br><br>Gains more immediate care for fighters<br><br>Gains medical supplies for fighters | Central African Republic, ISIS, Syria, Taliban |

*(continued)*

**TABLE 8.1** (CONTINUED)

| ACTS | POTENTIAL OBJECTIVES/LOGIC | EXAMPLES |
| --- | --- | --- |
| fighters (including abduction of health workers for that purpose); transporting weapons or fighters in ambulances; misusing emblem to disguise military operations; looting health supplies | | |
| Convenience: indiscriminate and disproportionate attacks; failing to warn before an attack; obstructing passage of, or shooting at ambulances. For arms sellers, failure to ensure that weapons and military assistance are not used to commit violations. | Compliance takes time and effort and may decrease operational efficiency<br><br>Avoids possible risks to one's own forces<br><br>Avoids military and diplomatic consequences of searching reviews of weapons sales that could damage relationships | Afghanistan, Israel, Saudi Arabia, U.S. in Raqqa, and U.S. and British weapons sales |
| Attacks on health workers and facilities as expression of hostility to governance. | Undermine government<br><br>Expressions of lack of trust and community anger<br><br>Force changes in practices | Democratic Republic of the Congo |

disinformation and conspiracy theories. It can also be a more spontaneous expression of fear and anger in communities generated by the health threat they face, the abandonment of their needs by government, corruption, and their lack of a voice. The two can be related, as community anger and violence is easily exploited by those with political agendas. This dimension of the logic was most apparent in the Democratic Republic of the Congo, but though not discussed here, was also evidenced in violence during the COVID-19 pandemic. These forms of logic are separate from, though often related to, cases where combatants inflict violence broadly on civilian populations, as in Liberia, which sweeps health care within the larger maelstrom. In some cases, the violence is both generalized and specifically targeted at health care, for example, the regime assaults on health care in Syria.

The response has to be to increase incentives and pressures from domestic and international constituencies to upset the logic by enhancing commitments to and implementation of norms in military operations and ratcheting up the consequences of noncompliance with the law. These steps remain challenging today.

## NORMS AT RISK

The flagrant, frequent violations of the Geneva Conventions have brought resolutions, declarations, and international summits that regularly, and often passionately, reaffirm commitments to protection of health care in war. The hypocrisy in many of these statements is evident, but the old adage that hypocrisy is the homage vice pays to virtue applies here: it is better to keep the norms alive and press for compliance with them than to dispense with them altogether. Far more problematic, though, is the slicing off of pieces of the norms. Commitments to norms of protection of health care don't of course guarantee protection, but without the commitment, respect for health care disappears—as is so clear in the conduct of ISIS.

The most insidious retrenchment, because it is rarely acknowledged, is the continuing vitality of Lieber's allowance for attacks on and interference with health care and civilians when combatants believe winning a just war quickly warrants it. Perhaps the most explicit defense of his approach comes from historian and legal scholar John Fabian Witt. He argues that the principle of humanity Dunant and his successors promoted only addresses one form of suffering, that experienced by people who are sick or wounded in war. Witt contends that Dunant takes no account of the suffering of a nation that is a product of the prolongation of war or the consequences of losing a just war. By contrast, Witt contends, Lieber adopted a "moral vision of the laws of war that held just ends to be more salient measures of the morality of war than human suffering."[10] For Lieber, the just end in the Civil War was ending the monstrosity of slavery. Witt cites President Truman's decision to drop the atomic bomb as another quintessential example of this reasoning. It caused apocalyptic death and suffering on the people of Hiroshima and Nagasaki but, Witt says, brought an end to a just war (for these purposes I put aside disputes on whether the bombings were in fact necessary to end the war). Invoking a more contemporary example, he points to the Israeli shelling of a school that housed more than thirteen hundred refugees during Operation Cast Lead in Gaza in 2009. According to a UN human rights report, Israel's shelling killed more than two dozen people, including children, and violated the Geneva Conventions by using means of attack that disproportionately harmed civilians in relation to the military objective. Israel answered that the attack was a justifiable response to Hamas's firing rockets from a nearby location. It also disputed the number of children killed.

Witt is not interested in adjudicating the facts or whether the attack met the legal requirements of proportionality, distinction, and precautions. Instead, he questions the relevance of those standards for making a moral judgment about the attack. He contends that Israel's conduct should not be assessed, as the Geneva Conventions would have it, by its conduct in each military act. Rather, he argues, it must be evaluated in light of the entire context, including Israel's claimed moral justification for the war, to stop Hamas's launching of rockets into Israel, especially in light of the difficult circumstances involved in fighting Hamas in densely populated Gaza. Echoing Lieber, Witt criticizes the Geneva Convention's "deep skepticism that even weighty ends justify grave means,"[11] arguing that Israel's conduct has to be judged by its legitimate need to end the firing of rockets that put Israelis at physical risk and traumatized them. He finds Lieber's invocation of military necessity by combatants helpful, in that it allows "highly contextual judgments about the circumstances in which they found themselves, even if those circumstances allowed terrible acts."[12]

Witt recognizes the slippery slope of his argument, conceding that relying on just ends to justify departure from the principle of humanity could lead "a nation to inflict massive and terrible suffering to achieve its ends in situations in which those ends did not in fact warrant such suffering."[13] He recalls that Lieber permitted siege warfare and executions of prisoners when considered militarily necessary. His answer is that inflicting terrible harms can undermine the claim that the war is indeed just. That approach is highly problematic, though. As Witt acknowledges, his approach admits of no hard and fast rules of conduct, nor does it provide concrete limits of permissible harm to the wounded and sick and other civilians. Without those limits, rationalizations for attacks that bring enormous harm come easily and judgments about the moral justifications of departure from norms could only be made after the fact. Most important of all, he does not consider that infliction of terrible harms does not necessarily refute a claim that a war was just. The strategic, incendiary bombing of populated cities in Germany and the city of Tokyo would properly be viewed today as war crimes, for which accountability is required, without questioning the justice of the war against Germany and Japan.

Witt's line of thinking is reflected, in more primitive fashion, in justifications by military officials for harming civilians in the name of counterterrorism. Then-Secretary of Defense James Mattis invoked military necessity in justifying civilian casualties in Raqqa. The loose interpretation of proportionality likely contributed to the shelling of a hospital used by ISIS to fire weapons even though it was filled with patients and staff. In a major speech in 2019, Paul Ney, then-general counsel of the Department of Defense in the Trump administration, defended the administration's opposition to proposals by the ICRC to restrict the use of indiscriminate explosive weapons with wide impacts in dense urban areas. He contended that the use of those weapons is justified if "the use of explosive weapons early in a campaign could prevent ISIS or other terrorist groups from seizing control of an urban area and using it as part of their tactical defense."[14]

In Witt's (and Lieber's) terms, he didn't contest the calamitous harm the explosive weapons cause by their indiscriminate nature, but argued that achieving the military objective of avoiding the taking of the city by terrorists allowed the tactic, as the cause was just. In the same speech, he also cited Lieber's claim that "[w]inning as quickly as possible can support humanitarian considerations."[15] There is no empirical basis for this claim.[16] The larger problem is, like Witt's argument, Ney subordinated standards of moral conduct in war to achieving military objectives. A few months after Ney's speech, the Department of Defense expressed this position in policy terms. It reversed a prior U.S. policy abjuring the use of indiscriminate cluster munitions and land mines, which are banned by international treaties that the U.S. had previously respected despite not ratifying them. The new policy allowed their use almost without limit when "necessary for mission success in major contingencies in extreme or exceptional circumstances,"[17] without mention of distinction and proportionality.

It is this kind of thinking that also supports the new counterterrorism laws, including criminalizing medical care to an alleged terrorist or enemy. In Witt's language, the "weighty end" of addressing the terrorist threat justifies the "grave means" of punishing health workers. As explained in chapter 3, many governments, especially in Europe, reject this thinking. But the U.S. is highly influential in interpreting the laws of war. Worse, its position provides encouragement and rationalizations to justify butchery by the likes of Assad. If there is a single step that can dramatically increase protection of health care in war and situations of political volatility, it is to recommit to the norm that security or military interests may never set aside commitments to immunity for the wounded and the sick and their caregivers from attack or punishment. As my colleague Alexandra Boivin of the ICRC put it so simply: "My enemy's doctor is not my enemy."[18]

A second contemporary challenge regarding norms concerns the obligations arising from governments and militaries increasingly supplying weapons, training, airpower, and technical support to military forces of other countries or friendly armed groups. Wars conducted by proxies and partners have become central to national security strategies of countries throughout the world. They can be a means to save resources or limit military commitments to achieve a military and political objective. Yet they carry enormous risks, including becoming entwined with forces that are corrupt, brutal, or incompetent, and may contribute to the escalation of conflicts and loosening compliance with the laws of war.[19] The transfer of weapons to Saudi Arabia, that were later used to bomb hospitals, is only one example of military supporters becoming enablers of attacks on health care. At the same time, governments that resist or circumvent domestic restrictions on arms sales to entities that attack civilians and other arms suppliers have declined to support a global arms treaty, all while distancing themselves from the conduct of their proxies and partners.

A strong case exists, though, to support the claim that the norms of the Geneva conventions impose a responsibility to ensure lawful behavior of proxies and partners. The first article of each of the four 1949 conventions impose the duty not only to respect their provisions but to "ensure respect" for them "in all circumstances." The elliptical phrase, *ensure respect*, does not answer the question, by whom? It is capable of profound or rather trivial meanings. The most expansive view is that all parties to the Conventions have a boundless responsibility to ensure that combatants throughout the world adhere to the conventions' requirements; the minimalist interpretation holds that the duty only means that a government must ensure that its own military forces adhere to the conventions. The controversy over its meaning has become of overriding importance in determining responsibility for the conduct of partners and proxies.

In 2016, the ICRC released a new commentary to the Geneva Conventions that took a fresh look at the phrase. It concluded that the obligation to "ensure respect" for the conventions imposes positive duties by parties to the conventions to take affirmative, concrete steps to employ their influence to bring a belligerent that is violating the conventions into compliance. The commentary, however, recognized that it made little sense to impose a duty on all parties to the conventions to be responsible for all conduct everywhere. Instead, the commentary called for a kind of sliding scale of duties that varies by the extent of military, diplomatic, and economic links to a party to the conflict. According to the commentary, the obligation is most stringent where a government or state military is engaged in joint operations with one or more belligerents or supports them through financing, equipment, arms, or training.[20] In such cases, the commentary states that the duty is not a "loose pledge," but a legal commitment. The ICRC's view has been recognized and accepted by authoritative bodies including the UN Security Council and General Assembly, the International Court of Justice, and many governments.[21] The commentary goes on to explain that the means of carrying out this duty can include protests, public criticisms, diplomatic consequences, and, importantly, a requirement "to refrain from transferring weapons if there is an expectation, based on factors or knowledge of past patterns, that such weapons would be used to violate the Conventions."[22]

In the past, the U.S. government supported the view that all parties to the convention are obligated to use their influence to secure compliance by others.[23] This interpretation has, however, been rejected by many of the governments that conduct or support wars by partner or proxy, including the United States and the United Kingdom. They interpret "ensure respect" only to apply to a nation's own troops and that, in any event, even with its sliding scale, the ICRC view imposes too broad and open-ended an obligation.[24] Underlying the disagreement, of course, is a more fundamental question about norms: whether responsibility to adhere to norms of humanity and dignity evaporate if war is outsourced. Officials never put it that way. They argue instead that while rejecting any legal obligation, their policy is to seek proxies' and partners' compliance with the Geneva Conventions, and they offer training and technical assistance to help them comply (they concede that other law applies if a government directs, aids, or assists another state in an intentionally wrongful act). As the Yemen experience demonstrates, the policy is clearly insufficient, as it leaves enormous room for evasion. Worse, the continuation of arms sales and military support sent a loud message about the weak, to the point of disappearing, enforcement of the norms. Health care cannot and will not be protected from violence in these circumstances unless the norms are not only embraced, but vigorously applied to partners or proxies. The consequence of major breaches of the law must be withdrawal of support. The norms themselves will become eviscerated if abdication in the form of distancing from the conduct of proxies and partners continues.

## PROTECTION AND AN END TO IMPUNITY

Aside from strengthening commitment to norms, reversing violence against health care requires action by domestic and international institutions and constituencies. Until deep into the second decade of the twenty-first century, strategies to prevent violence against health care were mostly left to health workers themselves and the organizations with which they were affiliated. Militaries adopted few rules and legislatures few laws to protect health care in conflict. The UN Security Council made no demands on governments or armed groups except general admonitions to comply with the law. The World Health Organization had no programs to study effective prevention methods, provide guidance on improving protection, or make demands of governments.

The record on ending impunity for violence against health care was equally shameful. Only one case involving an attack on a hospital was brought in an international criminal tribunal. Domestic investigations had an even worse record. Human Rights Watch conducted a study of investigations of twenty-five major incidents between 2013 and 2016 in which hospitals or health workers were attacked in ten countries—Afghanistan, Central African Republic, Iraq, Israel and the occupied Palestinian territory, Libya, South Sudan, Sudan, Syria, Ukraine, and Yemen. It found that at least sixteen of the episodes involved potential war crimes. Only five of the incidents—the Kunduz attack by the United States in Afghanistan, three attacks by Saudi Arabia in Yemen, and one in Gaza by Israel—were investigated and the results made public by military authorities. In only one of these, the Kunduz attack, did an investigation find wrongdoing and discipline soldiers, and in that case, no prosecutions were brought. In three of the twenty-five cases, authorities claimed to investigate incidents but released no findings. In the remaining seventeen cases, military and civilian authorities conducted no investigation at all, either denying responsibility, blaming another party, or claiming without review that the conduct was justified or warranted only minor discipline.[25]

These findings were depressingly consistent with other examinations of military and other domestic investigations of harms to civilians. One study looked at investigations of more than two hundred instances of civilian harm in U.S. operations in Afghanistan, Iraq, and other areas in the Middle East between 2004 and 2014. It showed a consistent pattern: the information gathered was incomplete and inadequate, usually relying only on internal records and eschewing interviews of civilian witnesses or site visits. The quality of the investigations depended almost entirely on the willingness of individual commanders to pursue them thoroughly, yet these individuals often had a conflict of interest because of their operational role on the ground. The results of the investigations were often opaque, and the entire process lacked transparency.[26]

Similarly, the Israeli human rights group B'Tselem reported that of the almost eight hundred complaints of human rights violations it submitted to Israeli military entities for investigation over twenty-five years, many accompanied by extensive documentation, more than 70 percent were dismissed or never investigated; in only 3 percent were charges brought. When investigations were conducted, they only addressed violations by lower-level soldiers, ignoring policies that may have contributed to the violations and decisions of senior commanders. Even in cases involving frontline soldiers, investigators only collected evidence from the complainant and the soldiers involved. In 2016, B'Tselem announced that the process was not only ineffective but also functioned as a means to protect perpetrators so it would no longer file complaints.[27]

In the second decade of the twenty-first century, momentum finally gathered toward global action on prevention of violence against health care and ending impunity. In 2011, I joined with sixteen organizations in asking then-WHO Director General Margaret Chan to engage the agency in addressing problems of violence against health care. She was receptive. Dr. Chan condemned attacks on health workers in her opening address to the World Health Assembly in May and ordered senior deputies to meet with representatives of our groups to discuss a role for the WHO in protecting health care from violence. Two months after her speech, the UN Security Council expanded the annual list of persistent perpetrators of grave violations of human rights against children in war (the list of shame) to include state military forces and armed groups that attack schools and hospitals. That summer, the ICRC published a report revealing more than 650 acts of violence against health care in sixteen countries in a two-and-a-half-year period.[28] The author of the report, Dr. Robin Coupland, a passionate and iconoclastic war surgeon, also persuaded the ICRC to launch an initiative that came to be called Health Care in Danger. The initiative employed the organization's formidable resources, long experience in health care in war, and access to high government and military officials, to raise the visibility of the problem and propose practical measures toward greater protection. The initiative complemented the NGO and academic center campaign I started that year, the Safeguarding Health in Conflict Coalition, to protect health care in conflict.

My view at the time was that, as in other areas of public health and human rights, one of the first steps needed was to move beyond reliance on episodic human rights reports and systematically collect data on attacks on health care. The strategy was based on the old adage, perhaps dating to the sixteenth century, that what gets measured gets done. Surveillance could be the foundation for understanding patterns and trends and then developing strategies to address them, just as epidemiological studies of disease contribute to prevention and treatment of them. Publication of data could also raise the visibility of the problem and, by doing so, stimulate political will toward prevention and accountability. I thought the task should be assigned to WHO as the leader in global health surveillance.[29] The Safeguarding Health in Conflict Coalition promoted the effort. In 2011, the Norwegian and U.S. governments, two of the powerhouses on the thirty-four-member executive board of the WHO, agreed to support an amendment to a pending resolution to require the agency to undertake the task. If approved by the board at its meeting in January 2012, it would be presented to the WHO's governing body, the World Health Assembly, consisting of all 194 member governments, when it met in May.

I spent much of an anxious week that January outside the executive board meeting pacing around the library of the WHO. I awaited breaks in the meeting to lobby governments on the amendment to consult with the sponsors about objections raised and to review proposed changes with them. It was far from a sure thing. Many of the WHO's own staff opposed taking on the task. They were concerned that collecting data on attacks on health facilities and personnel was too hot politically as it would require tracking misdeeds by the very governments that controlled the WHO's agenda and budget. What we did have, though, was the support of Dr. Bruce Aylward, who then ran the WHO's polio eradication initiative and its emergency division, in whose bailiwick responsibility for implementation would reside. Dr. Aylward considered collection of data by the WHO a necessary foundation to achieve respect for principles of impartial care and for the safety of health workers and infrastructure in conflict. He was unconcerned that member states that perpetrated attacks on health care would be offended and thought the WHO was up to the task. His views gave the resolution sponsors and his superiors at the WHO confidence to agree to support it.[30] The language on data collection survived, though in a watered-down version, and with about fifteen minutes left before mandatory adjournment of the meeting, it was approved and sent to the World Health Assembly. Five months later the assembly adopted it.[31]

After passage, though, bureaucratic resistance continued, and implementation faltered. Each year friendly governments put pressure on the WHO to follow through. Yet it took five-and-a-half years to launch a system, a result not only of internal resistance but the complications of designing a reporting structure. The system had to meet competing requirements of simplicity and comprehensiveness and to employ criteria designed to weed out questionable reports without eliminating valid ones. It had to gain cooperation from entities that gathered data in the field and send in reports. The system was finally put in place in 2018.[32] The WHO created a public dashboard on attacks and began speaking out about them. After three years in operation, the system had a mixed record, as it covered only a few countries, did not provide details about individual events or name perpetrators, and was not nearly as systematic as envisioned. Yet it was a start. Attention to the need for good data on the problem also stimulated academics and think tanks, NGOs, and the WHO itself, to wrestle with thorny methodological, conceptual, and pragmatic questions in tracking and reporting incidents of violence and their impacts, including the gender dimensions of violence against health care.[33]

Other initiatives began. The ICRC convened meetings of experts, military representatives, armed groups, and local health workers to develop pragmatic measures to enhance protection of health care.[34] The recommendations addressed matters such as conducting searches and operating checkpoints in a manner that will not unduly interfere with health care, protecting patient confidentiality, safely operating ambulance services, training health workers on their rights and responsibilities, and reforming domestic law. The Office of the High Commissioner for Human Rights began investigating attacks on health as part of its overall human rights monitoring. The UN Human Rights Council established independent commissions to examine violations of human rights and international humanitarian law in the occupied Palestinian territory, Syria, and later, Yemen, that included violence against health care within their mandates. The secretary-general's special representative on children in armed conflict began to investigate specific incidents of violence against health care.

The problem of violence against health care began appearing on the agendas of the governing bodies of the UN. In 2014, the government of Norway shepherded the first-ever resolution on the issue through the UN General Assembly. The resolution urged governments to take measures to prevent attacks, including adopting strong national legal frameworks that would enhance protection and data collection. In the wake of the U.S. bombing of an MSF hospital in Kunduz, Afghanistan, in 2015, Japan, Uruguay, Egypt, Spain, and New Zealand, all then nonpermanent members of the Security Council, drafted a resolution for the UN's most powerful body. By the time of its adoption in May 2016, Resolution 2286 had gained almost a hundred cosponsors. It contained tough language. It condemned attacks, reaffirmed the requirements of the Geneva

Conventions and human rights law, and warned of "the long-term consequences of such attacks for the civilian population and the health-care systems of the countries concerned." It departed from diplomatic niceties in condemning the "prevailing impunity for violations and abuses." It required that governments take "effective measures to prevent and address acts of violence, attacks and threats" through data collection, legal reform, and improvements in military training and operations. And it called for justice "to ensure that individuals responsible" for attacks "do not operate with impunity" and instead "are brought to justice." Toward that end, it required that governments conduct "full, prompt, impartial and effective investigations" and punish those found responsible.[35] The council also asked then-UN Secretary-General Ban Ki-Moon to report when medical aid was obstructed or subjected to violence, and to recommend specific actions to prevent attacks, increase protection of health care in conflict, and hold perpetrators accountable.

By summer's end the secretary-general sent ten pages of detailed recommendations to the Security Council. It was a truly comprehensive and even visionary document that addressed all the logics of violence against health care except the political uses of failed governance. Its immodest goal was to promote "a culture of respect" for health care in war.[36] The secretary-general asked that governments as well as the WHO and other UN agencies collect data on and document incidents of attacks on health care and share lessons learned from the country's experience. He provided details on specific reforms needed, starting with governments' putting their own houses in order. Domestic laws should incorporate the provisions of the Geneva Conventions, including prohibiting harassment, sanctions, or punishment of health workers for adhering to their ethical duties to treat all in need, whether friend or foe. Health workers should be trained on their rights and obligations. Military doctrine, rules of engagement, manuals, directives, standard operating procedures, and accompanying training (including for armed groups), should be reformed to protect health care. These include instituting precautionary measures for military operations and setting out responsibilities of officers and troops toward compliance with them. These precautions, he said, should encompass circumstances where a health facility is misused for military purposes so as to minimize harms to patients and staff. He urged cooperation in deconfliction procedures to map the locations of medical facilities and personnel as a means of ensuring that they remain off limits to attacks. He recommended bilateral and multilateral assistance for military training, and legislative and judicial reform. He recognized, too, that the UN had an important role to play, urging it review the role of peacekeepers in safe delivery of medical care, including through local capacity building and support for the security sector.

In addition to these prevention measures, Secretary-General Ban emphasized the need for accountability to end impunity. He called for mandatory reporting of potential violations to authorities and oversight bodies to monitor compliance, assess incidents, and to prevent future occurrences through adjustments in operational procedures. He recommended that governments create regular forums to allow affected communities to share their concerns about vulnerabilities of health care to attack and to suggest means of addressing them. Discipline and punishment of offenders was also central, both domestically and through international justice mechanisms. Secretary-General Ban called for strengthening domestic capacity for thorough, independent, and credible investigations into allegations of serious violations. He also said that international investigatory mechanisms should be invoked—and there many of them.[37] He called for greater support for the UN accountability mechanism to protect children in armed conflict so it could thoroughly address assaults on health care by state military forces and armed groups. He asked for reparations as well as medical and psychological support for victims.

These measures, he urged, must be accompanied by use of diplomatic, economic, and political levers to pressure parties to conflicts to comply with their obligations under international law. The key was to impose consequences on offenders for their violations. He recommended that governments review arms sales, and curtail them if the recipients would likely violate obligations of immunity of health care from attack. He urged the Security Council to use its power in appropriate cases to impose arms embargoes or economic sanctions on individuals, groups, and governments, and to refer cases to the International Criminal Court or to establish special tribunals. The secretary-general proposed an incentive for following through on the recommendations by suggesting that governments voluntarily report actions they take to implement all the steps needed. The reporting could help evaluate, compare, and adjust mechanisms for protection. It could also stimulate research on attacks on health care and the means of preventing them.

There was wide agreement among humanitarian, health, human rights organizations, and many governments that the measures the secretary-general recommended could, if implemented, dramatically increase protection of health care on the ground. Some of them were straightforward to accomplish, such as collecting data, education and support for health workers, reviewing and adjusting military doctrine, practice and training, strengthening procedures of domestic investigations, and holding soldiers to account through existing military justice mechanisms. Other proposals, such as forgoing arms sales to perpetrators, narrowing the scope of counterterrorism law to forbid punishing of health workers for treating alleged terrorists, using diplomatic and other pressures on rogue actors including the responsibility to protect, and invoking international justice, were more politically challenging. Nevertheless, there were good reasons to believe they could be implemented in at least some cases. As political scientists Peter Hoffman and Thomas Weiss show, the application of the responsibility to protect doctrine is subject to international politics, but when the politics are right, protection is possible.[38] Analysts have proposed sequenced steps for moving from incentives to comply to punitive measures in efforts to achieve compliance among military partners.[39]

The Security Council never brought the secretary-general's recommendations up for consideration. As his staff worked through the summer of 2016 to develop his recommendations, horrific assaults on health care were taking place, with ugly ramifications for further Security Council action. The Assad regime was in the midst of its offensive in Aleppo. In a single week in July, it launched six attacks on hospitals and many more followed. Many civilians wounded in the offensive were bereft of care as hospitals were left in rubble. In September, a convoy of eighteen trucks loaded with vital medical and humanitarian supplies was attacked in Aleppo, killing twenty people. In Yemen, after a cease-fire ended in August, renewed Saudi-led coalition airstrikes hit more hospitals and other civilian facilities on the no-strike list, including an MSF hospital in the city of Abs, killing nineteen people, even though the hospital's coordinates had been shared with the Saudis. It was the fourth attack on an MSF facility in a year, forcing MSF to withdraw from northern Yemen.

Against this violent background, the council was scheduled to review implementation of Resolution 2286 in September 2016. Everyone knew it was a test. I wrote at the time that the credibility of the Security Council was at stake and raised the question of "whether its commitment to the security of patients, doctors, nurses, emergency responders, vaccinators and other health workers extends beyond rhetoric."[40] The council invited Dr. Joanne Liu, then international president of MSF, and Peter Maurer, president of the ICRC, to brief it on developments since May. Dr. Liu could barely contain her anger. She told the council that hospitals, places of life, had been transformed into places of death, where "the doctors tell us they await their own deaths." She noted that four of the five permanent members of the Security Council were implicated in some way in these deaths. Dr. Liu castigated the council for failing to live up to its commitments, leaving norms and law to erode "almost beyond repair."[41] She demanded action.

The discussion among Security Council members that followed, however, consisted of little more than mutual recriminations. The U.S. and British representatives cited Russian and Syrian atrocities in Aleppo. The U.S. representative also defended support for Saudi Arabia in Yemen, arguing that the U.S. "had engaged the Saudi-led coalition" to emphasize the unacceptability of airstrikes on hospitals and other civilian structures. The British representative said his government took seriously violations of international humanitarian law in Yemen, including attacks on medical facilities, even as it continued to claim in court that it knew of none. Neither one acknowledged their ongoing military and weapons support for airstrikes against civilians. The Russian delegate, for his part, accused critics of fabrications and "provocative rhetoric" in pinning responsibility on

Russia for destruction of health facilities in Aleppo. He condemned the U.S. bombing of MSF's hospital in Afghanistan the year before and military assistance to the Saudi-led coalition.[42] Some Security Council members spoke in favor of the secretary-general's recommendations, but they were left in limbo when the session ended. The paralysis has lasted ever since.

In the years that followed, the Security Council annually discussed violence against health care but never acted on the recommendations. Nor did UN member states take action on the resolution itself. Four years after the adoption of Resolution 2286, in his relatively brief statement before the Security Council on protection of civilians in war, Peter Maurer made three separate pleas not to permit divisions in the council to impede effective action.[43] Without change in the power structure of the council, that was unlikely. The dysfunction of the Security Council, however, masked an equally disturbing fact: governments that purported to support actions recommended by Secretary Ban did not follow through domestically on his recommendations, even when they reaffirmed them in declarations and statements in other contexts. Each year the UN Secretary-General issued a report on civilian protection and the implementation of Resolution 2286. His staff searched for examples of good practice and actions by governments to prevent attacks on health care in conflict. Each year, the report cited only a pathetic handful of minor examples.

Even when attention to the problem of violence against health care was at an apex, opportunities for reform domestically were not pursued. In the aftermath of the Kunduz hospital attack, MSF pressured the Department of Defense to offer clearer instructions to troops in the field on protection of health care. Then-Secretary of Defense Ashton Carter sent a memorandum to all branches of the armed services regarding legal principles on protection of humanitarian organizations during conflict (he didn't address indigenous health providers) and requested that all the services engage in a prompt review of orders, rules of engagement, directives, regulations, policies, practices, and procedures to ensure that they were consistent with the principles.[44] Four years later, as there was no indication that the review had been conducted, Congress finally required one.

Progress in strengthening investigations and bringing perpetrators to justice, domestically or internationally, never got off the ground. In Syria, the stalemate at the Security Council led the UN General Assembly, which operates by majority vote but has much less power, to establish a special investigation mechanism to collect evidence of war crimes in Syria for future prosecutions. As yet, though, there is no tribunal authorized to receive the evidence. Milder forms of accountability remained stymied as well. Governments continued to avoid being named in the "list of shame" in the annex to the annual report of the secretary-general on children in armed conflict. In 2020, Saudi Arabia and Russia were not listed despite overwhelming evidence of their bombing of hospitals. Despite the report's finding that Afghanistan security forces were responsible for twenty-six attacks on hospitals and international forces (the U.S. was the only such force) for six assaults, they were not listed. Israel escaped listing as well, despite the secretary-general's finding that its military and security forces were responsible for almost two hundred incidents involving violence against hospitals.[45] Even the toothless International Humanitarian Fact-Finding Commission, established in Protocol 1 of the Geneva Conventions, which can only be invoked and release its findings with the consent of all parties, was never employed in connection with attacks on health care. When the Security Council authorized the secretary-general to prepare a report on the failure of deconfliction in northwest Syria, the mandate of the board of inquiry excluded findings of law or recommendations on legal liability, disciplinary action, or victim compensation.

During discussions at the Security Council and other international forums, many diplomats repeated the mantra that attacks on health care are unacceptable. Adopting the proposals to reduce the vulnerability of health care to violence developed in the second decade of the century would make them so. But inaction in the face of the violence suggested instead that governments would rather accept them than spend even the most modest amounts of political capital to prevent them or hold perpetrators to account. Looking back at the disregard of commitments to reduce violence against health care reminded me of two seemingly small moments at international meetings. One came during the negotiations of the resolution calling for the WHO to engage in systematic surveillance of attacks on health against health care in emergencies. Near the last minute, some governments demanded removing language that urged states to cooperate with the WHO in this work. The U.S. diplomat, who was my frequent interlocutor on the resolution, said that as time was running out, we should agree to the deletion. I concurred, thinking that the language was a throwaway, as the resolution was directed at the WHO, not member states. In retrospect, it turned out to be an ominous sign of the mismatch between governments' rhetorical support for protection and lack of willingness to take steps to achieve it. The second example came in 2015, when Switzerland introduced a resolution at the quadrennial meeting of the Red Cross and Red Crescent asking governments to approve an entirely voluntary mechanism to enhance accountability for alleged violations of the Geneva Conventions. The resolution didn't bind governments, nor even call for cooperation in the mechanism. It failed.

On the fifth anniversary of the Security Council's resolution, the monitoring group Insecurity Insight reported that, from 2016 through 2020, combatants engaged in more than four thousand incidents of violence against health care during armed conflicts. They damaged or destroyed almost one thousand health facilities through airstrikes, shelling, arson, and looting. They kidnapped or killed more than eleven hundred health workers.

# CONCLUSION

---

## Toward Humanity and Dignity

T
HE PARADOX OF the inaction in addressing violence against health care in war is that many governments and militaries, and a fair number of armed groups, view the imperative to protect health care from violence as essential to reflect their national or organizational values, instill pride in the forces, and demonstrate to others their embrace of global norms. The outrage they express about attacks is mostly genuine. Many governments spend significant resources on UN peacekeeping, humanitarian aid, and urging their militaries to comply with international humanitarian law. They speak up with passion in international forums to enable populations in need to access aid, and to train other countries' armed forces on compliance with the Geneva Conventions. Many of them resist sidelining norms of humanity and dignity to the counterterrorism paradigm and stand up for human rights.

The rhetoric and commitments, though, have not led to adoption of measures by governments to protect health care, many of which they have publicly supported. They hold back even when there is little political or military cost to doing so, such as undertaking reviews of military operations and adjusting practices in the field. In other cases, commitments are too easily subordinated to perceived, and sometimes misplaced or exaggerated, military, political, or diplomatic interests. In some instances, governments simply want to limit their obligations through unwarranted, crabbed views of their duties of proportionality and distinction, and to ensure respect for the Geneva Conventions, as well as the requirements of their own arms transfer laws. The ICRC, NGOs, and health providers do what they can to develop relationships with and persuade combatants to abide by humanitarian law. They also educate health workers about rights and responsibilities, develop practical measures to enhance protection, and push through modest legislative initiatives. But these steps, though valuable, inevitably remain somewhat at the margins. It is governments that have the greatest power to protect health care from violence.

What they must do has already been set out by the UN secretary-general, the ICRC, NGOs, and others. Some steps can be accomplished with some modest initiative and effort. Among them are reforming law and military doctrine, training soldiers, investigating potential breaches of the law and holding perpetrators to account, and abandoning thoughtless and destructive counterterrorism policy on health care. Others, like imposing diplomatic or economic consequences on military forces that show no respect for their obligations, stopping the transfer of weapons to perpetrators, and taking a more expansive view of the duty to ensure respect for the Geneva Conventions, may require the use of political capital. A third set of actions, such as reforming the structure of the UN Security Council and imposing no-fly or safe zones in the most egregious cases, require substantial political will, but need to be taken seriously if lives are to be saved.

As in other realms of human rights, leadership within militaries and governments and demands from civil society can stimulate action. During the second Intifada, Israel responded to pressure from monitoring and human rights groups, the media, and its own military officers to enable safe medical evacuation. When that pressure dissipated, so did reform. In the United States, investigations after the attack in Kunduz and changes in targeting procedures came as a result of MSF's global campaign, and as the campaign petered out, so did reforms. In Pakistan, heavy criticism for the widespread killing of community vaccinators led to increased police protection for them. In both the United States and the United Kingdom, political mobilization against arms sales, though facing strong resistance, exerted pressure to stop the transfers through legislative and judicial bodies. In the eastern DRC, pressures to empower communities in the Ebola response and to rein in security forces came late, but ultimately contributed to bringing the outbreak to an end. In the wake of military dawdling, in 2020, the U.S. Congress required the Department of Defense to report to it on changes in doctrine, instructions, and training to protect health care in military operations.[1]

One untapped resource to mobilize that pressure is the medical community itself. Millions of doctors, nurses, medics, pharmacists, and other health workers are well organized in national professional associations nationally and globally. Many are effective in lobbying both domestically and globally for better health care as well as for their own financial interests. International organizations of nurses and doctors have raised their voices, but they have limited influence at the domestic level. With some notable exceptions, however, health worker constituencies have rarely made protection of health care a priority domestically, where it is most needed. They could lobby governments, tell the stories of the risks to health workers, solicit support from the public, organize their members, and express solidarity with those who practice in dangerous, overwhelming circumstances.

A striking exception can be found in Turkey. For more than twenty-five years, the Turkish Medical Association stood up for members arrested and imprisoned by a powerful and repressive government. The members spoke out on behalf of their colleagues who were arrested for doing their ethical duty. Leaders of the association often paid a price, as they were subjected to threats and intimidation. Just as the minister of justice accused Dr. Fincancı of being an enemy of the state, the country's authoritarian president, Recep Tayyip Erdoğan, called the association "torture lovers." Despite the risks, it never backed down. In May 2019, eleven members of its governing body were sentenced to prison for saying that war is a public health problem. The association continued to speak out. It gained international support from medical groups, whose pressure on the Turkish government likely contributed to acquittals in some of the trials of doctors.

In other cases, the involvement by the medical community is critical, often when the risks to speaking out are low or nonexistent. In a different way, expatriate Syrian doctors supported their colleagues back home. They volunteered in understaffed hospitals in Syria, trained health workers in the treatment of complex traumatic injuries, lobbied donors for funding for salaries and security measures at hospitals, and raised the alarm about the catastrophe of health care in Syria. They did not succeed in stopping the bombing of hospitals but likely saved thousands of lives and enabled their colleagues to persevere.

The engagement of the health community should extend to ministries and departments of health as well. Leaders of health ministries in conflict-affected countries tend to take a hands-off view of violence. It is not all that surprising. Health ministries often lack clout within their governments and often fear further marginalization and loss of legitimacy within the government if they go out of their "lane" to discuss conduct of military forces, criticize the folly and outrageousness of including medical care as a form of support for terrorism, or interact with armed groups. In Afghanistan, high-level officials at the ministry have been reticent in doing more than raising concerns about abuses, refraining from direct contact with the Taliban. As Dr. Somse of the Central African Republic said, however, health leaders must see their mission as including the protection of patients, staff, and facilities, not just the provision of health services. They also need to be proactive in ensuring that communities have a voice in health programs, consulting them in a genuine, not a pro forma way. Fulfilling these obligations, it turns out, not only means better health care, but greater trust in government, which can result in greater security for health care.

Dr. Somse's work in the Central African Republic illustrates the potential role of health ministries. He saw that their mission was to embrace a role as "guardians of peace." He collaborated with security and peacekeeping forces, explaining to them why certain approaches to facility security will be helpful, and others not. He maintained relationships with armed groups his own government was fighting and condemned them when they inflicted violence on health care. He supported health workers in remaining safe and consoled them if attacked. There are other examples. Pakistan's National Emergency Operations Centre for Polio Eradication, run by the Ministry of Health in conjunction with other agencies and international partners, collaborated with security agencies to enhance protection of more than a quarter of a million frontline health workers.[2] Colombia's Ministry of Health and Social Protection for years actively promoted the protection of health workers. In South Sudan, the Ministry of Health collaborated with the country's doctors' union and ICRC on a policy to prohibit weapons in health facilities and agreed to reach out to the Ministry of Defense and Ministry of Interior to gain their cooperation. Health ministers can also train health workers in their rights and in coping with the challenges they confront, and demand and promote justice for the perpetrators.

Health activism is also critical at the global level. The World Health Organization has spoken out, usually gingerly. As a creature of its member states, who control its budget and select its director general, it has been reluctant to be bolder, as it immediately gets strong pushback when it criticizes governments or collects and releases data that reflects badly on them. Its tradition has been to induce and cajole governments, not confront and criticize them, which was illustrated in its restrained response when China withheld critical information in the early days of the COVID-19 outbreak. This diffidence is reflected in its action plan on protecting health care in war, which omitted references to accountability or ending impunity.[3] Its surveillance system on attacks on health care does not identify the perpetrators or reveal key details about the reported incidents. A senior official at the WHO told me that the organization was in no position to adjudicate the facts of particular incidents, and as a result it could not name names. But pressure from governments to limit its data collection resulted in silence even when the facts were clear. The WHO needs greater independence if it is to address the misconduct of its own members, but even now it could better maneuver in the space it has and would likely have allies among many of its powerful members.

Leadership, including by the health community, and political pressure won't end all the violence. Radical armed groups are not easily influenced

and butchers like Bashar al-Assad will not be dissuaded from their preda-
tions without vastly increasing the cost to them of their behavior. The global
mechanisms to end today's impunity are broken. Most notably, the structure of the UN Security Council, with the power to impose those costs or
adjust counterterrorism approaches, is probably the greatest obstacle to
account-ability, as all of its permanent members have a veto. The solution to
that obstacle involves politics well beyond the protection of health care. The
fact that there are tough cases, which require some structural change to
address, should not be a reason to refrain from taking any action. On the
contrary, it is essential, for the sake of the suffering wounded and the sick,
and the health workers who so often put their own safety and psychological well-being at risk to serve their patients.

As I was completing this book, accounts of frontline health workers
responding to the COVID-19 pandemic conveyed the grief from loss of
colleagues, exhaustion, fear for themselves and their families, depression,
and even the violence they sometimes experienced. They often lacked protective gear, confronted wrenching decisions about allocation of scarce
medical resources, had to forego normal triage protocols, or confront
angry patients and their families. Many experienced moral distress because
they were not able to save their patients' lives. Others were stigmatized or
subjected to violence. Hundreds of reports from around the world revealed
assaults and threats based on fear, misinformation, conspiracy theories and
political agendas. The health workers deserved support, and in many
countries received it from neighbors, people living in the vicinity of the
hospitals where they worked, from their professional societies, and from
the public.

It became conventional to call them heroes. The outpouring of appreciation reminded me of a passage in *A Memory of Solferino*, where Dunant
celebrated medical volunteers' "noble and compassionate spirits" that
lead them "to confront the same dangers as the warrior, of their own free
will, in a spirit of peace, for a purpose of comfort, from a motive of self-
sacrifice."[4] The reference to noble spirits and self-sacrifice was likely con-
siderably off base. The health workers whose stories appear in this book,
like many I have met, and probably those at Solferino, too, don't want to be

heroes, don't want to be considered noble, and are not motivated by self-sacrifice. Instead, they act in the belief that they have a moral and ethical duty, and see their job as providing medical care to those in need. Many would appreciate recognition for their steadfastness in the face of adversity, and for their perseverance, but they do not want to be martyrs. They want instead to be safe in their work, as the law entitles them to be.

Dunant's colleague J. H. C. Basting understood that the law should immunize health workers, along with the wounded and the sick, from attack. He persuaded Dunant to press convention delegates to protect them. Today, as they are denied that protection, they are being sacrificed. Their security is as uncertain and erratic today as it was on the field in Solferino, and the challenges are far more complicated than they were then. And as in the past, too, the seductiveness of Francis Lieber's idea that the claimed justice of a war and the desire to win quickly warrants departure from humanity puts health workers, and the patients they serve, at enormous risk. It will take supreme effort to counter these forces, but the costs in suffering and death are too great not to try.

# NOTES

## INTRODUCTION

1. Ezma Zecevic Cermerlic and Jane Green Schaller, "Human Wrongs: A Children's Hospital Destroyed," *Journal of the American Medical Association* 274, no. 5 (1995): 386. doi:10.1001/jama.1995.0353005003402.
2. Cermerlic and Schaller, "Human Wrongs."
3. Cermerlic and Schaller, "Human Wrongs."
4. Eric Stover and Richard Claude, *Medicine Under Siege in the Former Yugoslavia, 1991–1995* (Boston: Physicians for Human Rights, 1996). https://phr.org/wp-content/uploads/1996/05/medicine-under-siege-formerYugoslavia-1996.pdf.
5. Convention for the Amelioration of the Condition of the Wounded in Armies in the Field, Geneva (August 22, 1864), https://ihl-databases.icrc.org/ihl/INTRO/120?OpenDocument.
6. World Health Assembly, Resolution 46.39, Sanitary and Medical Services in Times of Armed Conflict, WHA46.39 (May 14, 1993), https://apps.who.int/iris/handle/10665/176491?search-result=true&query=wha46.39&scope=&rpp=10&sort_by=score&order=desc.
7. World Health Organization, Report by the Director General, Health and Medical Services in Times of Armed Conflict, A48/6 (February 27, 1995), https://apps.who.int/iris/bitstream/handle/10665/177483/WHA48_6_eng.pdf?sequence=1&isAllowed=y.
8. World Health Assembly, Resolution 55.13, The Protection of Medical Missions in Armed Conflict, WHA55.13 (May 18, 2002), https://apps.who.int/iris/bitstream/handle/10665/259364/WHA55-2002-REC1-eng.pdf?sequence=1&isAllowed=y.
9. Safeguarding Health in Conflict Coalition and Insecurity Insight, *Ineffective Past, Uncertain Future* (Safeguarding Health in Conflict Coalition and Insecurity Insight, 2021), https://bit.ly/3u2z3ic.

10. Sheri Fink, *War Hospital: A True Story of Surgery and Survival* (New York: Public Affairs, 2003), 151.

11. Paul H. Wise, "Epidemiologic Challenge to the Conduct of Just War: Confronting Indirect Civilian Casualties of War," *Daedalus* 146, no. 1 (Winter 2017): 139.

12. Mohammed Jawad, Thomas Hone, Eszter Vamos, Paul Roderick, Richard Sullivan, and Christopher Millet, "Estimating Indirect Mortality Impacts of Armed Conflict in Civilian Populations: Panel Regression Analyses of 193 Countries, 1990–2017," *BMC Medicine* 18 (2020): 266.

13. UN Office for Coordination of Humanitarian Affairs, "Humanitarian Needs Overview Afghanistan, Humanitarian Programme 2020," December 2019, 24, https://reliefweb.int/sites/reliefweb.int/files/resources/afg_humanitarian_needs_overview_2020.pdf.

14. Health Cluster Turkey Hub, "Health Cluster Bulletin," March 2020, https://www.humanitarianresponse.info/sites/www.humanitarianresponse.info/files/documents/files/turkey_health_cluster_bulletin_march_2020.pdf.

15. Katherine H. A. Footer, Emily Clouse, Diana Rayes, Zaher Sahloul, and Leonard S. Rubenstein, "Qualitative Accounts from Syrian Health Professionals Regarding Violations of the Right to Health, Including the Use of Chemical Weapons, in Opposition Held Syria," *BMJ Open* 8, no. 8 (August 2018): e021096.

16. Amol A. Verma, Marcia P. Jimenez, Rudolf H. Tangermann, S. V. Subramanian, and Fahad Razak, "Insecurity, Polio Vaccination Rates, and Polio Incidence in Northwest Pakistan," *Proceedings of the National Academy of Sciences* 115, no. 7 (2018): 1593.

17. Anton Camacho, Malika Bouhenia, and Reema Alyusfi et al., "Cholera Epidemic in Yemen, 2016–18: An Analysis of Surveillance Data," *Lancet Global Health* 6, no. 6 (June 2018): E680–90; Jonathan Kennedy, Andrew Harmer, and David McCoy, "The Political Determinants of the Cholera Outbreak in Yemen," *Lancet Global Health* 5, no. 10 (2017): E970–71.

18. Kate Cox, Richard Flint, Marina Favaro, Linda Slapakova, and Ruth Harris, *Researching Violence Against Health Care: Gaps and Priorities* (Rand Europe, ICRC, and Elrha, 2020), https://www.elrha.org/wp-content/themes/elrha/pdf/elrha-and-icrc-violence-against-health-care-full-report-010720-digital.pdf.

19. E.g., Abby Stoddard, *Necessary Risks: Professional Humanitarianism and Violence Against Aid Workers* (New York: Palgrave MacMillan, 2020); Jan Egeland, Anne Harmer, and Abby Stoddard, *To Stay and Deliver: Good Practice for Humanitarians in Complex Security Environments* (UN Office of Coordination of Humanitarian Affairs, 2011), https://www.unocha.org/sites/unocha/files/Stay_and_Deliver.pdf; Michael Neuman and Fabrice Weissman, eds., *Saving Lives and Staying Alive: Humanitarian Security in the Age of Risk Management* (London: Hurst, 2016); Larissa Fast, *Aid in Danger* (Philadelphia: University of Pennsylvania Press, 2014); Laura Hammond, "The Power of Holding Humanitarianism Hostage and the Myth of Protective Principles," in *Humanitarianism in Question*, ed. Michael N. Barnett and Thomas G. Weiss (Ithaca, NY: Cornell University Press, 2008).

20. A. Stoddard, P. Harvey, M. Czwarno, and M.-J. Breckenridge, *Aid Worker Security Report 2020: Contending with the Threats to Humanitarian Health Workers in the Age of Epidemics* (New York: Humanitarian Outcomes, 2020), https://www.humanitari anoutcomes.org/sites/default/files/publications/awsr2020_0_0.pdf.

21. Safeguarding Health in Conflict Coalition, *Health Workers at Risk: Violence Against Health Care* (Safeguarding Health in Conflict Coalition, 2019), https://www .safeguardinghealth.org/sites/shcc/files/SHCC2020final.pdf.

22. Fabrice Weissman, "Violence Against Aid Workers: The Meaning of Measuring," in Neuman and Weissman, *Saving Lives and Staying Alive*, 65.

## 1. PROTECTION OF HEALTH CARE IN WAR

1. John Fabian Witt, *Lincoln's Code* (New York: Free Press, 2012), 182.

2. Witt, *Lincoln's Code*, 182.

3. Andre Durand, "The Development of the Idea of Peace in the Thinking of Henri Dunant," *International Review of the Red Cross* no. 250 (1986): 16, 25.

4. Vincent Bernard, "Tactics, Techniques, Tragedies: A Humanitarian Perspective on the Changing Face of War," *International Review of the Red Cross* 97, no. 900 (December 2015): 959.

5. Peter W. Becker, "Prologue: Lieber's Place in History," in *Francis Lieber and the Culture of the Mind*, ed. Charles R. Mack and Henry H. Lesesne (Columbia: University of South Carolina Press, 2005), 1.

6. John Fabian Witt, "Two Conceptions of Suffering in War," in *Knowing the Suffering of Others: Legal Perspectives on Pain and its Meaning*, ed. Austin Sarat (Tuscaloosa: University of Alabama Press, 2014).

7. Witt, "Two Conceptions of Suffering in War."

8. Witt, *Lincoln's Code*, 176.

9. Becker, "Prologue."

10. Frank Friedel, "Francis Lieber, Charles Sumner, and Slavery," *Journal of Southern History* 9, no. 1 (1943): 79.

11. Paul Finkelman, "Lieber, Slavery, and the Problem of Free Thought in South Carolina," in *Francis Lieber and the Culture of the Mind*, ed. Charles R. Mack and Henry H. Lesesne (Columbia: University of South Carolina Press, 2005), 11.

12. Adjutant General's Office, General Orders No. 100: Instructions for the Government of Armies of the United States in the Field (1863) [Lieber Code], article 20, https://avalon .law.yale.edu/19th_century/lieber.asp.

13. Rotem Giladi, "A Different Sense of Humanity: Occupation in Francis Lieber's Code," *International Review of the Red Cross* 94, no. 885 (2012).

14. Witt, *Lincoln's Code*, 171–73.

15. Lieber Code. Henceforth, articles from the Lieber Code are cited within the text in parentheses.

16. Witt, "Two Conceptions of Suffering in War."

17. Lieber Code; Burrus M. Carnahan, "Lincoln, Lieber, and the Laws of War: The Origins and Limits of the Principle of Military Necessity," *American Journal of International Law* 92, no. 2 (1988): 213; Witt, *Lincoln's Code.*

18. Witt, *Lincoln's Code*, 234.

19. George S. Burkhardt, *Confederate Rage, Yankee Wrath: No Quarter in the Civil War* (Carbondale: Southern Illinois University Press, 2007).

20. Walt Whitman, *Memoranda During the War* (Camden, NJ: self-pub., 1875), 35.

21. Witt, *Lincoln's Code*, 252.

22. Witt, "Two Conceptions of Suffering in War," 142.

23. Paul Finkelman, "Francis Lieber and the Modern Law of War," review of *Lincoln's Code: The Laws of War in American History* by John Fabian Witt," *University of Chicago Law Review* 80, no. 4: 2071–132.

24. Frits Kalshoven and Liesbeth Zegveld, *Constraints on the Waging of War*, 4th ed. (Cambridge: Cambridge University Press, 2011), 10.

25. Convention (IV) Respecting the Laws and Customs of War, on Land, and Its Annex: Regulations Concerning the Laws and Customs of War on Land, The Hague (October 18, 1907), https://ihl-databases.icrc.org/ihl/INTRO/195.

26. Michael N. Schmitt, "Military Necessity and Humanity in International Humanitarian Law: Preserving the Delicate Balance," *Virginia Journal of International Law* 90, no. 4 (2010): 796, 800.

27. Kalshoven and Zegveld, *Constraints*, 12.

28. Witt, *Lincoln's Code*, 358.

29. Office of the General Counsel, Department of Defense, *United States Department of Defense, Law of War Manual* (2015), 3, https://dod.defense.gov/Portals/1/Documents/pubs/DoD%20Law%20of%20War%20Manual%20-%20June%202015%20Updated%20Dec%202016.pdf?ver=2016-12-13-172036-190.

30. Schmitt, "Military Necessity and Humanity," 838–39.

31. Sallie Morgenstern, "Henri Dunant and the Red Cross," *Bulletin of the New York Academy of Medicine* 55, no. 10 (1979): 949.

32. Morgenstern, "Henri Dunant and the Red Cross."

33. Henri Dunant, *A Memory of Solferino* (Geneva: International Committee of the Red Cross, 1959), 18.

34. Dunant, *Memory*, 19.

35. Dunant, *Memory*, 38.

36. Frits Kalshoven, "International Humanitarian Law and Violation of Medical Neutrality," in *Reflections on the Law of War: Collected Essays*, ed. Frits Alcove (Leiden: Brill, 2007), 1002.

37. Dunant, *Memory*, 41.

38. Dunant, *Memory*, 46.

39. Dunant, *Memory*, 46.

40. François Bugnion, "Birth of an Idea: The Founding of the International Committee of the Red Cross and of the International Red Cross and Red Crescent Movement; From Solferino to the Original Geneva Convention (1859–1864)," *International Review of the Red Cross* 94, no. 888 (2012): 1299.

41. Frank B. Berry, "Florence Nightingale's Influence on Military Medicine," *Bulletin of the New York Academy of Sciences* 32, no. 7 (1956): 547.

42. Dunant, *Memory*, 100.

43. Dunant, *Memory*, 101.

44. Dunant, *Memory*, 127.

45. Dunant, *Memory*, 173.

46. Hugo Slim, *Humanitarian Ethics: A Guide to the Morality of Aid in War and Disaster* (New York: Oxford University Press, 2015), 46; Stuart Gordon and Antonio Donini, "Romancing Principles and Human Rights: Are Humanitarian Principles Salvageable?," *International Review of the Red Cross* 97, no. 897/898 (2016): 77, 92; Alpaslan Özerdem and Gianni Rufini, "Humanitarianism and the Principles of Humanitarian Action in Post–Cold War Context," in Sultan Barakat, ed., *After the Conflict: Reconstruction and Development in the Aftermath of Conflict* (London: Palgrave Macmillan, 2005).

47. International Committee of the Red Cross, *Geneva Conventions of 12 August 1949, Commentary*, ed. Jean Pictet, 4 vols. (Geneva: International Committee of the Red Cross, 1959), 4: 136.

48. Slim, *Humanitarian Ethics*, 40–45.

49. UN Office of Coordination of Humanitarian Affairs, "What Are Humanitarian Principles?," June 2012, https://www.unocha.org/sites/dms/Documents/OOM-humanitarianprinciples_eng_June12.pdf.

50. Larissa Fast, "Unpacking the Principle of Humanity: Tensions and Implications," *International Review of the Red Cross* 97, no. 897–98 (February 2016): 111–31.

51. Dunant, *Memory*, 126.

52. Bugnion, "Birth of an Idea."

53. Bugnion, "Birth of an Idea."

54. John F. Hutchinson, *Champions of Charity: War and the Rise of the Red Cross* (Boulder, CO: Westview, 1996), 30; Kalshoven, "International Humanitarian Law and Violation of Medical Neutrality."

55. Frank Berry, "Florence Nightingale's Influence on Military Medicine."

56. Florence Nightingale, *Notes on Hospitals* (Mineola, NY: Dover, 2015), 24, 34–36; Christopher J. Gill and Gillian C. Gill, "Nightingale in Scutari: Her Legacy Reexamined," *Clinical Infectious Diseases* 40, no. 12 (2005): 1.

57. Nightingale, *Notes on Hospitals*.

58. Pierre Bossier, "Florence Nightingale and Henri Dunant," *International Review of the Red Cross* 13, no. 146 (1973): 227–38.

59. Bossier, "Florence Nightingale and Henri Dunant," 235.

60. Dunant, *Memory*, 121–22.

61. "U.S. Sanitary Commission: 1861," VCU Social Welfare History Project, https://socialwelfare.library.vcu.edu/programs/health-nutrition/u-s-sanitary-commission-1861.

62. Witt, *Lincoln's Code*, 340.

63. Hutchinson, *Champions of Charity*, 55.

64. Convention for the Amelioration of the Condition of the Wounded in Armies in the Field, Geneva (August 22, 1864), https://ihl-databases.icrc.org/ihl/INTRO/120?OpenDocument.

65. Michael Barnett, *Empire of Humanity: A History of Humanitarianism* (Ithaca, NY: Cornell University Press, 2011), 81–82.

66. Anisseh Van Engeland, "Differences and Similarities Between International Humanitarian Law and Islamic Humanitarian Law: Is There Ground for Reconciliation?" *Journal of Islamic Law and Culture* 10, no. 1 (2008): 81–99.

67. Dunant, *Memory*, 72.

68. Kalshoven, "International Humanitarian Law and Violation of Medical Neutrality," 1002.

69. Leonard Rubenstein, "A Way Forward in the Protection of Health in Conflict: Beyond the Humanitarian Paradigm," *International Review of the Red Cross* 95, no. 899 (2013): 331–40.

70. Bertrand Taithe, *Defeated Flesh: Welfare, Warfare and the Making of Modern France* (Manchester: Manchester University Press, 1999), 146–47, 162.

71. Tami Davis Biddle, "Strategic Bombing: Expectations, Theory, and Practice in the Early Twentieth Century," in *The American Way of Bombing: Changing Ethics and Legal Norms, from Flying Fortresses to Drones*, ed. Matthew Evangelista and Henry Shue (Ithaca, NY: Cornell University Press, 2014).

72. Duncan McLean, "Medical Care in Armed Conflict: Perpetrator Discourse in Historical Perspective," *International Review of the Red Cross* 101, no. 911 (2020): 771–803.

73. Andre Durand, *From Sarajevo to Hiroshima: History of the International Committee of the Red Cross* (Geneva: Henry Dunant Institute, 1984), 50.

74. Rainer Baudendistel, *Between Bombs and Good Intentions: The Red Cross and the Italo–Ethiopian War, 1935–36* (New York: Berghahn, 2006), 117.

75. Baudendistel, *Between Bombs and Good Intentions*, 126.

76. Marcel Junot, *Warrior Without Weapons* (Geneva: International Committee of the Red Cross, 1982), 50.

77. Junot, *Warrior*, 54–55.

78. McLean, "Medical Care in Armed Conflict."

79. Nicola Perugini and Neve Gordon, "Between Sovereignty and Race: The Bombardment of Hospitals in the Italo–Ethiopian War and the Colonial Imprint on International Law," *State Crime Journal* 8, no. 1 (2019): 104.

80. Richard Pankhurst, "Italian Fascist War Crimes in Ethiopia: A History of Their Discussion, from the League of Nations to the United Nations (1936–1949)," *Northeast African Studies*, New Series 6, no. 1/2 (1999): 83.

81. Richard Overy, *The Bombers and the Bombed: Allied Air War Over Europe, 1940–1945* (New York: Penguin, 2015), 52.

82. Hugo Slim, *Killing Civilians: Method, Morality and Madness in War* (Oxford: Oxford University Press, 2010).

83. Overy, *The Bombers and the Bombed.*

84. Biddle, "Strategic Bombing," 44.

85. John Hersey, "Hiroshima," *New Yorker*, August 24, 1946, https://www.newyorker.com /magazine/1946/08/31/hiroshima.

86. Overy, *The Bombers and the Bombed*, 431.

87. François Bugnion, *The International Committee of the Red Cross and the Protection of War Victims* (Oxford: Macmillan, 2003).

88. Convention (I) for the Amelioration of the Condition of the Wounded and Sick in Armed Forces in the Field, Geneva (August 12, 1949), Article 18, https://ihl-databases .icrc.org/applic/ihl/ihl.nsf/Treaty.xsp?documentId=4825657B0C7E6BF0C12563CD002 D6B0B&action=openDocument.

89. Convention (IV) Relative to the Protection of Civilians in Times of War, Geneva (August 12, 1949), article 16, https://ihl-databases.icrc.org/applic/ihl/ihl.nsf/Treaty.xsp ?documentId=AE2D398352C5B028C12563CD002D6B5C&action=openDocument.

90. Schmitt, "Military Necessity and Humanity."

91. Giovanni Mantilla, "Origins and Evolution of the 1949 Geneva Conventions and the 1977 Additional Protocols," in Evangelista and Tannenwald, *Do the Geneva Conventions Matter?*

92. Sahr Conway-Lanz, "The Ethics of Bombing Civilians After World War II: The Persistence of Norms Against Targeting Civilians in North Korea," *Asia Pacific Journal* 12, no. 37 (2014): Article ID 4180.

93. Conway-Lanz, "The Ethics of Bombing."

94. Lindesay Parrot, "379 Planes Rip Foe's New Capital Below Manchuria," *New York Times*, November 9, 1950, 1, https://timesmachine.nytimes.com/timesmachine/1950/11 /09/88420344.html?pageNumber=1.

95. Sahr Conway-Lanz, "The Struggle to Fight a Humane War: The United States, the Korean War, and the 1949 Geneva Conventions," in *Do the Geneva Conventions Matter?* ed. Matthew Evangelista and Nina Tannenwald (New York: Oxford University Press, 2017).

96. Austin Stevens, "U.S. Counters Red Charges Napalm Is Used on Civilians," *New York Times*, August 19, 1952, 1.

97. Charles Armstrong, "The Destruction and Reconstruction of North Korea, 1950–1960," *Asia Pacific Journal* 7 (2009): Article ID 3460.

98. Conway-Lanz, "The Struggle to Fight a Humane War."

99. Stevens, "U.S. Counters Red Charges."

100. Conway-Lanz, "The Ethics of Bombing."

101. Convention (IV) Relative to the Protection of Civilians in Time of War, Geneva, (August 12, 1949), Commentary of 1958, article 18, https://ihl-databases.icrc.org/applic /ihl/ihl.nsf/Treaty.xsp?action=openDocument&documentId=AE2D398352C5B028C1 2563CD002D6B5C&SessionID=DVAV558YJ0.

102. Nick Turse, *Kill Anything That Moves: The Real American War in Vietnam* (New York: Henry Holt, 2013).

103. Neta C. Crawford, "Targeting Civilians and U.S. Strategic Bombing Norms: Plus Ca Change, Plus c'est la Meme Chose?" in Evangelista and Shue, *The American Way of Bombing*.

104. "Civilian Casualties Resulting from ROLLING THUNDER PROGRAM in North Vietnam," CIA (1967), https://www.cia.gov/library/readingroom/docs/CIA -RDP78T02095R000600020001-0.pdf.

105. W. Hays Parks, "Rolling Thunder and the Law of War," *Air University Review* 33, no. 2 (January–February 1982): 2–23.

106. Telford Taylor, *Nuremburg and Vietnam: An American Tragedy* (New York: Quadrangle, 1970), 142.

107. Crawford, "Targeting Civilians and U.S. Strategic Bombing Norms," 71–72.

108. Crawford, "Targeting Civilians and U.S. Strategic Bombing Norms," 72–73.

109. Telford Taylor, "Hanoi Under the Bombing: Sirens Shelters, Rubble, and Death," *New York Times*, January 6, 1973, https://www.nytimes.com/1973/01/07/archives/hanoi-under -the-bombing-sirens-shelters-rubble-and-death-a-regular.html.

110. W. Hays Parks, "Linebacker and the Law of War," *Air University Review* 34, no. 2 (January–February 1983): 2–30.

111. Mantilla, "Origins and Evolution."

112. Mantilla, "Origins and Evolution."

113. Protocol Additional to the Geneva Conventions of 12 August 1949, and Relating to the Protection of Victims of International Armed Conflicts (Protocol I) (June 8, 1977), https://ihl-databases.icrc.org/ihl/INTRO/470. Articles from the protocols cited within the text in parenthesis.

114. International Committee of the Red Cross, Protocol Additional to the Geneva Conventions of 12 August 1949, and Relating to the Protection of Victims of International Armed Conflict (Protocol 1) (June 8, 1977), *Commentary of 1987*, General Protection of Medical Duties, Article 16, https://ihl-databases.icrc.org/applic/ihl/ihl .nsf/Comment.xsp?action=openDocument&documentId=C63B87837232A165C1256 3CD00430C81.

115. International Committee of the Red Cross, Protocol Additional to the Geneva Conventions of 12 August 1949, and Relating to the Protection of Victims of International Armed Conflict, (Protocol 2) (June 8, 1977), Article 7, https://ihl-databases.icrc.org/applic /ihl/ihl.nsf/INTRO/475.

116. Jean-Marie Henckaerts and Louise Doswald-Beck, *Customary International Humanitarian Law*, vol. 1 (Cambridge: Cambridge University Press, 2005), Rule 26.

117. Sigrid Mehring, *First Do No Harm: Medical Ethics in International Humanitarian Law* (Boston: Brill, 2014); Dustin A. Lewis, Naz K. Modirzadeh, and Gabriella Blum, *Medical Care in Armed Conflict: International Humanitarian Law and State Responses to Terrorism* (Harvard Law School Program on International Law and Armed Conflict, 2015), https://pilac.law.harvard.edu/medical-care-in-armed-conflict-report.

118. UN Security Council Resolution 2286, S/Res/2286 (2016), https://digitallibrary.un.org /record/827916/files/S_RES_2286%282016%29-EN.pdf.

119. Human Rights Watch, "Bahrain: Injured People Denied Medical Care," press release, March 17, 2011, https://www.hrw.org/news/2011/03/17/bahrain-injured-people-denied-medical-care.

120. Physicians for Human Rights, *Do No Harm: A Call for Bahrain to End Systematic Attacks on Doctors and Patients* (Cambridge, MA: Physicians for Human Rights, 2011), https://phr.org/wp-content/uploads/2011/04/bahrain-do-no-harm-2011.pdf; Human Rights Watch, "Bahrain: Arbitrary Arrests Escalate," May 4, 2011, https://www.hrw.org/news/2011/05/04/bahrain-arbitrary-arrests-escalate.

121. Bahrain Independent Commission of Inquiry, *Report of the Bahrain Independent Commission of Inquiry* (2011), Paragraph 678, http://www.bici.org.bh/BICIreport EN.pdf.

122. Physicians for Human Rights, "Bahrain Appeals Court Decision Corrects Some Injustices, but Others Remain," March 28, 2013, https://phr.org/news/bahrain-appeals-court-decision-corrects-some-injustices-but-others-remain/.

123. Brian Dooley, "Stories from Bahrain's crackdown: Dr. Ali Al Ekri," Human Rights First (blog), March 17, 2014, https://www.humanrightsfirst.org/blog/stories-bahrains-crackdown-dr-ali-al-ekri.

124. Leonard Rubenstein and Katherine Footer, "WHO Steps Up and Addresses Issue of Attacks on Health Workers, *PLOS* Blog (May 19, 2011), https://blogs.plos.org/speakingofmedicine/2011/05/19/who-steps-up-and-addresses-the-issue-of-attacks-on-health-workers-and-facilities/.

125. John Zarocostas, "Rise in Attacks on Health Personnel and Facilities Is 'Not Acceptable,' WHO Assembly Hears," *BMJ* 342, no. 7808 (2011): 342:d3265, https://doi.org/10.1136/bmj.d3265.

126. Egyptian Initiative for Personal Rights, "Field Doctors Bear Witness to the Targeting of Field Hospitals in Tahrir Square by Security Forces and Military Police," press release, December 1, 2011, https://eipr.org/en/press/2011/12/egyptian-initiative-personal-rights-field-doctors-bear-witness-targeting-field.

127. Sophie Roborgh, "Beyond Medical Humanitarianism: Politics and Humanitarianism in the Figure of Mīdānī Physician," *Social Science and Medicine* 211 (2018): 321.

128. Kathryn Sikkink, *Evidence for Hope: Making Human Rights Work in the 21st Century* (Princeton, NJ: Princeton University Press, 2017).

129. Mary Ann Glendon, *A World Made New: Eleanor Roosevelt and the Universal Declaration of Human Rights* (New York: Random House, 2001).

130. United Nations, Universal Declaration of Human Rights (1948), https://www.un.org/en/universal-declaration-human-rights/.

131. United Nations, Human Rights Instruments, Compilation of General Comments and General Recommendations Adopted by Human Rights Treaty Bodies, HRI\GEN\1\Rev.8 (1994), https://digitallibrary.un.org/record/576098?ln=cn; Cyprus v. Turkey, App. No. 2578q/94, European Court of Human Rights (2001), paragraph 154, https://www.asylumlawdatabase.eu/en/content/ecthr-cyprus-v-turkey-application-no-2578194-10-may-200.

132. UN General Assembly, Report of the Special Rapporteur on the Right to the Highest Attainable Standard of Physical and Mental Health A/68/297 (2013), http://undocs.org /A/68/297; Office of the High Commissioner of Human Rights, *International Legal Protection of Human Rights in Armed Conflicts* (2011), https://www.ohchr.org/Documents /Publications/HR_in_armed_conflict.pdf; UN General Assembly, Report of the Special Rapporteur of the Human Rights Council on Extrajudicial, Summary or Arbitrary Executions, Saving Lives Is Not a Crime, A/73/314, https://www.ohchr.org/Documents /Issues/Executions/A_73_42960.pdf.

133. UN General Assembly, Report of the Special Rapporteur on the Right to the Highest Attainable Standard of Physical and Mental Health.

134. UN Economic and Social Council, Committee on Economic, Social and Cultural Rights, General Comment 14, the Right to the Highest Attainable Standard of Physical and Mental Health, E/C.12/2000/14 (2000), para. 28, 34, https://undocs.org/E/C.12 /2000/4.

135. UN General Assembly, Report by the Special Rapporteur of the Human Rights Council on Extrajudicial, Arbitrary and Summary Executions.

136. Office of the High Commissioner for Human Rights, "Letter on Mandates of the Working Group on Arbitrary Detention," 2017, https://spcommreports.ohchr.org /TMResultsBase/DownLoadPublicCommunicationFile?gId=23180.

137. Bahrain Independent Commission of Inquiry, *Report*, para. 846, 847.

138. Bahrain Independent Commission of Inquiry, para. 842, 843, 848.

139. International Court of Justice, "Legal Consequences of the Construction of a Wall in the Occupied Palestinian Territory," Advisory Opinion, 2004, https://www.icj-cij.org /files/case-related/131/131-20040709-ADV-01-00-EN.pdf; Amrei Müller, *The Relationship Between Economic, Social and Cultural Rights and International Humanitarian Law* (Leiden: Martinus Nijhoff, 2013).

140. UN General Assembly, Report of the Special Rapporteur on the Right to the Highest Attainable Standard of Physical and Mental Health, para. 15.

141. Müller, *Relationship*, 230.

142. Müller, *Relationship*, 235–36.

143. UN General Assembly, Report of the Special Rapporteur on the Right to the Highest Attainable Standard of Physical and Mental Health, para. 15.

144. Albekov and Others v. Russia, No. 68216, European Court of Human Rights (2008), https://www.refworld.org/cases,ECHR,490ac3cc2.html.

145. De La Cruz-Flores v. Peru, Inter-American Court of Human Rights, Separate Opinion of Judge Sergio Garcia Ramirez, 2004, https://www.corteidh.or.cr/docs/casos/articulos /seriec_115_ing.pdf.

146. David Luban, "Human Rights Thinking and the Law of War," in *Theoretical Boundaries of Armed Conflict and Human Rights*, ed. Jens David Ohlin (Cambridge: Cambridge University Press, 2016), 23. Fast, "Unpacking the Principle of Humanity"; Jean Pictet, "The Fundamental Principles of the Red Cross: Commentary,"

*International Review of the Red Cross*, no. 210 (1979), 141; Protocol 2 Additional to the Geneva Conventions.

147. Giladi, "A Different Sense of Humanity."

148. "Mass Atrocity Endings: El Salvador," World Peace Foundation (blog), August 7, 2015, https://sites.tufts.edu/atrocityendings/2015/08/07/el-salvador/.

149. "El Salvador Civil War," *Encyclopedia Britannica*, https://www.britannica.com/place/El -Salvador/Civil-war.

150. Alfred Gellhorn, "Medical Mission Report on El Salvador," *New England Journal of Medicine* 308 (1983): 1043.

151. Gellhorn, "Medical Mission Report."

152. Charles Clements, *Witness to War: An American Doctor in El Salvador* (New York: Bantam, 1984).

153. Jack Geiger, Carola Eisenberg, Stephen Gloyd, José Quiroga, Thomas Schlenker, Nevin Scrimshaw, and Julia Devin, "A New Medical Mission to El Salvador," *New England Journal of Medicine* 321 (1989): 1136–40; Physicians for Human Rights, *El Salvador: Health Care Under Siege; Violations of Medical Neutrality in the Civil Conflict* (Somerville, MA: Physicians for Human Rights, 1990).

154. Leonard Rubenstein and Melanie Bittle, "Responsibility for Protection of Medical Workers and Facilities in Armed Conflict," *Lancet* 375, no. 9711 (2010): 329–40.

155. Richard M. Garfield, Thomas Frieden, and Sten H. Vermund, "Health-Related Outcome of War in Nicaragua," *American Journal of Public Health* 77, no. 5 (1987): 615.

## 2. DENYING CARE TO ENEMIES

1. Khassan Baiev, with Ruth Daniloff and Nicholas Daniloff, *The Oath* (New York: Walker, 2003), 298–99.

2. Baiev, *The Oath*, 302.

3. Leonard Rubenstein, Doug Ford, Ondrej Mach, and Allison Cohen et al., *Endless Brutality: War Crimes in Chechnya* (Boston: Physicians for Human Rights, 2001), 79, https://s3.amazonaws.com/PHR_Reports/chechnya-endless-brutality-report2001.pdf.

4. Baiev, *The Oath*, 280

5. Baiev, *The Oath*, 283.

6. Rubenstein et al., *Endless Brutality*.

7. "AMA Principles of Medical Ethics (2016)," American Medical Association, https://www.ama-assn.org/about/publications-newsletters/ama-principles-medical -ethics.

8. David Barton Smith, *Health Care Divided: Race and Healing a Nation* (Ann Arbor: University of Michigan Press, 1999).

9. "Code of Medical Ethics Opinion 1.1.2," American Medical Association, https://www .ama-assn.org/delivering-care/ethics/prospective-patients.

10. "WMA Regulations in Times of Armed Conflict and Other Situations of Violence," World Medical Association, revised 2012, https://www.wma.net/policies-post/wma -regulations-in-times-of-armed-conflict-and-other-situations-of-violence/.

11. "The ICN Code of Ethics for Nurses (2012)," International Council of Nurses, https://www .icn.ch/sites/default/files/inline-files/2012_ICN_Codeofethicsfornurses_%20eng.pdf.

12. Chiara Lepora, Marion Davis, and Alan Wertheimer, "No Exceptionalism Needed to Treat Terrorists," *American Journal of Bioethics* 9, no. 10 (2009): 53–54.

13. Benjamin Gesundheit, Nachman Ash, Shraga Blazer, and Avraham I. Rivkind, "Medical Care for Terrorists—Yes to Treat!" *American Journal of Bioethics* 9, no. 10 (2009): W3.

14. Michael Davis, "Terrorists and Just Patients," *American Journal of Bioethics* 9, no. 10 (2009): 56.

15. Ari Zivotofsky, "Medical Care for Terrorists Is Beyond the Letter of the Law," *American Journal of Bioethics* 9, no. 10 (2009): 43.

16. Beth Schwartzapfel, "Tending to Tsarnaev," Interview with Dr. Stephen Odom, Marshall Project, March 11, 2015, https://www.themarshallproject.org/2015/03/11/tending -to-tsarnaev.

17. C. S. Sperry, "The Revisions of the Geneva Conventions, 1906," *Proceedings of the American Political Science Association* 3 (1906): 33–57.

18. Protocol Additional to the Geneva Conventions of 12 August 1949, and Relating to the Protection of Victims of International Armed Conflicts (Protocol I) (June 8, 1977), article 8(a), https://ihl-databases.icrc.org/applic/ihl/ihl.nsf/Treaty.xsp?documentId=D9E6 B6264D7723C3C12563CD002D6CE4&action=openDocument; Protocol Additional to the Geneva Conventions of 12 August 1949, and Relating to the Protection of Victims of International Armed Conflicts (Protocol I) (June 8, 1977), Commentaries of 1987, para 4637, https://ihl-databases.icrc.org/applic/ihl/ihl.nsf/Comment.xsp?action=openDocu ment&documentId=CB507989C1767179C12563CD0043A5D3.

19. Michael Gross, *Bioethics and Armed Conflict: Moral Dilemmas of Medicine and War* (Cambridge, MA: MIT Press, 2006), 197, 209–10.

20. Leonard Rubenstein, "Medicine and War," *Hastings Center Report* 34, no. 6 (November–December 2004).

21. International Committee of the Red Cross, *Commentary to Geneva Convention*, ed. Jean Pictet (1952), Convention 1, article 18, page 193, https://www.loc.gov/rr/frd/Military_ Law/pdf/GC_1949-I.pdf.

22. S. De Dycker, K. T. Druckman, K. Abdou Djabarma, and A. Aronovitz et al., *Legal Opinion on the Obligation of Healthcare Professionals to Report Gunshot Wounds* (Swiss Institute of Comparative Law, 2019), https://www.isdc.ch/media/1834/17-120-final -nov19.pdf.

23. Alexander Breitegger, "The Legal Framework Applicable to Insecurity and Violence Affecting the Delivery of Health Care in Armed Conflicts and Other Emergencies," *International Review of the Red Cross* 95, no. 889 (2013): 83; Hernan Reyes, "Confidentiality Subject to National Law," *Medische Neutraliteit, Medisch Beroepsgeheim Jaargang* 51 (8 November 1996): MC NR 45 1456.

24. *Commentary of 1987: General Protection of Medical Duties*, commentary on Protocol Additional to the Geneva Convention of 12 August 1949, and Relating to the Protection of Victims of Non-International Armed Conflicts (Protocol II), 8 June 1977, para. 688, https://ihl-databases.icrc.org/applic/ihl/ihl.nsf/Comment.xsp?action=openDocument&documentId=1E86B663DA082F6AC12563CD0043A78E.

25. Amrei Müller, *The Relationship Between Economic, Social, and Cultural Rights and International Humanitarian Law* (Leiden: Martinus Nijhoff, 2013), 231–32.

26. ICRC, *Protecting Health Care: Guidance for Armed Forces* (Geneva: International Committee of the Red Cross, 2020), 65, https://shop.icrc.org/protecting-healthcare-guidance-for-the-armed-forces-pdf-en.

27. Mark Kramer, "Russia, Chechnya, and the Geneva Conventions, 1994–2006," in Matthew Evangelista and Nina Tannenwald, eds., *Do the Geneva Conventions Matter?* (New York: Oxford University Press, 2017).

28. Kramer, "Russia, Chechnya, and the Geneva Conventions."

29. Jane Buchanan, *Who Will Tell Me What Happened to My Son* (New York: Human Rights Watch, 2009), https://www.hrw.org/sites/default/files/reports/russia0909web_0.pdf.

30. James Goldgeier and Michael McFaul, *Power and Purpose: U.S. Policy Toward Russia After the Cold War* (Washington, DC: Brookings Institution, 2003), 275.

31. Congressional Research Service, *Renewed Chechnya Conflict: Developments in 1999–2000* (Washington, DC: Congressional Research Service, 2000), https://www.everycrsreport.com/files/20000503_RL30389_b07a1ae0bcc930af080588e41416a9bb7985794d.pdf.

32. Leonard Rubenstein, "U.S. Evasions on Chechnya Crimes," *Boston Globe*, April 24, 2000.

33. World Bank, *Progress in the Face of Insecurity: Improving Health Outcomes in Afghanistan* (Washington, DC: World Bank, 2018), https://documents.worldbank.org/curated/en/330491520002103598/; Jean-Francois Trani, Praveen Kumar, Ellis Ballard, and Tarani Chandola, "Assessment of Progress Towards Universal Health Coverage for People with Disabilities in Afghanistan: A Multilevel Analysis of Repeated Cross-Sectional Surveys," *Lancet Global Health* 5, no. 8 (2017): e828–37.

34. "Message from Minister," Government of Afghanistan, Ministry of Public Health, https://moph.gov.af/en.

35. Mujib Mashal, "Hospital Raid by Afghan Forces Said to Kill 3," *New York Times*, February 16, 2016, https://www.nytimes.com/2016/02/19/world/asia/hospital-raid-afghan-forces-nato-wardak-province.html%20https://www.nytimes.com/2016/02/25/world/asia/swedish-committee-for-afghanistan-hospital-raid.html.

36. United Nations Assistance Mission in Afghanistan, *Quarterly Report on the Protection of Civilians in Armed Conflict, 1 January 2019 to 30 September 2019* (October 19, 2019), https://unama.unmissions.org/sites/default/files/unama_protection_of_civilians_in_armed conflict_-_3rd_quarter_update_2019.pdf; Human Rights Watch, "Afghanistan: Special Forces Raid Medical Clinic," July 12, 2019, https://www.hrw.org/news/2019/07/12/afghanistan-special-forces-raid-medical-clinic.

37. Patty Grossman, *"They've Shot Many Like This": Abusive Raids by CIA-Backed Afghan Strike Forces* (New York: Human Rights Watch, 2019).

38. United Nations Assistance Mission in Afghanistan, *Midyear Update on the Protection of Civilians in Armed Conflict: 1 January 2019 to 30 June 2019* (2019), https://unama.unmissions .org/sites/default/files/unama_poc_midyear_update_2019_-_30_july_english.pdf.

39. Breitegger, "The Legal Framework," 117–18.

40. International Committee of the Red Cross, *Promoting Military Operational Practice that Ensures Safe Access to and Delivery of Health Care* (Geneva: ICRC, 2014), http:// healthcareindanger.org/wp-content/uploads/2015/09/icrc-002-4208-promoting-military -op-practice-ensures-safe-access-health-care.pdf.

41. Ayaz Gal, "Taliban Shuts 42 Swedish-Run Clinics in Afghanistan," *Voice of America*, July 17, 2019, https://www.voanews.com/south-central-asia/taliban-shuts-42-swedish -run-health-clinics-afghanistan.

42. International Committee of the Red Cross, *Promoting Military Operational Practice*.

43. Xavier Crombé and Joanna Kuper, "War Breaks Out: Interpreting Violence on Health-care in the Early Stage of the South Sudanese Civil War," *Journal of Humanitarian Affairs* 1, no. 2 (2019): 4–12; Vincent Iacopino, Martina W. Frank, Allen S. Keller, Sheri L. Fink, Daniel J. Pallin, and Ronald Waldman et al., *War Crimes in Kosovo: A Population-Based Assessment of Human Rights Violations Against Kosovar Albanians* (Boston: Physicians for Human Rights, 1999), https://phr.org/wp-content/uploads/1999/08 /kosovo-war-crimes-1999.pdf.

44. Iacopino et al., *War Crimes in Kosovo*.

45. Jason Cone and Françoise Duroch, "Don't Shoot the Ambulance," *World Policy Journal* 30, no. 3 (2013): 65–77; Crombé and Kuper, "War Breaks Out."

46. Christine Monaghan, *"Everything and Everyone Is a Target": The Impact on Children of Attacks on Health Care and Humanitarian Access in South Sudan* (New York: Watchlist on Children in Armed Conflict, 2018), 17, https://watchlist.org/wp-content/uploads /watchlist-field_report-southsudan-web.pdf.

47. ICRC, *Protecting Health Care: Guidance for Armed Forces*, 63–68.

48. John Sutherland, Rick Baillergeon, and Tim McKane, "Cordon and Search Operations—'A Deadly Game of Hide and Seek,'" *Air and Sea Bulletin* no. 2010–3 (2010): 4–10.

49. "COMISAF Directive on Medical Facilities Revision 2," Headquarters, International Security Assistance/United States Forces Afghanistan, October 31, 2011.

50. Department of Defense, *Law of War Manual* (2016), section 7.3.3.3, https://dod.defense .gov/Portals/1/Documents/pubs/DoD%20Law%20of%20War%20Manual%20-%20 June%202015%20Updated%20Dec%202016.pdf?ver=2016-12-13-172036-190.

51. Special Inspector General for Afghanistan Reconstruction, *Reconstructing the Afghan National Defense and Security Forces: Lessons from the U.S. Experience in Afghanistan* (2017), https://www.sigar.mil/pdf/lessonslearned/SIGAR-17-62-LL.pdf#page=133.

52. Sahr Muhammedally and Marc Garlasco, "Reduction of Civilian Harm in Afghanistan: A Way Forward," *Just Security*, February 20, 2020, https://www.justsecurity.org /68810/reduction-of-civilian-harm-in-afghanistan-a-way-forward/.

53. Thomas Gibbons-Neff, Eric Schmitt, and Adam Goldman, "A Newly Assertive CIA Expands Its Taliban Hunt in Afghanistan," *New York Times*, October 22, 2017,

https://www.nytimes.com/2017/10/22/world/asia/cia-expanding-taliban-fight
-afghanistan.html.

54. United Nations Assistance Mission in Afghanistan and United Nations Human Rights, Afghanistan, *Protection of Civilians in Armed Conflict, Annual Report 2018–2019*, 41, https://unama.unmissions.org/sites/default/files/unama_annual_protection_of_civilians_report_2018_-_23_feb_2019_-_english.pdf.

55. United Nations Mission in Afghanistan and United Nations Office of the High Commissioner of Human Rights, *Afghanistan: Protection of Civilians in Armed Conflict, Annual Report 2019*, https://unama.unmissions.org/sites/default/files/afghanistan_protection_of_civilians_annual_report_2019_-_22_february.pdf.

56. United Nations Assistance Mission in Afghanistan, *Quarterly Report on Protection of Civilians in Armed Conflict: 1 January 2019–31 March 2019*, 5, https://unama.unmissions.org/sites/default/files/unama_protection_of_civilians_in_armed_conflict_-_first_quarter_report_2019_english_.pdf.

57. United Nations Assistance Mission in Afghanistan, *Quarterly Report on Protection of Civilians in Armed Conflict*.

58. United Nations Assistance Mission in Afghanistan, "UN Urges Parties to Heed Call from Afghans: Zero Casualties," 2019, https://unama.unmissions.org/un-urges-parties-heed-call-afghans-zero-civilian-casualties.

59. Muhammedally and Garlasco, "Reduction of Civilian Harm in Afghanistan."

60. Grossman, *"They've Shot Many Like This"*; Astri Suhrke and Antonio De Lauri, "The CIA's 'Army': A Threat to Human Rights and an Obstacle to Peace in Afghanistan," Watson Institute of International Affairs, Brown University, 2019, https://watson.brown.edu/costsofwar/files/cow/imce/papers/2019/Costs%20of%20War%2C%20CIA%20Afghanistan_Aug%2021%2C%202019.pdf.

61. Joanne Liu, "Whose Lives Matter?," Cleveringa Lecture, Leiden University, November 25, 2016, https://www.universiteitleiden.nl/en/news/2016/11/doctors-and-citizens-under-fire-in-conflict-zones.

62. Xavier Crombé with Michiel Hofman, "Afghanistan: Regaining Leverage," in *Humanitarian Negotiations Revealed*, ed. Clare Magone, Michael Neuman, and Fabrice Weissman (New York: Columbia University Press, 2011), 59.

63. Katherine H. A. Footer, Sarah Meyer, Susan G. Sherman, and Leonard Rubenstein, "On the Frontline of Eastern Myanmar's Chronic Conflict: Listening to the Voices of Local Health Workers," *Social Science and Medicine* 120 (2014): 378.

64. Medicines Sans Frontiers, "Prevented from Working, the French Section of MSF Leaves Myanmar (Burma)," press release, March 30, 2006, https://www.doctorswithoutborders.org/what-we-do/news-stories/news/prevented-working-french-section-msf-leaves-myanmar-Myanmar.

65. Bill Davis and Kim Joliffe, *Achieving Health Equity in Contested Areas of Southeastern Myanmar* (Yangon: Asia Foundation, 2016), https://asiafoundation.org/wp-content/uploads/2016/07/Achieving-health-equity-in-contested-corner-of-southeast-myanmar_ENG.pdf.

66. Karen Human Rights Group, *Attacks on Education and Health Facilities and Related Personnel: Trends and Recent Incidents from Eastern Myanmar* (2011), https://khrg.org/2011/12/khrg1105/attacks-health-and-education-trends-and-incidents-eastern-Myanmar-2010-2011; ICRC, "Myanmar: ICRC Denounces Major and Repeated Violations of International Humanitarian Law," ICRC, press release, June 29, 2007, https://www.icrc.org/en/doc/resources/documents/news-release/2009-and-earlier/myanmar-news-290607.htm; UN General Assembly, *Children in Armed Conflict: Report of the Secretary-General*, A/65/820–S/2011/250 (2011), https://reliefweb.int/sites/reliefweb.int/files/resources/Children%20in%20armed%20conflict.pdf.

67. Davis and Joliffe, *Achieving Health Equity.*

68. Thailand Myanmar Border Consortium, "Displacement and Poverty in South East Myanmar/Myanmar," 2011, 17, http://www.refworld.org/docid/4ea7e9652.html.

69. Norwegian Refugee Council, Global IDP Project, *Myanmar: Displacement Continues Unabated in One of the World's Worst IDP Situations* (Geneva: Norwegian Refugee Council, 2005); Heather Rae, "Internal Displacement in Eastern Myanmar," *Forced Migration Review* 28 (2007): 45; Mary P. Callahan, *Making Enemies: War and State Building in Myanmar* (Ithaca, NY: Cornell University Press, 2003).

70. International Crisis Group, *Instruments of Pain (II): Conflict and Famine in South Sudan, Policy, Crisis Group Africa Briefing No. 124* (Nairobi/Brussels: International Crisis Group 2017), 2, https://d2071andvipowj.cloudfront.net/b124-instruments-of-pain-ii.pdf.

71. Back Pack Health Worker Team, *Provision of Primary Healthcare Among the Internally Displaced Persons and Vulnerable Populations of Myanmar, 2012 Annual Report*, 48, http://backpackteam.org/wp-content/uploads/2014/06/2012-BPHWT-Annual-Report.pdf.

72. Chris Beyrer, Juan Carlos Villar, Voravit Suwanvanichkij, Sonal Singh, Stefan Baral, and Edward Mills, "Neglected Diseases, Civil Conflicts, and the Right to Health," *Lancet* 370, no. 9587 (2008): P619–27.

73. Anne Decobert, *The Politics of Aid to Myanmar: A Humanitarian Struggle on the Thai–Burmese Border* (London: Routledge, 2015).

74. Luke C. Mullany, Catherine I. Lee, Lin Yone, Palae Paw, Eh Kalu Shwe Oo, Cynthia Maung, Thomas J. Lee, and Chris Beyer, "Access to Essential Maternal Health Interventions and Human Rights Violations Among Vulnerable Communities in Eastern Myanmar," *PLOS Medicine* 23, no. 12 (2008): 1969; Luke C. Mullany, Adam K. Richards, and Catherine I. Lee et al., "Population-Based Survey Methods to Quantify Associations Between Human Rights Violations and Health Outcomes Among Internally Displaced Persons in Eastern Myanmar," *Journal of Epidemiology and Community Health* 61, no. 10 (2007): 908.

75. Davis and Joliffe, *Achieving Health Equity.*

76. Decobert, *The Politics of Aid.*

77. Davis and Joliffe, *Achieving Health Equity.*

78. Back Pack Health Worker Team, *Provision of Primary Healthcare*, 48.

79. Decobert, *The Politics of Aid*, 171.

80. "Interview with Backpack-Medic Mahn Mahn (part 2)," RFA Burmese, November 2, 2011, English translation by Sandra Hsu Hnin Mon, https://www.youtube.com/watch?v=RcNfdXiFbRc.

81. Decobert, *The Politics of Aid.*

82. Footer et al., "On the Frontline."

83. Footer et al., "On the Frontline."

84. Footer et al., "On the Frontline."

85. Footer et al., "On the Frontline."

86. Footer et al., "On the Frontline."

87. Footer et al., "On the Frontline."

88. William W. Davis et al., "Militarization, Human Rights Violations and Community Responses as Determinants of Health in Southeastern Myanmar," *Conflict and Health* 9 (2015): Article 32; Ashley South, Malin Perhult, and Nils Carstensen, "Conflict and Survival: Self-Protection in South-East Myanmar," Asia Programme Paper: ASP PP 2010/04 (London: Chatham House, 2010), https://www.local2global.info/wp-content/uploads/Executive-Summary-Conflict-and-Survival-Self-Protection-in-South-East-Burma.pdf.

89. Karen Human Rights Group, *Self-Protection Under Strain: Targeting of Civilians and Local Responses in Northern Karen State* (Karen Human Rights Group, 2010), https://khrg.org/2010/08/self-protection-under-strain-targeting-civilians-and-local-responses-northern-karen-state.

90. Back Pack Health Worker Team, *Provision of Primary Healthcare*, 4.

91. Lieber Code: Adjutant General's Office, General Orders No. 100: Instructions for the Government of Armies of the United States in the Field (1863), article 23, emphasis added, https://avalon.law.yale.edu/19th_century/lieber.asp.

92. Lieber Code, article 24.

93. Decobert, *The Politics of Aid*, 196.

94. Bahrain Independent Commission of Inquiry, *Report of the Bahrain Independent Commission of Inquiry* (Manama, 2011), 214, 216–17.

95. Hugo Slim, *Killing Civilians: Method, Madness, and Morality in War* (New York: Columbia University Press, 2008), ch. 5.

96. Nils Meltzer, *Interpretative Guidance on the Notion of Direct Participation in Hostilities Under International Humanitarian Law* (Geneva: International Committee of the Red Cross, 2009).

97. Protocol Additional to the Geneva Conventions of 12 August 1949, and Relating to the Protection of Victims of International Armed Conflicts (Protocol I) (June 8, 1977), article 13, https://ihl-databases.icrc.org/ihl/INTRO/470.

98. Sophie Roborgh, "Beyond Medical Humanitarianism: Politics and Humanitarianism in the Figure of the *Midāni* Physicians," *Social Science and Medicine* 211 (2018): 321.

99. Egyptian Initiative for Personal Rights, "Field Doctors Bear Witness to the Targeting of Field Hospitals in Tahrir Square by Security Forces and Military," http://eipr.org/node/1314; S. F. Hamdy and S. Bayoumi, "Egypt's Popular Uprising and the Stakes of Medical Neutrality," *Culture, Medicine, and Psychiatry* 40, no. 2 (2015): 223–41.

100. Roborgh, "Beyond Medical Humanitarianism."

101. Rohini Haar, *Intimidation and Persecution: Sudan's Attacks on Peaceful Protestors and Physicians* (New York: Physicians for Human Rights, 2019).

102. Adrienne Fricke, *"Chaos and Fire": An Analysis of Sudan's June 3, Khartoum Massacre* (New York: Physicians for Human Rights, 2020), https://phr.org/our-work/resources /chaos-and-fire-an-analysis-of-sudans-june-3-2019-khartoum-massacre/.

103. "Statement on Sudan by the WHO Regional Director for the Eastern Mediterranean," World Health Organization, June 7, 2019, reliefweb.int/report/sudan/statement -sudan-who-regional-director-eastern-mediterranean-dr-ahmed-al-mandhari -enar.

104. Jonathan Pedneault, "Police Targeting Street Medics at U.S. Protests," press release, Human Rights Watch, June 17, 2020, https://www.hrw.org/news/2020/06/17/police -targeting-street-medics-us-protests; Kathryn Hampton, Michele Heisler, and Donna McKay, *"Now They Seem to Just Want to Hurt Us": Dangerous Use of Crowd-Control Weapons Against Protestors and Medics in Portland, Oregon* (New York: Physicians for Human Rights, 2020), https://phr.org/our-work/resources/now-they-just-seem-to-want-to-hurt -us-portland-oregon/.

## 3. COUNTERTERRORISM

1. Vincent Iacopino, Michelle Heisler, and Robert J. Rosoff, *Torture in Turkey and Its Unwilling Accomplices: The Scope of State Persecution and the Coercion of Physicians* (Boston: Physicians for Human Rights, 1996).

2. Vincent Iacopino, Michelle Heisler, S. Pishevar, and Robert H. Kirschner, "Physician Complicity in Misrepresentation and Omission of Evidence of Torture in Post-Detention Medical Examinations in Turkey," *Journal of the American Medical Association* 276, no. 5 (1996): 396; Iacopino et al., *Torture in Turkey*.

3. Government of Turkey, Law on Fight Against Terrorism of Turkey, Act no. 3713 (1991, as amended through 2010), https://www.ilo.org/dyn/natlex/natlex4.detail?p_lang =en&p_isn=22104&p_country=TUR&p_count=801&p_classification=01.04&p_class count=30.

4. Amnesty International, *Healing the Healers*, AI Index: ACT 75/02/00 (London: Amnesty International, 2000), https://www.amnesty.org/download/Documents/132000 /act750022000en.pdf.

5. Amnesty International, *Medical Letter Writing Action, Prosecution of Doctors, Dr. H. Zeki Uzun, Turkey*, AI Index EUR 44/24/00 (2000), https://www.amnesty.org/en/documents /EUR44/024/2000/en/.

6. International Helsinki Federation for Human Rights, *Annual Report on Human Rights* (2000), 373, https://www.refworld.org/publisher,IHF,ANNUALREPORT,T UR,469241c90,0.html.

7. Amnesty International, *Medical Letter Writing Action*.

8. Council of Europe, European Commission for Democracy Through Law, *Penal Code of Turkey* (2016), Section 220, https://www.legislationline.org/download/id/6453/file /Turkey_CC_2004_am2016_en.pdf.

9. Ola Claësson, "Doctors Urged to Condemn Turkey's Emergency Care Law," *Lancet* 383, no. 9921 (2014): P941.

10. Christine Mehta and Önder Özkalipci, *Southeastern Turkey: Health Care Under Siege* (New York: Physicians for Human Rights, 2016), 19, https://s3.amazonaws.com/PHR _Reports/southeastern-turkey-health-care-under-siege.pdf.

11. Vincent Iacopino, Vivian Nathanson, Otmar Kloiber, and Julian Sheather et al., "Call for the Turkish Government to Respect Medical Workers' Duty to Provide Medical Care to Those in Need," *British Medical Journal* 347 (2014): f7472.

12. Office of the High Commissioner for Human Rights, "Need for Transparency, Investigations, in Light of 'Alarming' Reports of Major Violations in South-East Turkey— Zeid," press release, May 10, 2016, https://www.ohchr.org/SP/NewsEvents/Pages /DisplayNews.aspx?NewsID=19937&LangID=E.

13. Human Rights Watch, "Turkey: Mounting Security Operations Deaths," press release, December 22, 2015, https://www.hrw.org/news/2015/12/22/turkey-mounting-security -operation-deaths.

14. Mehta and Özkalipci, *Southeastern Turkey*.

15. Mehta and Özkalipci, *Southeastern Turkey*.

16. Christina Mehta, "A Doctor's Trial in a Turkish Border Town," *New York Times*, May 29, 2017, https://www.nytimes.com/2017/05/29/opinion/a-doctors-trial-in-a-turkish-border -town.html.

17. Stockholm Center for Freedom, *Turkey Cracks Down on Health Care Professionals* (Stockholm: Stockholm Center for Freedom, 2007), https://stockholmcf.org/wp -content/uploads/2017/12/Turkey-Cracks-Down-On-Health-Care-Professionals _report_06.12.2017.pdf.

18. Marine Buissonnière, Sarah Woznick, and Leonard Rubenstein, *The Criminalization of Health Care* (Essex: University of Essex, Center for Public Health and Human Rights at the Johns Hopkins Bloomberg School of Public Health, Safeguarding Health in Conflict Coalition, 2018), Appendix, Country Profiles, https://www1.essex.ac.uk/hrc /documents/criminalization-of-healthcare-country-profiles-v2.pdf.

19. Tansu Pişkin, "Şebnem Korur Fincancı, Gençay Gürsoy acquitted," *Bianet*, July 20, 2020, http://bianet.org/english/freedom-of-expression/227010-sebnem-korur-Fincancı -gencay-gursoy-acquitted.

20. UN General Assembly, "Situation of the Human Rights in Kosovo," A/RES/49/204 (1994), https://www.un.org/documents/ga/res/49/a49r204.htm.

21. Leonard Rubenstein, Jennifer Leaning, Luan Jaha, Doug Ford, Laurie Vollen, and Allison Cohen, *Perilous Medicine: The Legacy of Oppression and Conflict in Kosovo* (Cambridge, MA: Physicians for Human Rights, 2009), 24n40, https://s3.amazonaws.com /PHR_Reports/perilous-medicineKosovo-legacy.pdf.

22. Rubenstein et al., *Perilous Medicine* (2009), 25.

23. Rubenstein et al., *Perilous Medicine* (2009), 22.

24. Vincent Iacopino et al., *War Crimes in Kosovo: A Population-Based Assessment of Human Rights Violations Against Kosovar Albanians* (Boston: Physicians for Human Rights, 1999), https://phr.org/wp-content/uploads/1999/08/kosovo-war-crimes-1999.pdf.

25. Rubenstein et al., *Perilous Medicine* (2009), 24.

26. Iacopino et al., *War Crimes in Kosovo*, 105–10.

27. Rubenstein et al., *Perilous Medicine* (2009), 32.

28. Iacopino et al., *War Crimes in Kosovo*, 99–100.

29. Iacopino et al., *War Crimes in Kosovo*, 98, 103–7.

30. British Medical Association, *The Medical Profession and Human Rights: Handbook for a Changing Agenda* (London: Zed, 2001), 242.

31. Rubenstein et al., *Perilous Medicine* (2009), 39.

32. Rubenstein et al., *Perilous Medicine* (2009), 41.

33. Rubenstein et al., *Perilous Medicine* (2009), 40.

34. D. Bloom, I. Hoxha, D. Sambunjak, and E. Sondorp, "Ethnic Segregation in Kosovo's Post-War Health Care System," *European Journal of Public Health* 17, no. 5 (October 2007): 430–36.

35. U.S. Department of State, "Serbia-Montenegro Report on Human Rights Practices for 1998," https://1997-2001.state.gov/global/human_rights/1998_hrp_report/serbiamo.html; U.S. Department of State, "Serbia-Montenegro Report on Human Rights Practices for 1999," U.S. Department of State Country Reports Human Rights Practices for 1999, Serbia Montenegro, https://1997-2001.state.gov/global/human_rights/1999_hrp_report/serbiamo .html; U.S. Department of State Country Reports Human Rights Practices for 1995—Turkey, https://1997-2001.state.gov/global/human_rights/1996_hrp_report/turkey.html.

36. Laxmi Vilas Ghimire and Matiram Pun, "Health Effects of Maoist Insurgency in Nepal," *Lancet* 368, no. 9546 (2006): 1494.

37. U.S. Department of Justice, Executive Office of Immigration Review, Board of Immigration Appeals, in re: BT, File A098 415 637 (2008), unpublished.

38. Buissonnière et al., *Criminalization*, Appendix, 41.

39. Human Rights First, *Denial and Delay: The Impact of the Immigration Law's "Terrorism Bars" on Asylum Seekers and Refugees in the United States* (New York: Human Rights First, 2008), 20, https://www.humanrightsfirst.org/resource/denial-and-delay-report.

40. UN Security Council Resolution 1373, S/Res/1373 (2001), https://www.unodc.org/pdf /crime/terrorism/res_1373_english.pdf.

41. Alice Debarre, *Safeguarding Medical Care and Humanitarian Action in the UN Counterterrorism Framework* (New York: International Peace Institute, 2018), https://www .ipinst.org/wp-content/uploads/2018/09/1809_Safeguarding-Medical-Care.pdf.

42. Debarre, *Safeguarding Medical Care*; Emanuela-Chiara Gillard, *Recommendations for Reducing Tensions in the Interplay Between Sanctions, Counterterrorism Measures, and Humanitarian Action* (London: Chatham House, 2017), https://www.chathamhouse.org /publication/recommendations-reducing-tensions-interplay-between-sanctions -counterterrorism-measures.

43. Dustin A. Lewis, Naz K. Modirzadeh, and Gabriella Blum, *Medical Care in Armed Conflict: International Humanitarian Law and State Responses to Terrorism* (Harvard Law School Program on International Law and Armed Conflict, 2015), http://ssrn.com /abstract=2657036.

44. Elena Pokalova, "Legislative Responses to Terrorism: What Drives States to Adopt New Counterterrorism Legislation?" *Terrorism and Political Violence* 27, no. 3 (2015): 474, 477.

45. Buissonnière et al., *Criminalization*, Appendix, Country Profiles, https://www1.essex .ac.uk/hrc/documents/criminalization-of-healthcare-country-profiles-v2.pdf.

46. Buissonnière et al., *Criminalization*, Appendix, 40.

47. Buissonnière et al., *Criminalization*, Appendix, 5.

48. Holder v. Humanitarian Law Project, 561 U.S. 1 (2010).

49. Buissonnière et al., *Criminalization*.

50. Safeguarding Health in Conflict Coalition, *Violence on the Front Line: Attacks on Health Care in 2017* (2018), https://www.safeguardinghealth.org/sites/shcc/files /SHCC2018final.pdf.

51. Human Rights Watch, "Iraq: Displacement, Detention of Suspected 'ISIS Families,'" March 5, 2017, https://www.hrw.org/news/2017/03/05/iraq-displacement-detention -suspected-isis-families.

52. Shah v. United States, 474 F. Supp. 2d 492, 493 (S.D.N.Y. 2007), affirmed *United States v. Farhane*, 634 F.3d 127, 132 (2d Cir. 2011).

53. Lewis, Modirzadeh, and Blum, *Medical Care in Armed Conflict*, 129n123.

54. Victor de Currea-Lugo, "Protecting the Health Sector in Colombia: A Step to Make the Health Sector Less Cruel," *International Review of the Red Cross* 83, no. 844 (2001); ICRC, "Colombia: Poor Access to Health Care and Violations Against Medical Personnel and Services," October 10, 2013, https://www.icrc.org/en/doc/resources/documents /feature/2013/07-10-colombia-report-health-hcid.htm.

55. Ekaterina Ortiz Linares and Marisela Silva Chau, "Reflections on the Colombian Case Law on the Protection of Medical Personnel Against Punishment," *International Review of the Red Cross* 95, no. 980 (2013): 251, citing Supreme Court of Justice of Colombia, Criminal Cassation Chamber, Case No. 27227 of May 21, 2009.

56. "Doctors Working for FARC: Medical Mix-Up?," *Semana*, February 13, 2009, http:// www.semana.com/international/print-edition/articulo/doctors-working-for-farc -medical-mix-up/100099-3.

57. Buissonnière et al., *Criminalization*.

58. Naz Modirzadeh, Statement at International Peace Institute, "Safeguarding the Space for Principled Humanitarian Action in Counterterrorism," May 23, 2018, online video, https://www.ipinst.org/2018/05/poc-counterterrorism-contexts#2.

59. Naz Modirzadeh, "International Law and Armed Conflict in Dark Times: A Call for Engagement," *International Review of the Red Cross* 96, no. 895/896 (2014): 737; Naz Modirzadeh, Statement at International Peace Institute.

60. Center for Protection of Civilians in Conflict, "Counter-Terrorism Is Devouring International Law," Interview with UN Special Rapporteur, 2018, https://www.civicus.org

/index.php/media-resources/news/interviews/3657-un-special-rapporteur-counter
-terrorism-is-devouring-international-law.

61. Alberto J. Gonzales, "Memorandum to the President," Subject: Decisions re Application of the Geneva Convention on Prisoners of War to the Conflict with Al Qaeda and the Taliban, January 25, 2002, https://nsarchive2.gwu.edu//NSAEBB/NSAEBB127/02.01.25.pdf.

62. CIA, "Office of Medical Services Guidelines on Medical and Psychological Support for Detainee Rendition, Interrogation, and Rendition (2004)," https://www.cia.gov/library/readingroom/docs/0006541536.pdf.

63. Steven Miles, *Oath Betrayed: America's Torture Doctors*, 2nd ed. (Berkeley: University of California Press, 2009); U.S. Senate, Select Committee on Intelligence, *Report of the Senate Select Committee on Intelligence Committee Study of the Central Intelligence Agency's Detention and Interrogation Program* (2014), https://www.intelligence.senate.gov/sites/default/files/publications/CRPT-113srpt288.pdf; Institute on Medicine as a Profession, Columbia University, *Ethics Abandoned: Medical Professionalism and Detainee Abuse in the War on Terrorism* (New York: Institute on Medicine as a Profession, 2013), http://hrp.law.harvard.edu/wp-content/uploads/2013/11/IMAP-EthicsTextFinal2.pdf; Leonard Rubenstein, "From Complicity to Impunity: Medical Participation and the Definition of Torture at the Central Intelligence Agency," in *Torture and Its Definition in International Law*, ed. Metin Basoglu (Oxford: Oxford University Press, 2017).

64. Zackery Berger, Leonard Rubenstein, and Matthew DeCamp, "Clinical Care and Complicity with Torture," *British Medical Journal* 360 (2018): k449.

65. ICRC, personal communication.

66. Debarre, *Safeguarding Medical Care*; Norwegian Refugee Council, *Principles Under Pressure: The Impact of Counterterrorism Measures and Preventing/Countering Violent Extremism On Principled Humanitarian Action* (Norwegian Refugee Council, 2018), https://www.nrc.no/globalassets/pdf/reports/principles-under-pressure/nrc-principles_under_pressure-report-2018-screen.pdf; Ashley Jackson and Steven A. Zyck, *Presence and Proximity: To Deliver Five Years On* (UN OCHA, Norwegian Refugee Council, and Jindal School of International Affairs, 2017), https://www.unocha.org/sites/unocha/files/Presence%20and%20Proximity.pdf.

67. Yves Daccord, Statement at International Peace Institute, "Safeguarding the Space for Principled Humanitarian Action in Counterterrorism," May 23, 2018, online video, https://www.ipinst.org/2018/05/poc-counterterrorism-contexts#2.

68. Norwegian Refugee Council, *Principles Under Pressure*, 23. Mark Bradbury, *State-Building, Counterterrorism, and Licensing Humanitarianism in Somalia* (Medford, MA: Feinstein International Center, Tufts University, 2010), https://fic.tufts.edu/wp-content/uploads/state-building-somalia.pdf.

69. Norwegian Refugee Council, *Principles Under Pressure*, 23.

70. Norwegian Refugee Council, *Principles Under Pressure*.

71. Laura Hammond and Hanna Vaughan-Lee, *Humanitarian Space in Somalia: A Scarce Commodity*, HPG Working Paper (London: Overseas Development Institute, 2012), 15,

http://www.odi.org.uk/publications/6430-humanitarian-space-somalia-aid-workers
-principles.

72. Kate Mackintosh and Patrick Duplat, *Study of the Impact of Donor Counter-Terrorism Measures on Principled Humanitarian Action* (UN Office for the Coordination of Humanitarian Action and Norwegian Refugee Council, 2013), 82, https://www.unocha.org/sites/unocha/files/CounterTerrorism_Study_Full_Report.pdf.

73. Mackintosh and Duplat, *Study of the Impact*, 103.

74. Muhammad Bello, "MSF Fingered in 'Secret Backing' of Boko Haram," *Leadership Newspaper*, May 19, 2017, https://leadership.ng/2017/05/19/msf-fingered-secret-backing-boko-haram/.

75. Stephanie Busari, "UNICEF: Boko Haram Has Kidnapped More Than 1,000 Children in Nigeria," *CNN*, April 13, 2018, https://www.cnn.com/2018/04/13/africa/boko-haram-children-abduction-intl/index.html; Joel R. Charny, "Counter-Terrorism and Humanitarian Action: The Perils of Zero Tolerance," *War on the Rocks* (blog), March 20, 2019, https://warontherocks.com/2019/03/counter-terrorism-and-humanitarian-action-the-perils-of-zero-tolerance/.

76. Ben Parker, "UK Keeps Limits on Cash Aid Over Counter-Terrorism Fears," *New Humanitarian*, May 16, 2019, https://www.thenewhumanitarian.org/news/2019/05/16/uk-keeps-limits-cash-aid-syria-over-counter-terror-fears.

77. Obi Anyadike, "Aid Workers Question USAID Counter-Terrorism Clause in Nigeria," *New Humanitarian*, November 3, 2019, https://www.thenewhumanitarian.org/news-feature/2019/11/05/USAID-counter-terror-Nigeria-Boko-Haram.

78. Leonard Rubenstein, "Global health and Security in the Age of Counterterrorism," *Journal of the Royal Society of Medicine* 108, no 2 (2015): 49–52.

79. Mark Mazzetti, *The Way of the Knife* (New York: Penguin, 2013), 282.

80. Alexander Mullaney and Syeda Amna Hassan, "He Led the CIA to bin Laden—and Unwittingly Fueled a Vaccine Backlash," *National Geographic*, February 27, 2015, https://www.nationalgeographic.com/news/2015/02/150227-polio-pakistan-vaccination-taliban-osama-bin-laden/.

81. Mazzetti, *The Way of the Knife*, 283.

82. "Pakistani Doctor Jailed for Helping Find bin Laden Faces More Trouble, Moved to Higher-Security Prison," *Fox News.com*, April 28, 2018, https://www.foxnews.com/world/pakistani-doctor-jailed-for-helping-find-bin-laden-faces-more-trouble-moved-to-higher-security-prison.

83. Monica Martinez-Bravo and Andreas Stegmann, *In Vaccines We Trust? The Effects of the CIA's Vaccine Ruse on Immunization in Pakistan* (CEMFI, 2020), https://www.cemfi.es/~martinez bravo/mmb/Research_files/MS_Vaccines_20200814.pdf.

84. Arsla Jawaid, "Pakistan's Army and Lady Health Workers Are at the Center of the Global Effort to Eradicate Polio. How Successful Have They Been?" *Foreign Policy*, October 22, 2015, http://foreignpolicy.com/2015/10/22/the-polio-capital-of-the-world/.

85. Jonathan Kennedy, "How Drone Strikes and a Fake Vaccination Campaign Have Inhibited Polio Eradication: An Analysis of National-Level Data," *International Journal of Global Health* 47, no. 4 (2017): 807.

86. Letter from Lisa Monaco, Assistant to the President for Homeland Security and Counterterrorism, to Deans of Public Health, May 16, 2014, https://www.jhsph.edu/news/news-releases/2014/White%20House%20Letter%20on%20Vaccine%20Workers.pdf.

87. La Cruz-Flores v. Peru, Merits, Reparations, and Costs, Judgment, Inter-Am. Ct. H.R. (ser. C) No. 115, para. 57(c) (2004).

88. Gillard, *Recommendations for Reducing Tensions.*

89. Debarre, *Safeguarding Medical Care.*

90. Debarre, *Safeguarding Medical Care.*

91. Buissonnière et al., *Criminalization.*

92. UN General Assembly, Resolution on Terrorism and Human Rights, A/Res/73/174 (2019), https://documents-dds-ny.un.org/doc/UNDOC/GEN/N18/449/62/PDF/N1844962.pdf ?OpenElement.

93. United States Mission to the United Nations, "Explanation of Position at a Third Committee Plenary Meeting on Human Rights and Terrorism," December 17, 2018, https://usun.usmission.gov/explanation-of-position-at-a-third-committee-plenary-meeting-on-human-rights-and-terrorism/.

94. Security Council Report, "Combatting Financing of Terrorism Open Debate," What's in Blue, Security Council Report, May 27, 2019, https://www.securitycouncilreport.org/whatsinblue/2019/03/combatting-financing-of-terrorism-open-debate.php.

95. UN Security Council Resolution 2462, S/Res/2462 (2019), http://undocs.org/en/S/RES/2462(2019).

96. UN Security Council, Statement by the President of the Council, S/PRST/2021/1 (2021), https://www.securitycouncilreport.org/atf/cf/%7B65BFCF9B-6D27-4E9C-8CD3-CF6E4FF96FF9%7D/s_prst_2021_1.pdf.

# 4. HEALTH CARE AS A STRATEGIC TARGET

1. Julie Cliff and Razak Noormahomed, "Health as a Target: South Africa's Destabilization of Mozambique," *Social Science and Medicine* 27, no. 7 (1988): 717–22.

2. Paul Brentlinger, "Health Sector Response to Security Threats During the Civil War in El Salvador," *British Medical Journal* 313, no. 7070 (1996): 1470.

3. Xavier Crombé and Joanna Kuper, "War Breaks Out: Interpreting Violence on Healthcare in the Early Stage of the South Sudanese Civil War," *Journal of Humanitarian Affairs* 1, no. 2 (2019): 4–12.

4. Leonard Rubenstein, Kathleen Fallon, Dr. Zaher Sahloul, and Hazem Rihawi et al., *Syrian Medical Voices from the Ground: The Ordeal of Syria's Healthcare Professionals* (Baltimore: Center for Public Health and Human Rights, Johns Hopkins Bloomberg School of Public Health, and Washington, DC: Syrian American Medical Society, 2015),

https://www.sams-usa.net/wp-content/uploads/2016/09/Syrian-Medical-Voices-from
-the-Ground_F.pdf.

5. Robert Worth, *A Rage for Order: The Middle East in Turmoil from Tahrir Square to ISIS* (New York: Farrar, Straus and Giroux 2016); Hugo Slim and Lorenzo Trombetta, *Syria Common Context Analysis* (IASC Inter-Agency Humanitarian Evaluations Steering Group as part of the Syria Coordinated Accountability and Lessons Learning Initiative, 2014), https://interagencystandingcommittee.org/system/files/syria_crisis_common_context_analysis_june_2014.pdf.

6. Sam Dagher, *Assad or We Burn the Country: How One Family's Lust for Power Destroyed Syria* (New York: Little Brown, 2019).

7. "UN Human Rights Chief Urges Immediate Action on Syria as Death Toll Passes 3000," *UN News*, October 14, 2011, https://news.un.org/en/story/2011/10/391512-un-human-rights-chief-urges-immediate-action-syria-death-toll-passes-3000.

8. "As Syrian Death Toll Tops 5,000, UN Human Rights Chief Warns about Key City," *UN News*, December 11, 2011, https://news.un.org/en/story/2011/12/398082-syrian-death-toll-tops-5000-un-human-rights-chief-warns-about-key-city.

9. UN Human Rights Council, *Assault on Medical Care in Syria*, Independent International Commission of Inquiry on the Syrian Arab Republic, Conference Room Paper, A/HRC/24/CRP.2 (2013), https://www.ohchr.org/EN/HRBodies/HRC/RegularSessions/Session24/Documents/A-HRC-24-CRP-2.doc.

10. UN Human Rights Council, *Report of the Independent International Commission of Inquiry on the Syrian Arab Republic*, A/HRC/S-17/2/Add. (2011), https://documents-dds-ny.un.org/doc/UNDOC/GEN/G11/170/97/PDF/G1117097.pdf?OpenElement; Amnesty International, *Health Crisis: Syrian Governments Targets the Wounded and Health Workers* (London: Amnesty International, 2011), https://www.amnesty.org/download/Documents/32000/mde2405920011en.pdf.

11. MSF, "Syria: Medicine as a Weapon of Persecution," *MSF Press Dossier*, February 8, 2012, https://msf.lu/sites/default/files/in-syria-medicine-as-a-weapon-of-persecution.pdf; Amnesty International, *Health Crisis*; Abdulrazzaq Al-Saiedi and Richard Sollom, *Syria: Attacks on Doctors, Patients and Hospitals* (Boston: Physicians for Human Rights, 2011), https://phr.org/wp-content/uploads/2011/12/syria-attacks-on-drs-patients-hospitals-final-2011-1.pdf.

12. UN Human Rights Council, *Assault on Medical Care*.

13. UN Human Rights Council, *Assault on Medical Care*.

14. Slim and Trombetta, *Syria Common Context Analysis*.

15. UN Human Rights Council, *Assault on Medical Care*.

16. Violations Documentation Center in Syria, *Special Report on Counter-Terrorism Law no. 19 and the Counter-Terrorism Court in Syria* (2015), http://www.vdc-sy.info/pdf/reports/1430186775-English.pdf.

17. Amnesty International, "Urgent Action, Syrian Protest Detainees at Risk," March 23, 2011, https://www.amnesty.org/download/Documents/32000/mde2401320011en.pdf; International Federation of Human Rights, "Assault and Arrest of Dozens of Family

Members of Human Rights Defenders and Prisoners of Conscience," March 16, 2011, http://www.pacificfreepress.com/2011/03/26/opinion/an-urgent-crisis-now-political -prisoners-in-syria.html.

18. Carola C. Schubert and Raija-Leena Punamäki, "Torture and PTSD: Prevalence, Sequelae, Protective Factors, and Therapy," in *Comprehensive Guide to Post-Traumatic Stress Disorder*, ed. Colin Martin, Victor Preedy, and Vinood Patel (New York: Springer, 2015).

19. Rubenstein et al., *Syrian Medical Voices from the Ground*. The findings of the interviews, along with those conducted in the latter chemical attack were later published in a journal. Katherine H. A. Footer, Emily Clouse, Diana Rayes, Zaher Sahloul, and Leonard S. Rubenstein, "Qualitative Accounts from Syrian Health Professionals Regarding Violations of the Right to Health, Including the Use of Chemical Weapons, in Opposition Held Syria," *BMJ Open* 8 (2018): e021096.

20. UN Human Rights Council, *Assault on Medical Care*; Abdulrazzaq Al-Saiedi and Richard Sollom, *Syria: Attacks on Doctors, Patients and Hospitals* (Cambridge, MA: Physicians for Human Rights, 2011), https://phr.org/wp-content/uploads/2011/12/syria -attacks-on-drs-patients-hospitals-final-2011-1.pdf.

21. Physicians for Human Rights, "Map of Attacks on Hospitals in Syria," http://syriamap .phr.org/#/en/attacks/1; "Syria: Hama Hospitals 'Closed After Army Attacks,'" *BBC News*, August 1, 2011, https://www.bbc.com/news/world-middle-east-14519969.

22. UN Human Rights Council, *Assault on Medical Care in Syria*.

23. WHO, Syrian Arab Republic, *Revised Syrian Humanitarian Assistance Response Plan, Jan.–Dec. 2013*, https://www.who.int/hac/Revision_2013_Syria_HARP.pdf.

24. UN Human Rights Council, *Assault on Medical Care in Syria*.

25. Physicians for Human Rights, *Syria's Medical Community Under Assault* (New York: Physicians for Human Rights, 2014), https://s3.amazonaws.com/PHR_other/Syria%27s -Medical-Community-Under-Assault-October-2014.pdf.

26. World Health Organization, *Snapshots on MoH Public Hospitals, 2nd quarter 2014*, http://www.emro.who.int/images/stories/syria/documents/Snapshot_MoH_Public _Hospitals_2ndQ_190814.pdf?ua=1.

27. Debarati Guha-Sapir, Benjamin Schlüter, Jose Manuel Rodriguez-Llanes, Louis Lillywhite, and Madelyn Hsiao-Rei Hicks, "Patterns of Civilian and Child Deaths Due to War-Related Violence in Syria: A Comparative Analysis from the Violation Documentation Center Dataset, 2011–16," *Lancet Global Health* 6, no. 1 (2018): e103.

28. Zaher Sahloul, Adam Coutts, Fouad M. Fouad, Sawsan Jabri, Rola Hallam, Fuad Azrak, and Wasim Maziak, "Health Response System in Syria: Beyond the Official Narrative," *Lancet* 383, no. 9915 (2014): P407; Annie Sparrow, "Syria's Polio Epidemic: The Suppressed Truth," *New York Review of Books*, February 20, 2014, https://www .nybooks.com/articles/2014/02/20/syrias-polio-epidemic-suppressed-truth/.

29. UN Office of Coordination of Humanitarian Affairs, *2015 Humanitarian Overview, Syrian Arab Republic*, November 2014, https://www.documentcloud.org/documents /2774832-2015-Humanitarian-Needs-Overview.html.

30. World Health Organization, *The Syrian Arab Republic Fact Sheet*, March 2014, https://www.who.int/hac/crises/syr/sitreps/syria_country_fact_sheet_13march2014_final.pdf.

31. Jonathan Kennedy and Domna Michailidou, "Civil War, Contested Sovereignty, and the Limits of Global Health Partnerships: A Case Study of the Syrian Polio Outbreak of 2013," *Health Policy and Planning* 32, no. 5 (2017): 690; Assistance Coordination Unit, "Conclusion of the Eight Vaccination Campaigns Against Poliomyelitis with a 99% Coverage Rate and a Lack of Medical Errors in All Governates," 2015, https://www.acu-sy.org/en/conclusion-of-the-eighth-vaccination-campaign-against-poliomyelitis-with-a-99-coverage-rate-and-a-lack-of-medical-errors-in-all-governorates/; Sparrow, "Syria's Polio Epidemic."

32. Abdulkarim Ekzayez, "Analysis: A Model for Rebuilding Infrastructure in Northwestern Syria," *News Deeply*, February 19, 2018, https://www.newsdeeply.com/peacebuilding/articles/2018/02/19/analysis-a-model-for-rebuilding-infrastructure-in-northwestern-syria; Zedoun Alzoubi, Khaled Iyad, Mamoun Othman, Houssam Alnahhas, and Omar Abdulaziz Hallaj, *Reinventing State: Health Governance in Syrian Opposition-Held Areas* (MIDMAR and Friedrich Ebert Stichting, 2019), https://www.fes-syria.org/publications/.

33. Rubenstein et al., *Syrian Medical Voices from the Ground*.

34. James Smith, "Difficult Decision-Making, Compromise, and Moral Distress in Medical Humanitarian Response," in *Humanitarian Action and Ethics*, ed. Ayesha Ahmad and James Smith (London: Zed, 2018); Sofia Nilsson, Misa Sjöberg, Kjell Kallenberg, and Gerry Larsson, "Moral Stress in International Humanitarian Aid and Rescue Operations: A Grounded Theory Study," *Ethics and Behavior* 21, no. 1 (2011): 49; Center for Public Health and Human Rights et al., *Reality Makes Our Decisions: Ethical Challenges in Humanitarian Health in Situations of Extreme Violence* (Center for Public Health and Human Rights and Center for Humanitarian Health, Johns Hopkins Bloomberg School of Public Health, Syrian American Medical Society, International Rescue Committee, 2019), http://hopkinshumanitarianhealth.org/assets/documents/LR_XViolenceReport_2019_final.pdf.

35. Rubenstein et al., *Syrian Medical Voices from the Ground*.

36. Human Rights Watch, "Barrage of Barrel Bombs," news release, July 30, 2014, https://www.hrw.org/news/2014/07/30/syria-barrage-barrel-bombs.

37. Guha-Sapir et al., "Patterns of Civilian and Child Deaths."

38. Footer et al., "Qualitative Accounts."

39. Aleppo City Medical Council, *Third Annual Report*, March 2014, https://www.slideshare.net/FadiHakim2/acmc-3rd-medical-report-50048760.

40. Rubenstein et al., *Syrian Medical Voices from the Ground*.

41. Rubenstein et al., *Syrian Medical Voices from the Ground*.

42. Footer et al., "Qualitative Accounts."

43. MSF, "Review of Attack on Al Quds hospital in Aleppo City," 2016, https://www.msf.org/sites/msf.org/files/al_quds_report.pdf; Center for Public Health et al., *Reality Makes Our Decisions*.

44. David Nott, *War Doctor: Surgery on the Front Line* (London: Picador, 2019), 304–10.

45. Center for Public Health et al., *Reality Makes Our Decisions*.

46. Center for Public Health et al., *Reality Makes Our Decisions*; Cindy Sousa and Amy Hagopian, "Conflict, Health Care, and Professional Perseverance: A Qualitative Study in the West Bank," *Global Public Health* 6, no. 5 (2011): 520–33.

47. Justine Namakula and Sophie Witter, "Living Through Conflict and Post-Conflict: Experiences of Health Workers in Northern Uganda and Lessons for People-Centred Health Systems," *Health Policy and Planning* 29, Supp. 2 (2014): ii-6–ii14.

48. UN Human Rights Council, *Assault on Medical Care*.

49. Guha-Sapir et al., "Patterns of Civilian and Child Deaths."

50. Atlantic Council, *Breaking Aleppo, Hospital Attacks* (Washington, DC: Atlantic Council 2017), http://www.publications.at/lanticcouncil.org/br'eakingaleppo/hospital-attacks/.

51. C. Hayes Wong and Christine Yen-Ting Chen, "Ambulances Under Siege in Syria," *BMJ Global Health* 3, no. 6 (2018): e001003, https://gh.bmj.com/content/3/6/e001003.

52. Abdulkarim Ekzayez and Ammar Sabouni, "Targeting Healthcare in Syria: Military Tactic or Collateral Damage?," *Journal of Humanitarian Affairs* 2, no. 2 (2020): 3–12.

53. Center for Public Health et al., *Reality Makes Our Decisions*.

54. Wong and Chen, "Ambulances Under Siege."

55. Syrian American Medical Society, *Saving Lives Underground: The Case for Underground Hospitals in Syria* (Washington, DC: Syrian American Medical Society, 2017), https://www.sams-usa.net/wp-content/uploads/2017/05/Saving-Lives-Underground -report.pdf.

56. Syrian American Medical Society, *Saving Lives Underground*.

57. Letter dated October 26, 2017 from the Secretary-General Addressed to the President of the Security Council, 7th Report of Organisation for the Prohibition of Chemical Weapons-United Nations Joint Investigative Mechanism (see annex), S/2017/904 (2017), https://www.securitycouncilreport.org/atf/cf/%7B65BFCF9B-6D27-4E9C-8CD3 -CF6E4FF96FF9%7D/s_2017_904.pdf.

58. Chaza Akik, Aline Semaan, Linda Shaker-Berbari, Zeina Jamaluddine, Ghada E. Saad, Katherine Lopes, Joanne Constantin, Abuldkarim Ekzyayez, Neha S. Singh, Karl Blanchet, Jocelyn DeJong, and Hala Ghattas, "Responding to Health Needs of Women, Children and Adolescents Within Syria During Conflict: Intervention Coverage, Challenges and Adaptations," *Conflict and Health* 14 (2020): Article no. 37.

59. Rubenstein et al., *Medical Voices from the Ground*.

60. Center for Public Health et al., *Reality Makes Our Decisions*.

61. Center for Public Health et al., *Reality Makes Our Decisions*.

62. Footer et al., "Qualitative Accounts."

63. Footer et al., "Qualitative Accounts."

64. Reinoud Leenders and Kholoud Mansour, "Humanitarianism, State Sovereignty, and Authoritarian Regime Maintenance in the Syrian War," *Political Science Quarterly* 133, no. 3 (2018): 225; Annie Sparrow, "How UN Humanitarian Aid Has Propped up Assad," *Foreign Affairs*, September 20, 2018, https://www.foreignaffairs.com/articles/syria/2018 -09-20/how-un-humanitarian-aid-has-propped-assad.

65. Letter from Dr. Imad al-Kabbani to Dr. Tedros Adhanom Ghebreyesus, Director General, World Health Organization, December 15, 2017, https://www.hrw.org/sites/default/files/supporting_resources/syria_eastern_ghouta_doctors.pdf.

66. Amnesty International, "Syria: 'Flagrant War Crimes' Being Committed in Eastern Ghouta," February 21, 2018, https://www.amnesty.org.uk/press-releases/syria-flagrant-war-crimes-being-committed-eastern-ghouta.

67. Syrian American Medical Society, "Thirteen Targeted Attacks on Hospitals in East Ghouta in 48 Hours: Medics Describe the Situation as 'Catastrophic,'" press release, February 20, 2018, https://www.sams-usa.net/press_release/thirteen-targeted-attacks-hospitals-east-ghouta-48-hours-medics-describe-situation-catastrophic/.

68. United Nations Human Rights Council, "The Siege and Recapture of Eastern Ghouta," conference room paper of the Independent International Commission of Inquiry on the Syrian Arab Republic, June 20, 2018, https://www.ohchr.org/EN/HRBodies/HRC/IICISyria/Pages/IndependentInternationalCommission.aspx.

69. Identical letters dated July 16, 2018 from the Permanent Representative of the Syrian Arab Republic to the United Nations addressed to the Secretary-General and President of the Security Council, S/2019/572 (2019), https://www.securitycouncil-report.org/atf/cf/%7B65BFCF9B-6D27-4E9C-8CD3-CF6E4FF96FF9%7D/s_2019_572.pdf.

70. UN Office of Coordination of Humanitarian Affairs, Under-Secretary-General for Humanitarian Affairs and Emergency Relief Coordinator Mark Lowcock, Briefing to the Security Council on the Humanitarian Situation in Syria, July 31, 2019, https://reliefweb.int/sites/reliefweb.int/files/resources/ERC_USG%20Mark%20Lowcock%20Statement%20to%20the%20SecCo%20on%20Syria-%2031July2019%20-%20as%20delivered.pdf.

71. Leonard Rubenstein and Zaher Sahloul, "In Syria, Doctors Become the Victims," *New York Times*, November 19, 2014, https://www.nytimes.com/2014/11/20/opinion/in-syria-doctors-become-the-victims.html

72. Peter J. Hoffman and Thomas G. Weiss, *Humanitarianism, War, and Politics: Solferino to Syria and Beyond* (Lanham, MD: Rowman & Littlefield, 2017), 156.

73. Hoffman and Weiss, *Humanitarianism, War, and Politics*, 154.

74. Nathalie Weizmann, "Trump's 'Safe Areas' in Syria—An Explainer on International Law," *Just Security*, January 27, 2017, https://www.justsecurity.org/36889/trumps-safe-areas-syria-explainer-international-law/.

75. Rony Brauman, *Humanitarian Wars? Lies and Brainwashing, in Conversation with Régis Meyran* (London: Hurst, 2019).

76. Josh Rogin, "Obama Asks Pentagon for Syria-Fly Zone War Plan," *Daily Beast*, May 28, 2013, https://www.thedailybeast.com/obama-asks-pentagon-for-syria-no-fly-zone-plan.

77. Ben Rhodes, *The World as It Is: A Memoir of the Obama White House* (New York: Penguin Random House, 2018), 235.

78. Rhodes, *The World as It Is*.

79. Susan Rice, "In Syria, the U.S. Had No Good Options," *Atlantic*, October 7, 2019, https://www.theatlantic.com/ideas/archive/2019/10/susan-rice-how-obama-found-least-bad-syria-policy/599296/.

80. Dexter Filkins, "A Russian-Backed Offensive in Syria Makes a Mockery of Trump," *New Yorker*, July 7, 2018, https://www.newyorker.com/news/news-desk/a-russian-backed-offensive-in-syria-makes-a-mockery-of-trump.

81. "Syrian American Medical Society (SAMS) and 11 Humanitarian Organizations Share Hospital Coordinates," April 18, 2018, press release, https://www.sams-usa.net/press_release/sams-11-humanitarian-organizations-share-hospital-coordinates/.

82. UN Secretary-General, "Note to Correspondents: Transcript of Press Stakeout by United Nations Senior Adviser, Jan Egeland," September 20, 2018, https://www.un.org/sg/en/content/sg/note-correspondents/2018-09-20/note-correspondents-transcript-press-stakeout-united.

83. Ben Parker, "What Is Humanitarian Deconfliction?," *New Humanitarian*, November 13, 2018, https://www.irinnews.org/analysis/2018/11/13/what-humanitarian-deconfliction-syria-yemen?utm_source=twitter&utm_medium=irinsocial&utm_campaign=irin updates.

84. Parker, "What Is Humanitarian Deconfliction?"

85. Malachy Browne, Christiaan Triebert, Evan Hill, Whitney Hurst, Gabriel Gianordoli, and Dmitriy Khavin, "Hospitals and Schools Are Being Bombed in Syria: A UN Inquiry Is Limited; We Took a Deeper Look," *New York Times*, December 31, 2019, https://www.nytimes.com/interactive/2019/12/31/world/middleeast/syria-united-nations-investigation.html.

86. Richard Hall and Borzou Daragahi, "Doctors in Idlib Will No Longer Share Coordinates of Hospitals with UN After Repeated Attacks from Russian and Syrian Forces," *Independent*, June 3, 2019, https://www.independent.co.uk/news/world/middle-east/syria-hospital-bombings-idlib-un-doctors-russia-assad-attack-a8942076.html.

87. UN Office of Coordination of Humanitarian Affairs, Briefing to the Security Council.

88. Michelle Bachelet, "Opening Statement by UN High Commissioner Michelle Bachelet," United Nations Office of the High Commissioner for Human Rights Press Conference, September 4, 2019, https://www.ohchr.org/EN/NewsEvents/Pages/DisplayNews.aspx?NewsID=24945&LangID=E.

89. Browne et al., "Hospitals and Schools are being Bombed"; Belkis Wille and Richard Weir, *"Targeting Life in Idlib": Syrian and Russian Strikes on Civilian Infrastructure* (New York: Human Rights Watch, 2020), https://www.hrw.org/sites/default/files/media_2020/10/syria1020_0.pdf; Amnesty International, *"Nowhere Is Safe for Us": Unlawful Attacks and Mass Displacement in North-West Syria* (London: Amnesty International, 2020), https://www.amnesty.org/download/Documents/MDE2420892020ENGLISH.PDF.

90. Wille and Weir, *"Targeting Life in Idlib,"* 49.

91. "Inside Idlib's Bombed-Out Hospitals and Clinics," *New Humanitarian*, January 13, 2020, https://www.thenewhumanitarian.org/photo-feature/2020/1/13/Syria-Idlib-ceasefire-healthcare-hospitals.

92. "Health Cluster Bulletin March 2020," World Health Organization, Health Cluster Hub, https://www.humanitarianresponse.info/sites/www.humanitarianresponse.info/files/documents/files/turkey_health_cluster_bulletin_march_2020.pdf; Amnesty International, *"Nowhere Is Safe for Us."*

93. Mark Lowcock, "Statement on Northwest Syria," UN Undersecretary-General for Humanitarian Affairs and Emergency Relief Coordinator Mark Lowcock, February 17, 2020, https://reliefweb.int/sites/reliefweb.int/files/resources/Statement%20on%20Northwest%20Syria.pdf.

94. "Summary by the Secretary-General of the Report of the United Nations Headquarters Board of Inquiry Into Certain Incidents in Northwest Syria Since 7 September 2018 Involving Facilities on the United Nations Deconfliction List and United Nations Supported Facilities," United Nations, https://www.un.org/sg/sites/www.un.org.sg/files/atoms/files/NWS_BOI_Summary_06_April_2020.pdf.

95. Rice, "In Syria, the U.S. Had No Good Options."

96. UN Human Rights Council, *Report of the Independent International Commission of Inquiry on the Syrian Arab Republic*, A/HRC/44/61, July 2, 2020, https://www.ohchr.org/en/hrbodies/hrc/iicisyria/pages/independentinternationalcommission.aspx.

97. International Rescue Committee, *A Decade of Destruction: Attacks on Health Care in Syria* (New York: International Rescue Committee, 2021), https://www.rescue.org/sites/default/files/document/5648/adecadeofdestructionattacksonhealthcareinsyria.pdf.

## 5. RECKLESSNESS

1. MSF, *Healthcare Under Siege in Taiz* (Amsterdam: MSF, 2017), https://www.msf.org/yemen-healthcare-under-siege-taiz.

2. OCHA Yemen, *Deteriorating Humanitarian Crisis, Situation Report No. 9 (as of 29 May 2015)*, https://reliefweb.int/sites/reliefweb.int/files/resources/OCHA%20Situation%20Report_No.9_EN_final.pdf.

3. Rajat Madhok and Eman Al Sharafi, "In Yemen, Conflict and Poverty Exacerbate Child Malnutrition," UNICEF, January 30, 2017, https://www.unicef.org/stories/yemen-conflict-and-poverty-exacerbate-child-malnutrition.

4. Paul B. Spiegel, Ruwan Ratnayake, Nora Hellman, and Daniele S. Lantagne et al., *Cholera in Yemen: A Case Study of Epidemic Preparedness and Response* (Baltimore: Johns Hopkins Center for Humanitarian Health, 2018), http://www.hopkinshumanitarianhealth.org/assets/documents/CHOLERA_YEMEN_REPORT_LONG_Low_Res_Dec_4_2018.pdf.

5. Jonathan Kennedy, Andrew Harmer, and David McCoy, "The Political Determinants of the Cholera Outbreak in Yemen," *Lancet Global Health* 5, no. 10 (2017): e970.

6. World Health Organization, Regional Office for the Eastern Mediterranean, "Cholera Situation in Yemen," August 2019, http://applications.emro.who.int/docs/EMROPub _2019_cholera_August_yemen_EN.pdf?ua=1.

7. "Cholera Cases Reported by Year and by Continent, 1989–2015," infographic, World Health Organization, https://www.who.int/gho/epidemic_diseases/cholera /cholera_005.jpg.

8. International Crisis Group, "Yemen at War," March 28, 2015, https://www.crisisgroup .org/middle-east-north-africa/gulf-and-arabian-peninsula/yemen/yemen-war.

9. Micah Zenko, "Make No Mistake, the United States Is at War in Yemen," *Foreign Policy*, March 30, 2015, https://foreignpolicy.com/2015/03/30/make-no-mistake-the -united-states-is-at-war-in-yemen-saudi-arabia-iran/.

10. Andrew Exum, "What's Really at Stake for American in Yemen's Conflict," *Atlantic*, April 14, 2017, https://www.theatlantic.com/international/archive/2017/04/yemen-trump -aqap/522957/.

11. Robert Malley and Stephen Pomper, "Yemen Cannot Afford to Wait," *Atlantic*, April 5, 2019, https://www.theatlantic.com/ideas/archive/2019/04/us-culpable-yemens-tragedy /586558/; Robert Malley and Stephen Pomper, "Accomplice to Carnage, How America Enables War in Yemen," *Foreign Affairs*, March/April 2021, https://www.foreignaffairs .com/articles/united-states/2021-02-09/how-america-enables-war-yemen.

12. David Kirkpatrick and Kareem Fahim, "Saudi Leaders Have High Hopes for Yemen Airstrikes, but Houthi Attacks Continue," *New York Times*, April 2, 2015, https://www .nytimes.com/2015/04/03/world/middleeast/yemen-al-qaeda-attack.html.

13. Michaël Neuman, "No Patients, No Problems: Exposure of Risk of Medical Personnel Working in MSF Projects in Yemen's Governate of Amran," *Journal of Humanitarian Assistance*, February 14, 2014.

14. Michaël Neuman, "The Case of 'Dangerous Patients' in Yemen's Governate of Amran," in *Saving Lives and Staying Alive*, ed. Michael Neuman and Fabrice Weissman (London: Hurst, 2016).

15. Mwatana for Human Rights and Physicians for Human Rights, *"I Ripped the IV Out and Started Running": Attacks on Health Care in Yemen* (Mwatana for Human Rights and Physicians for Human Rights, 2020), https://phr.org/wp-content/uploads/2020/03/ PHR-Mwatana-March-2020-Report-Attacks-on-Health-Care-in-Yemen -ENGLISH.pdf.

16. Kate Kizer, "Hitting Iran Where It Doesn't Hurt: Why U.S. Intervention in Yemen Will Backfire," *Just Security*, March 8, 2017, https://www.justsecurity.org/38543/hitting -iran-doesnt-hurt-u-s-intervention-yemen-backfire/.

17. MSF, "The Steady Bleed: MSF Briefs on the Collapse of Healthcare in War-Torn Yemen," press release, August 2015, https://www.msf.org/report-steady-bleed-msf -briefs-collapse-healthcare-war-torn-yemen.

18. UN Security Council, Letter Dated 22 January 2016 from Panel of Experts on Yemen Established Pursuant to Security Council Resolution 2140 (2014) Addressed to the

President of the Security Council, January 26, 2016, S/2016/73, https://reliefweb.int/sites/reliefweb.int/files/resources/N1600299.pdf.

19. "Saudi FM on Civilian Casualties in Yemen: 'This Is Warfare,'" *CBS News*, September 30, 2015, https://www.cbsnews.com/news/saudi-foreign-minister-adel-al-jubeir-airstrikes-in-yemen-civilian-casualties/.

20. UN News, "Yemen: Amid 'Massive' Humanitarian Crisis, UN Reports Civilian Death Toll Now Exceeds 1,500," July 7, 2015, https://news.un.org/en/story/2015/07/503632-yemen-amid-massive-humanitarian-crisis-un-reports-civilian-death-toll-now.

21. World Health Organization, "Health System in Yemen Close to Collapse," *Bulletin of the World Health Organization* 93, no. 10 (Oct. 2015): 670.

22. United Nations Information Center, Sana'a, Statement Attributable to the Spokesman for the Secretary-General on Yemen, September 28, 2015, https://sanaa.sites.unicnetwork.org/2015/09/29/statement-attributable-to-the-spokesman-for-the-secretary-general-on-yemen-12/.

23. World Health Organization, "Health System in Yemen Close to Collapse."

24. Letter dated 22 January 2016 from the Panel of Experts on Yemen Established Pursuant to Security Council Resolution 2140 (2014) Addressed to the President of the Security Council, S/2016/73 (2016), https://www.securitycouncilreport.org/atf/cf/%7B65BFCF9B-6D27-4E9C-8CD3-CF6E4FF96FF9%7D/s_2016_73.pdf.

25. Kareem Shaheen, "MSF Accuses Saudi-Led Coalition of Bombing Clinic in Yemen," *Guardian*, December 4, 2015, https://www.theguardian.com/world/2015/dec/04/msf-accuses-saudi-led-coalition-of-bombing-clinic-in-yemen.

26. UN Human Rights Council, *Annual Report of the United Nations High Commissioner for Human Rights and Reports of the Office of the High Commissioner and the Secretary-General*, A/HRC/30/31 (2015), https://undocs.org/A/HRC/30/31.

27. World Health Organization, "Health System in Yemen Close to Collapse."

28. UNICEF, *Children on the Brink: The Impact of Violence and Conflict on Yemen and Its Children* (UNICEF, 2016), https://www.unicef.org/yemen/sites/unicef.org.yemen/files/2019-05/yem-children-on-the-brink-2016-en.pdf.

29. UNICEF, *Children on the Brink.*

30. Charbel El Bcheraoui, Aisha O. Jumaan, Michael L. Collison, Farah Daoud, and Ali H. Mokdad, "Health in Yemen: Losing Ground in Time of War," *Globalization and Health* 14, no. 1 (2018): 42.

31. UN Humanitarian Country Team, Yemen, *Humanitarian Response Plan, January–December 2016*, https://www.humanitarianresponse.info/sites/www.humanitarianresponse.info/files/documents/files/2016_hrp_yemen_20160217_0.pdf.

32. Shatha Elnakib, Sarah Elaraby, Fouad Othman, Huda BaSaleem, Nagiba A. Abdulghani AlShawafi, and Iman Ahmed Saleh et al., "Providing Care Under Extreme Adversity: The Impact of the Yemen Conflict on the Personal and Professional Lives of Health Workers," *Social Science and Medicine* 272 (2012): 113751.

33. International Crisis Group, "Is Peace Possible," Crisis Middle East Report No. 167, February 9, 2016, https://d2071andvipowj.cloudfront.net/167-yemen-is-peace-possible.pdf.

34. Yara Bayoumy, Noah Browning, and Mohammed Ghobari, "How Saudi Arabia's War in Yemen Has Made al Qaeda Stronger—and Richer," *Reuters*, April 8, 2016, https://www.reuters.com/investigates/special-report/yemen-aqap/.

35. April Longley Alley, "Quick Thoughts: April Longley Alley on the Yemen Conflict," International Crisis Group, July 31, 2015, https://www.crisisgroup.org/middle-east-north-africa/gulf-and-arabian-peninsula/yemen/quick-thoughts-april-longley-alley-yemen-conflict.

36. Malley and Pomper, "Yemen Cannot Afford to Wait."

37. Malley and Pomper, "Yemen Cannot Afford to Wait."

38. Reuters, "UPDATE 2—U.S. Speeds Up Arms to Saudi-led Coalition Against Yemen's Houthis," *Reuters Commodity News*, April 7, 2015, https://af.reuters.com/article/commoditiesNews/idAFL6N0X43602015040 7.

39. Stockholm International Peace Research Institute, *International Arms Transfers*, https://www.sipri.org/research/armament-and-disarmament/arms-transfers-and-military-spending/international-arms-transfers.

40. Campaign Against the Arms Trade, "UK Export Licenses, Export Licenses Approved," 2014, https://www.caat.org.uk/resources/export-licences/dashboard?date_from=2014-01&date_to=2014-12&region=Saudi+Arabia; Campaign Against the Arms Trade, "UK Export Licenses, Export Licenses Approved," 2015, https://www.caat.org.uk/resources/export-licences/dashboard?date_from=2015-01&date_to=2015-12&region=Saudi+Arabia.

41. Stephen Castle, "Britain Says It Will Resume Arms Sales to Saudi Arabia," *New York Times*, July 7, 2020, https://www.nytimes.com/2020/07/07/world/europe/britain-arms-sales-saudi-arabia.html.

42. Arron Merat, "'The Saudis Couldn't Do It Without Us': The True UK Role in Yemen's Deadly War," *Guardian*, June 21, 2019, https://www.theguardian.com/world/2019/jun/18/the-saudis-couldnt-do-it-without-us-the-uks-true-role-in-yemens-deadly-war.

43. Michael Newton, "An Assessment of the Legality of Arms Sales to the Kingdom of Saudi Arabia, in the Context of the Conflict in Yemen," Vanderbilt University Law School Legal Studies Research Paper Series Working Paper Number 17–26, May 19, 2017, https://papers.ssrn.com/sol3/papers.cfm?abstract_id=2971208; Daniel Mahanty and Annie Shiel, *With Great Power: Modifying U.S. Arms Sales to Reduce Civilian Harm* (Washington, DC: Center for Civilians in Conflict and Stimson Center, 2018).

44. Warren Strobel and Jonathan Landay, "Exclusive: As Saudis Bombed Yemen, U.S. Worried About Legal Blowback," *Reuters*, October 10, 2016, https://www.reuters.com/article/us-usa-saudi-yemen/exclusive-as-saudis-bombed-yemen-u-s-worried-about-legal-blowback-idUSKCN12A0BQ.

45. Letter from Representative Ted Lieu to Joseph Dunford, Chair of the Joint Chiefs of Staff, September 29, 2015, hosted on the website of the *New York Times*, https://www

.nytimes.com/interactive/2015/09/29/world/middleeast/document-ted-lieus-letter-to-jcs-chairman-dunford-on-yemen.html.

46. Samuel Oakford, "As Saudis Block a Human Rights Inquiry in Yemen, America Stays Quiet," *Vice News*, October 1, 2015, https://www.vice.com/en_us/article/xw3yjn/as-saudis-block-a-human-rights-inquiry-in-yemen-the-us-stays-quiet.

47. Dr. Matthew Offord, "Yemen: Military Intervention: Written Question, July 13, 2015," UK Parliament, https://www.parliament.uk/business/publications/written-questions-answers-statements/written-question/Commons/2015-07-13/6862/.

48. Caroline Mortimer, "Government Quietly Admits It Was Wrong to Say Saudi Arabia Is Not Targeting Civilians or Committing War Crimes," *Independent*, July 22, 2016, https://www.independent.co.uk/news/uk/politics/saudi-arabia-war-crimes-human-rights-uk-british-government-yemen-saudi-correction-philip-hammond-a7150761.html.

49. Secretaries of State for International Trade, Defence, Foreign and Commonwealth Affairs, and International Development, "First Joint Report of the Business, Innovation and Skills and International Development Committees of Session 2016–17, The Use of UK-Manufactured Arms in Yemen, Response of the Secretaries of State for International Trade, Defence, Foreign and Commonwealth Affairs, and International Development," November 2016, https://assets.publishing.service.gov.uk/government/uploads/system/uploads/attachment_data/file/568299/57524_Cm_9349_PRINT_v0.2.pdf.

50. Rowena Mason, "David Cameron Boasts of 'Brilliant' UK Arms Exports to Saudi Arabia," *Guardian*, February 25, 2016, https://www.theguardian.com/world/2016/feb/25/david-cameron-brilliant-uk-arms-exports-saudi-arabia-bae.

51. Malley and Pomper, "Accomplice to Carnage."

52. Larry Lewis, *Reducing and Mitigating Civilian Casualties: Enduring Lessons* (Joint and Coalition Operational Analysis, 2013), https://info.publicintelligence.net/JCOA-Reducing CIVCAS.pdf.

53. Françoise Bouchet-Saulnier and Jonathan Whittall, "An Environment Conducive to Mistakes? Lessons Learnt from the Attack on the Médecins San Frontières Hospital in Kunduz, Afghanistan," *International Review of the Red Cross* 100, nos. 1–2–3 (2018): 227.

54. "Department of Defense Press Briefing by General Campbell via Teleconference From Afghanistan," Department of Defense, November 25, 2015, https://www.defense.gov/Newsroom/Transcripts/Transcript/Article/631359/department-of-defense-press-briefing-by-general-campbell-via-teleconference-fro/.

55. Larry Lewis, *Promoting Civilian Protection During Security Assistance: Learning from Yemen* (Arlington, VA: CNA, 2019).

56. Exum, "What's Really at Stake."

57. Somini Sengupta, "United Nations Chief Exposes Limits to His Authority by Citing Saudi Threat," *New York Times*, June 9, 2016, https://www.nytimes.com/2016/06/10/world/middleeast/saudi-arabia-yemen-children-ban-ki-moon.html.

58. Ewen MacAskill and Paul Torpey, "One in Three Saudi Air Raids on Yemen Hit Civilian Sites, Data Shows," *Guardian*, September 16, 2016, https://www.theguardian

.com/world/2016/sep/16/third-of-saudi-airstrikes-on-yemen-have-hit-civilian-sites
-data-shows; Paul Torpey, Pablo Gutierrez, Glenn Swann, and Cath Levett, "What
Is Happening in Yemen and How Are Saudi Arabia's Airstrikes Affecting Civilians—
Explainer," *Guardian*, September 16, 2016, https://www.theguardian.com/world/ng
-interactive/2016/sep/16/how-saudi-arabias-airstrikes-have-hit-civilian-life-in
-yemen.

59. Samantha Power (@ambpower44), Twitter, April 16, 2016, 6:53 p.m., https://twitter.com
/AmbPower44/status/765682969520418817.

60. "Joint Incidents Assessment Team (JIAT) on Yemen Responds to Claims on Coalition
Forces' Violations in Decisive Storm Operations," *Saudi Press Agency* (2016), https://
www.spa.gov.sa/viewstory.php?lang=en&newsid=1524799.

61. UN Human Rights Council, *Annual Report of the United Nations High Commissioner for
Human Rights and reports of the Office of the High Commissioner and the Secretary-General,
Situation of Human Rights in Yemen, Including Violations and Abuses since September 2014*,
Annex 3, A/HRC/39/43 (2018), https://undocs.org/en/A/HRC/39/43.

62. UN Human Rights Council, *Situation of Human Rights in Yemen, Including Violations
and Abuses since September 2014, Report of the Group of Eminent International and Regional
Expert as Submitted to the United Nations High Commissioner for Human Rights since September 2014*, A/HRC/42/417 (2019), https://documents-dds-ny.un.org/doc/UNDOC
/GEN/G19/240/87/PDF/G1924087.pdf?OpenElement.

63. "Statement by NSC Spokesperson Ned Price on Yemen," White House, Office of the
Press Secretary, October 8, 2015, https://obamawhitehouse.archives.gov/the-press
-office/2016/10/08/statement-nsc-spokesperson-ned-price-yemen.

64. Patrick Wintour, "Labour Calls for UK to Withdraw Support for Saudi-led Coalition
in Yemen Fails," *Guardian*, October 28, 2016, https://www.theguardian.com/world
/2016/oct/26/labour-call-for-uk-to-withdraw-support-for-saudi-led-coalition-in-yemen
-fails.

65. "Saudi Arabia, Blanket Order Training," Defense Security Cooperation Agency, press
release, June 5, 2017, https://www.dsca.mil/press-media/major-arms-sales/saudi-arabia
-blanket-order-training.

66. Ministry of Foreign Affairs, *Saudi Arabia and the Yemen Conflict, 2017 Report*, https://
www.saudiembassy.net/sites/default/files/WhitePaper_Yemen_April2017_0.pdf.

67. Saudi Arabia Ministry of Media, Center for International Communication, "JIAT
Clears Arab Coalition from Responsibility for Many Bombings," March 6, 2018,
https://cic.org.sa/2018/03/jiat-clears-arab-coalition-responsibility-many-bombings/.

68. Kate Gilmore, United Nations Deputy High Commissioner for Human Rights, "Intro-
duction," in *Country Reports/Briefings/Updates of the Secretary-General and the High
Commissioner, March 21 and 22, 2018*, https://www.ohchr.org/en/NewsEvents/Pages
/DisplayNews.aspx?NewsID=22884&LangID=E.

69. Yemen Data Project, *Three Years of Saudi-led Air War: Yemen Data Project Full Data Summary*, 2018, https://us16.campaign-archive.com/?u=1912a1b11cab332fa977d3a6a&id=b39
e674ae7.

70. UN Human Rights Council, *Situation of Human Rights in Yemen, including Violations and Abuses Since September 2014, Report of the United Nations High Commissioner for Human Rights Containing the Findings of the Group of Independent Eminent International and Regional Experts and a Summary of Technical Assistance Provided by the Office of the High Commissioner to the National Commission of Inquiry*, A/HRC/39/53 (August 18, 2018), https://www.ohchr.org/EN/HRBodies/HRC/Pages/NewsDetail.aspx?NewsID=23479 &LangID=E.

71. "Yemen Could be 'Worst' Humanitarian Crisis in 50 years," *Al Jazeera*, January 5, 2018, https://www.aljazeera.com/news/2018/01/yemen-worst-humanitarian-crisis-50-years -180105190332474.html.

72. "Yemen Crisis Overview," United Nations Office for the Coordination of Humanitarian Affairs, July 2018, https://www.unocha.org/yemen/crisis-overview.

73. Robert F. Worth, "Behind the Reporting: How the War in Yemen Became a Bloody Stalemate," *New York Times Magazine*, November 2, 2018, https://www.nytimes.com /interactive/2018/10/31/magazine/yemen-war-saudi-arabia.html?module=inline.

74. Nikki Haley, "The UN's Uncomfortable Truths About Iran," op-ed, *New York Times*, February 17, 2018, https://www.nytimes.com/2018/02/17/opinion/nikki-haley-united -nations-iran.html.

75. "General Votel Exchange with Senator Angus King Concerning U.S. Support to Saudi-Led Coalition," *C-SPAN*, March 13, 2018, https://www.c-span.org/video /?c4753259/general-votel-exchange-senator-angus-king-support-saudi-led-coalition.

76. "CENTCOM Commander General Votel on Yemen Targeting," *C-SPAN*, March 13, 2018, https://www.c-span.org/video/?c4718576/centcom-commander-gen-joseph-votel -yemen-targeting.

77. *SFRC Hearing on Yemen, Mr. Robert Karem, Assistant Secretary of Defense for Policy, Before the Senate Foreign Relations Committee*, April 17, 2018, https://www.foreign.senate .gov/imo/media/doc/041718_Karem_Testimony.pdf.

78. "Senate Foreign Relations Committee Hearing on Yemen," *C-SPAN*, April 17, 2018, at 37:00 and following and 1:35:00 and following, https://www.c-span.org/video/?444089 -1/senators-express-concern-saudi-campaign-yemen.

79. *Testimony of Joseph Dunford, Chairman of the Joint Chiefs of Staff, Before the United States Senate, Committee on Armed Services, Hearing to Receive Testimony of the Department of Defense Budget Posture in Review of the Defense Authorization Request for Fiscal Year 2019 and the Future Years Defense Program*, April 26, 2018, https://www.armed-services.senate .gov/imo/media/doc/18-44_04-26-18.pdf.

80. Office of the Inspector General, United States Department of State, *Review of the Department of State's Role in Arms Transfer to the Kingdom of Saudi Arabia and the United Arab Emirates,* August 2020, note 23, https://www.stateoig.gov/system/files/isp-i-20-19.pdf.

81. Nima Elbagir, Salma Abdelaziz, Ryan Browne, Barbara Arvanitidis, and Laura Smith-Spark, "Bomb That Killed 40 Children in Yemen Was Supplied by the U.S.," *CNN*, August 17, 2018, https://edition.cnn.com/2018/08/17/middleeast/us-saudi-yemen-bus -strike-intl/index.html.

82. Samuel Oakford, "One American's Failed Quest to Protect Civilians in Yemen," *Atlantic*, August 17, 2018, https://www.theatlantic.com/international/archive/2018/08/yemen-saudi-airstrike-school-bus/567799/.

83. Memorandum of Justification Regarding Certification Pursuant to Section 1290 of the John S. McCain National Defense Authorization Act for Fiscal Year 2019 (P.L. 115–232), September 10, 2018, https://assets.documentcloud.org/documents/4873723/Pompeo-Certification-Under-NDAA-for-Saudi-Arabia.pdf.

84. Larry Lewis, "Grading the Pompeo Certification on Yemen War and Civilian Protection: Time for Serious Reconsideration," *Just Security*, September 18, 2018, https://www.justsecurity.org/60766/grading-pompeo-certification-yemen-war-civilian-protection-time-reconsideration/.

85. Office of Inspector General, *Review of the Department of State's Role in Arms Transfers to the Kingdom of Saudi Arabia and the United Arab Emirates*, August 2020, https://www.stateoig.gov/system/files/isp-i-20-19.pdf.

86. Jeremy Hunt, "Yemen Crisis Won't Be Solved by Arms Exports Halt," *Politico*, March 26, 2019, https://www.politico.eu/article/conflict-war-un-yemen-crisis-wont-be-solved-by-uk-arms-exports-halt/.

87. The Queen on Application of Campaign Against Arms Trade et al. v. The Secretary of State for International Trade, [2019] EWCA Civ 1020, https://www.judiciary.uk/wp-content/uploads/2019/06/CAAT-v-Secretary-of-State-and-Others-Open-12-June-2019.pdf.

88. Parliament, UK, Trade Update: Written Statement HCWS339 (2020), https://www.parliament.uk/business/publications/written-questions-answers-statements/written-statement/Commons/2020-07-07/HCWS339/.

89. Malley and Pomper, "Yemen Cannot Afford to Wait"; Malley and Pomper, "Accomplice to Carnage."

90. Jeremy Sharp, Christopher Blanchard, and Sarah Collins, *Congress and the War in Yemen Oversight and Legislation 2015–2020* (Congressional Research Service, Updated, June 19, 2020), https://crsreports.congress.gov/product/pdf/R/R45046.

91. Ruhan Nagra and Brynne O'Neal, *Day of Judgment: The Role of U.S. and Europe in Civilian Death, Destruction, and Trauma in Yemen* (Mwatana for Human Rights, University Network for Human Rights, and PAX, 2019), and sources in note 31, https://drive.google.com/file/d/1QlhNzzOrOVCCv4NClKeRJfhkGz8bwCOo/view.

92. Ryan Goodman, "The Law of Aiding Abetting (Alleged) War Crimes: How to Assess U.S. and UK Support for Saudi Air Strikes in Yemen," *Just Security*, September 1, 2016, https://www.justsecurity.org/32656/law-aiding-abetting-alleged-war-crimes-assess-uk-support-saudi-strikes-yemen; Oona A. Hathaway, Aaron Haviland, Srinath Reddy Kethireddy, and Alyssa Yamamoto, "Yemen: Is the U.S. Breaking the Law?," *Harvard National Security Journal* 10, no. 1 (2019): 1, https://harvardnsj.org/wp-content/uploads/sites/13/2019/02/Yemen-Is-the-U.S.-Breaking-the-Law.pdf.

93. Oona Hathaway, Alexandria Francis, Alyssa Yamamoto, Srinath Reddy Kethireddy, and Aaron Haviland, "Common Article 1 and the Duty to Ensure Respect for the

Geneva Conventions, in Yemen," *Just Security*, April 26, 2018, https://www.justsecurity
.org/55415/common-article-1-u-s-duty-ensure-respect-geneva-conventions-yemen/.

94. UN Human Rights Council, *Report of the Eminent International and Regional Experts as Submitted to the United Nations High Commissioner for Human Rights*, A/HRC/42/17, 2019, https://documents-dds-ny.un.org/doc/UNDOC/GEN/G19/240/87/PDF/G1924087.pdf ?OpenElement.

95. UN Human Rights Council, *Report of the Eminent International and Regional Experts as Submitted to the United Nations High Commissioner for Human Rights*, A/HRC/45/6, 2020, https://www.securitycouncilreport.org/atf/cf/%7B65BFCF9B-6D27-4E9C-8CD3 -CF6E4FF96FF9%7D/A_HRC_45_6.pdf.

96. Melissa Dalton, Jenny McAvoy, Daniel Mahanty, Hijab Shah, Kelsey Hampton, and Julie Snyder, *The Protection of Civilians in Partnered Operations* (Center for Strategic and International Studies, Center for Civilians in Conflict, and InterAction, 2018), https:// civiliansinconflict.org/wp-content/uploads/2018/10/USProgram_PartneredOperations .pdf.

97. National Defense Authorization Act of 2018, Pub L. No. 115–91, 131 STAT. 1283, Section 1209, https://www.congress.gov/bill/115th-congress/house-bill/2810/text.

98. Dalton et al., *The Protection of Civilians in Partnered Operation*; Lewis, *Promoting Civilian Protection During Security Assistance*.

99. "Financial Value of the Global Arms Trade," Stockholm International Peace Research Institute, https://www.sipri.org/databases/financial-value-global-arms-trade.

100. "Global Arms Trade: USA Increases Dominance; Arms Flows to the Middle East Surge, says SIPRI," Stockholm International Peace Research Institute press release, March 11, 2019, https://www.sipri.org/media/press-release/2019/global-arms-trade-usa -increases-dominance-arms-flows-middle-east-surge-says-sipri.

101. Oliver Pamp, Lukas Rudolph, Paul W. Thurner, Andreas Mehltretter, and Simon Primus, "The Build-up of Coercive Capacities: Arms Imports and the Outbreak of Violent Intrastate Conflicts," *Journal of Peace Research* 55, no. 4 (2018): 430–44, http://journals .sagepub.com/doi/10.1177/0022343317740417.

102. UN Security Council, Letter dated January 2016 from the Panel of Experts on South Sudan Established Pursuant to Security Council Resolution 2206 (2015) Addressed to the President of the Security Council, S/2016/70 (2016), https://undocs.org/S/2016 /70; Letter Dated 21 August 2015 from the Panel of Experts on South Sudan Established Pursuant to Security Council Resolution 2206 (2015) Addressed to the President of the Security Council S/2015/656, https://digitallibrary.un.org/record/800180 ?ln=en.

103. UN Security Council, Letter dated 23 July 2018 from the Panel of Experts on the Central African Republic Established Pursuant to Security Council Resolution 2399 (2018) Addressed to the President of the Security Council, S/2018/729 (2018) Annex 6, https:// www.undocs.org/S/2018/729.

104. James M. Blake, "Yemen's Triple Emergency," *Lawfare* (blog), August 24, 2020, https:// www.lawfareblog.com/yemens-triple-emergency.

105. Bethan McKernan, "Yemen: In a Country Stalked by Disease, Covid Barely Registers," *Guardian*, November 27, 2020, https://www.theguardian.com/global-development/2020/nov/27/yemen-disease-covid-war.

## 6. OBSTRUCTION

1. Geneva Convention IV, article 4, article 10; Protocol 1, article 10; Protocol 2, article 7; Geneva Convention I (on Wounded and Sick Combatants), article 15, states the obligation in different words, that the belligerents must, "without delay, take all possible measures to search for and collect the wounded and sick."
2. Convention I, article 35; Protocol 1, article 21; Protocol 2, article 11. Henckaerts and Doswald-Beck, *Customary International Humanitarian Law*, vol. 1, rule 29.
3. Alexander Breitegger, "The Legal Framework Applicable to Insecurity and Violence Affecting the Delivery of Health Care in Armed Conflicts and Other Emergencies," *International Review of the Red Cross* 95, no. 889 (2013): 115.
4. HCJ 4764/04 Physicians for Human Rights v. IDF Commander in Gaza [2004] IsrSC 58(5) 385; [2004] IsrLR 200; see also HCJ 2936/02 Physicians for Human Rights v. IDF Commander in West Bank [19], at pp. 4–5 {37}; Physicians for Human Rights v. IDF Commander in West Bank [6], at 29.
5. B'Tselem, *Wounded in the Field: Impeding Medical Treatment and Firing at Ambulances by IDF Soldiers in the Occupied Territories* (Jerusalem: B'Tselem, 2002), https://www.btselem.org/download/200203_medical_treatment_eng.pdf.
6. B'Tselem, *Wounded in the Field*.
7. B'Tselem, *Wounded in the Field*.
8. Cited in B'Tselem, *Wounded in the Field*.
9. Yoram Schweitzer, "The Rise and Fall of Suicide Bombings in the Second Intifada," *Strategic Assessment* 10, no. 3 (Oct. 2010): 39–48.
10. "Death of UN worker," UNRWA Statement, November 22, 2002, https://web.archive.org/web/20040314230638/https://www.un.org/unrwa/news/releases/pr-2002/stat-22nov02.html.
11. Thomas Gregory, "Dangerous Feelings: Checkpoints and the Perception of Hostile Intent," *Security Dialogue* 50, no. 2 (2019): 131–47.
12. B'Tselem, *Trigger Happy: Unjustified Gunfire and the IDF's Open-Fire Regulations During the Al-Aqsa Intifada* (Jerusalem: B'Tselem, 2002), https://www.btselem.org/sites/default/files/sites/default/files2/publication/200203_trigger_happy_eng.pdf.
13. B'Tselem, *Wounded in the Field*.
14. Leonard Rubenstein to the Honorable Binyamin Ben-Eliezer, Minister of Defense, April 1, 2002, in "Physicians for Human Rights (USA) Urgent International Medical Call to Action for Israel and the Occupied Territories," press release, ReliefWeb, https://reliefweb.int/report/israel/physicians-human-rights-usa-urgent-international-medical-call-action-israel-and.

15. David Kretzmer, *The Occupation of Justice: The Supreme Court of Israel and the Occupied Territories* (Albany: SUNY Press, 2002).

16. Physicians for Human Rights v. the Commander of the IDF Forces in the West Bank HCJ 2941/02, April 8, 2002, http://www.asser.nl/upload/documents/DomCLIC/Docs/NLP/Israel/Physicians_SC_Judgment_8-4-2002.pdf.

17. Physicians for Human Rights v. the Commander of the IDF Forces in the West Bank.

18. Physicians for Human Rights v. the Commander of the IDF Forces in the West Bank.

19. Leonard Rubenstein to The Honorable Binyamin Ben-Eliezer.

20. Michael Gross, *Bioethics and Armed Conflict: Moral Dilemmas of Medicine and War* (Cambridge, MA: MIT Press, 2006), 193.

21. Fadawa 'abd al Salem et al. v. Minister of Defense, HCJ 7517/99, 1999.

22. Catherine Bertini, Personal Humanitarian Envoy of the Secretary-General, *Mission Report, 11–19 August 2002*, https://www.un.org/unispal/document/auto-insert-196666/.

23. Bertini, *Mission Report.*

24. B'Tselem, *No Way Out: Medical Implications of Israel's Siege Policy* (Jerusalem: B'Tselem, 2001).

25. B'Tselem, *No Way Out.*

26. Bertini, *Mission Report.*

27. "About Us," Machsom Watch, last retrieved on February 6, 2021, https://machsomwatch.org/en/about.

28. Shlomi Swisa, *Harm to Medical Personnel: The Delay, Abuse and Humiliation of Personnel by Israeli Security Forces* (B'Tselem and Physicians for Human Rights Israel, 2003).

29. Israel Ministry of Foreign Affairs, "Palestinian Misuse of Ambulances for Terrorist Activities," press release, October 13, 2004, https://mfa.gov.il/mfa/aboutisrael/state/law/pages/palestinian%20misuse%20of%20medical%20services%20and%20ambulances%20for%20terrorist%20activities%2013-oct-2004.aspx.

30. Eyal Ben-Ari, Meirev Maymon, Nir Gazit, and Ron Shatzberg, *From Checkpoints to Flowpoints: Sites of Friction Between the Israel Defense Forces and Palestinians* (Jerusalem: Harry S. Truman Research institute for the Advancement of Peace, Hebrew University of Jerusalem, 2005).

31. Ben-Ari et al., *From Checkpoints to Flowpoints*, 25.

32. Devorah Manekin, "Violence Against Civilians in the Second Intifada: The Moderating Effect of Armed Group Structure on Opportunistic Violence," *Comparative Political Studies* 46, no. 1 (2013): 1273; Erella Grassiani, "Moral Othering at the Checkpoint: The Case of Israeli Soldiers and Palestinian Civilians," *Critique of Anthropology* 35, no. 4 (2015): 373.

33. Oded Na'aman, "The Checkpoint," *Boston Review*, November 13, 2012, http://bostonreview.net/world/checkpoint-oded-naaman.

34. Na'aman, "The Checkpoint."

35. Ben-Ari et al., *From Checkpoints to Flowpoints*, 12.

36. Samy Cohen, "Between Humanitarian Logic and Operational Effectiveness: How the Israeli Army Faced the Second Intifada," *Democracies at War Against Terrorism: A Comparative Perspective*, ed. Samy Cohen (New York: Palgrave MacMillan, 2008), 153.

37. International Committee of the Red Cross, *Violent Incidents Affecting the Delivery of Health Care January 2012 to December 2014* (Geneva: International Committee of the Red Cross, 2015), https://shop.icrc.org/download/ebook?sku=4237/002-ebook.

38. Larry Lewis, *Reducing and Mitigating Civilian Casualties: Enduring Lessons* (Joint and Coalition Operational Analysis, 2013), https://info.publicintelligence.net/JCOA -ReducingCIVCAS.pdf.

39. Victor de Currea Lugo, "Protecting the Health Sector in Colombia: A Step to Make the Health Sector Less Cruel," *International Review of the Red Cross* 83, no. 844 (2001): 1111–26; personal communication, 2020.

40. Human Rights Watch, "Ukraine: Danger, Unnecessary Delays at Crossing Points," February 17, 2017, https://www.hrw.org/news/2017/02/17/ukraine-dangers-unnecessary -delays-crossing-points#.

41. Christine Monaghan, *"Everything and Everyone Is a Target": The Impact on Children of Attacks on Health Care and Humanitarian Access in South Sudan* (New York: Watchlist on Children in Armed Conflict, 2018), https://watchlist.org/wp-content/uploads/watchlist -field_report-southsudan-web.pdf.

42. Shatha Elnakib, Sarah Elaraby, Fouad Othman, Huda BaSaleem, Nagiba A. Abdulghani AlShawafi, and Iman Ahmed Saleh et al., "Providing Care Under Extreme Adversity: The Impact of the Yemen Conflict on the Personal and Professional Lives of Health Workers," *Social Science and Medicine* 272 (2012): 113751.

43. "Panel Recommends Code of Conduct for IDF Checkpoints," *Haaretz*, August 25, 2004, https://www.haaretz.com/1.4832560; B'Tselem, *Ground to a Halt: Denial of Palestinians' Freedom of Movement in the West Bank* (2007), http://www.hamoked.org /files/2012/9260_eng(1).pdf; Eyal Weitzman, *Hollow Land: Israel's Architecture of Occupation* (London: Verso, 2007), chapter 6.

44. Weitzman, *Hollow Land*, chapter 6.

45. Irus Braverman, "Checkpoint Watch: Bureaucracy and Resistance at the Israeli/Palestinian Border," *Social and Legal Studies* 21, no. 3 (2012): 297–320.

46. Weitzman, *Hollow Land*.

47. Braverman, "Checkpoint Watch."

48. Minister (Hon.) Pär Stenbäck, Independent Monitor Appointed by the International Committee of the Red Cross (ICRC) and the International Federation of Red Cross and Red Crescent Societies, *Interim Report on the Implementation of the Memorandum of Understanding and the Agreement on Operational Arrangements Dated 28 November 2005 Between Magen David Adom in Israel and Palestine Red Crescent Society*, January 26, 2011, https://www.icrc.org/en/doc/assets/files/red-cross-crescent-movement/31st -international-conference/31-int-conference-mou-report-january-2011-en.pdf.

49. World Health Organization, *Crossing Barriers to Access Health Care in the Occupied Palestinian territory, 2013*, http://www.emro.who.int/images/stories/palestine/documents /WHO_-_RTH_crossing_barriers_to_access_health.pdf?ua=1.

50. 33rd International Conference of the Red Cross and Red Crescent, *Implementation of the Memorandum of Understanding and Agreement on Operational Arrangements Dated 28*

*November 2005 Between Magen David Adom in Israel and the Palestine Red Crescent Society*, 2019, https://rcrcconference.org/app/uploads/2019/12/33IC-R8-MoU_CLEAN_ADOPTED_en.pdf.

51. Maren Johanne Heilskov Rytter, Anne-Lene Kjældgaard, Henrik Brønnum-Hansen, and Karin Helweg-Larsen, "Effects of Armed Conflict on Access to Emergency Health Care in Palestinian West Bank: Systematic Collection of Data in Emergency Departments," *BMJ* 332, no. 7550 (2006): 1122–24.

52. B'Tselem, *Ground to a Halt*.

53. World Health Organization, *Crossing Barriers*.

54. World Health Organization, *Report by the Director-General, Health Conditions in the Occupied Palestinian Territory, Including East Jerusalem, and in the Occupied Syrian Golan*, A72/33, 2019, https://apps.who.int/gb/ebwha/pdf_files/WHA72/A72_33-en.pdf.

55. Minister (Hon.) Pär Stenbäck, *Interim Report*.

56. UN Office for the Coordination of Humanitarian Affairs, West Bank, *Closure Count and Analysis* (2006), https://www.ochaopt.org/content/west-bank-closure-count-and-analysis-september-2006.

57. B'Tselem, *Ground to a Halt*; B'Tselem, "Restrictions on Movement," November 11, 2017, https://www.btselem.org/freedom_of_movement.

58. Cindy Sousa and Amy Hagopian, "Conflict, Health Care, and Professional Perseverance: A Qualitative Study in the West Bank," *Global Public Health* 6, no. 5 (2011): 520–33.

59. Sousa and Hagopian, "Conflict, Health Care, and Professional Perseverance."

60. Amal Jamal, *The Rise of "Bad" Civil Society in Israel: Nationalist Civil Society Organizations and the Politics of Delegitimization* (German Institute for International and Security Affairs, 2018), https://www.swp-berlin.org/fileadmin/contents/products/comments/2018C02_jamal.pdf; Policy Working Group, *NGO Monitor: Shrinking Space; Defaming Human Rights Organizations that Criticize the Israeli Occupation* (Policy Working Group, 2018), http://policyworkinggroup.org.il/report_en.pdf.

61. Office of the UN High Commissioner for Human Rights, Israel/OPT, "UN Experts Call on Israel to Ensure Equal Access to COVID-19 Vaccines for Palestinians," January 14, 2021, https://www.ohchr.org/EN/NewsEvents/Pages/DisplayNews.aspx?NewsID=26655&LangID=E.

62. ICRC, *Promoting Military Operational Practice That Ensures Safe Access to and Delivery of Healthcare* (Geneva: International Committee for the Red Cross, 2015), https://shop.icrc.org/promoting-military-operational-practice-that-ensures-safe-access-to-and-delivery-of-health-care-pdf-en; ICRC, *Protecting Health Care: Guidance for Armed Forces* (Geneva: International Committee of the Red Cross, 2020), https://shop.icrc.org/protecting-healthcare-guidance-for-the-armed-forces-pdf-en.

63. Lawrence Wright, "Letter from Gaza: Captives," *New Yorker*, November 1, 2009, https://www.newyorker.com/magazine/2009/11/09/captives-2.

64. Merav Sarig, "Striking Medics in Gaza Temporarily Return to Work After Talks with Hamas," *British Medical Journal* 335, no. 7626 (2007): 904.

65. World Bank, "Cash-Strapped Gaza and an Economy in Collapse Put Palestinian Basic Needs at Risk," press release, September 25, 2018, https://www.worldbank.org/en/news /press-release/2018/09/25/cash-strapped-gaza-and-an-economy-in-collapse-put -palestinian-basic-needs-at-risk.

66. World Health Organization, Regional Office for the Eastern Mediterranean, *Situation Report #2*, December 27, 2015, http://www.emro.who.int/images/stories/palestine /documents/WHO_Sitrep_on_oPt__health_attacks_12.2015_-_final.pdf.

67. Jeannie Sowers and Erika Weinthal, "How Targeting Infrastructure Undermines Live-lihoods in the West Bank and Gaza," *International Affairs* 95, no. 2 (2019): 319–40.

68. ICRC, "Gaza: ICRC Demands Urgent Access to Wounded as Israeli Army Fails to Assist Wounded Palestinians," press release, January 8, 2009, https://www.icrc.org/en /doc/resources/documents/news-release/2009-and-earlier/palestine-news-080109.htm.

69. ICRC, "Gaza: ICRC Demands Urgent Access."

70. ICRC, "Gaza: Life-Saving Ambulances Must Be Given Unrestricted Access to the Wounded," press release, January 8, 2009, https://www.icrc.org/en/doc/resources /documents/news-release/2009-and-earlier/palestine-israel-news-080109.htm.

71. Taghreed El-Khodary and Isabel Kershner, "For Arab Clan, Days of Agony in a Cross-Fire," *New York Times*, January 9, 2009, https://www.nytimes.com/2009/01/10/world /middleeast/10gaza.html?hp.

72. Sebastian Van As, Alicia Vacas Moro, Ralf Syring, Jørgen Lange Thomsen, and Shab-bir Ahmed Wadee, *Final Report: Independent Fact-Finding Mission into Violations of Human Rights in the Gaza Strip During the Period 27.12.2008–18.01.2009* (Brussels: Physicians for Human Rights Israel and Palestinian Medical Relief Society, 2009), 19, https://reliefweb.int/sites/reliefweb.int/files/resources/608DA2F894A3DEF2C1257590 00415319-Full_Report.pdf.

73. World Health Organization/Health Cluster, *Gaza: Initial Needs Assessment*, https:// www.who.int/hac/crises/international/wbgs/gaza_early_health_assessment_16feb09 .pdf; Amnesty International, Israel/Gaza, *Operation 'Cast Lead': 22 Days of Death and Destruction* (London: Amnesty International, 2009), https://www.amnesty.org /download/Documents/48000/mde150152009en.pdf.

74. Physicians for Human Rights v. Prime Minister, Supreme Court Sitting as High Court, HC 201/09 (2009), https://www.asser.nl/upload/documents/DomCLIC/Docs/NLP /Israel/Physicians_v_PM_SC_Judgment_19-1-09_EN.pdf.

75. Physicians for Human Rights v. Prime Minister.

76. State of Israel, *The Operation in Gaza: Factual and Legal Aspects*, 2009, https://mfa.gov .il/mfa/foreignpolicy/terrorism/palestinian/pages/operation_in_gaza-factual_and _legal_aspects.aspx.

77. State of Israel, *The Operation in Gaza*.

78. "Conclusions of Investigations into Central Claims and 2009 Issues in Operation Cast Lead," in "IDF Investigations Refute Major Claims of Wrongdoing," *Middle East Analysis* April 22, 2009, http://middle-east-analysis.blogspot.com/2009_04_19 _archive.html.

79. UN Human Rights Council, *Report of the United Nations Fact-Finding Mission on the Gaza Conflict*, paragraph 474, A/HRC/12/48 (2009), paragraph 119, and note 328, https://www2.ohchr.org/english/bodies/hrcouncil/docs/12session/A-HRC-12-48.pdf.

80. State of Israel, *The Operation in Gaza*, paragraphs 223–25.

81. Breaking the Silence, *Soldiers' Testimonies from Operation Cast Lead, Gaza, 2009*, testimony 9, https://www.breakingthesilence.org.il/wp-content/uploads/2011/02/Operation _Cast_Lead_Gaza_2009_Eng.pdf.

82. Breaking the Silence, *Soldiers' Testimonies*, testimony 10.

83. Breaking the Silence, *Soldiers' Testimonies*, testimony 7.

84. Breaking the Silence, *Soldiers' Testimonies*, testimony 7, 8, 21.

85. Breaking the Silence, *Soldiers' Testimonies*, testimony 31.

86. Breaking the Silence, *Soldiers' Testimonies*, testimony 26.

87. Breaking the Silence, *Soldiers' Testimonies*, testimony 18.

88. UN Human Rights Council, *Report of the United Nations High Commissioner for Human Rights on the Implementation of Human Rights Council Resolutions S-9/1 and S-12/1, Addendum, Concerns Related to Adherence to International Human Rights and International Humanitarian Law in the Context of the Escalation Between the State of Israel, the De Facto Authorities in Gaza, and Palestinian Armed Groups in Gaza that Occurred From 14 to 21 November 2012*, A/HRC/22/35/Add. 1 (2013), https://documents-dds-ny.un.org/doc /UNDOC/GEN/G13/154/84/PDF/G1315484.pdf?OpenElement.

89. Health Cluster in the Occupied Palestinian Territories, *Gaza Strip Joint Health Sector Assessment Report 2014*, https://www.ecoi.net/en/file/local/1208443/1930_1466061945 _joint-health-sector-assessment-report-gaza-sept-2014-final.pdf.

90. Jutta Bachmann, Laurel Baldwin-Ragaven, Hans Petter Hougen, Jennifer Leaning, Karen Kelly, Önder Özkalipci, Louis Reynolds, and Alicia Vacas, *Findings of an Independent Medical Fact-Finding Mission* (Physicians for Human Rights Israel, Al Mezan Center for Human Rights—Gaza, Gaza Community Health Program, Palestinian Center for Human Rights—Gaza, 2014), 48, https://www.humanitarianre-sponse.info/sites/www.humanitarianresponse.info/files/assessments/Findings%20 of%20an%20Independent%20Medical%20Fact-Finding%20Mission%20Gaza%20 2014.pdf.

91. Bachmann et. al, *Findings of an Independent Medical Fact-Finding Mission*, 48.

92. Al Mezan Center for Human Rights, Lawyers for Palestinian Rights, Medical Aid for Palestinians, *No More Impunity: Gaza's Health Sector Under Attack* (Al Mezan Center for Human Rights, Lawyers for Palestinian Rights, Medical Aid for Palestinians, 2015).

93. Breaking the Silence, *This Is How We Fought in Gaza: Soldiers' Testimonies and Photographs from Operation "Protective Edge" (2014)* (Jerusalem: Breaking the Silence, 2015), https://www.breakingthesilence.org.il/pdf/ProtectiveEdge.pdf; Raphael S. Cohen et al., *From Cast Lead to Protective Edge: Lessons from Israel's War in Gaza*, RAND, 2017, 155.

94. UN Human Rights Council, *Report of the Detailed Findings of the Independent Commission of Inquiry Established Pursuant to Human Rights Council Resolution S-21/1*,

A/HRC/29/CRP.4 (2014), paragraph 458, https://reliefweb.int/report/occupied -palestinian-territory/report-detailed-findings-independent-commission-inquiry.

95. B'Tselem, "Ambulance Driver Rami 'Ali Recounts Attacks that Killed Paramedic 'Aaed al-Bura'i and Injured Team Sent to Rescue Him, Both Despite Coordination with Red Crescent," press release, July 27, 2014, https://www.btselem.org/testimonies/20140727_ gaza_ambulance_driver_rami_ali; International Committee of the Red Cross, "ICRC Condemns killing of Red Crescent Volunteer," press release, July 25, 2014.

96. ICRC, "No Wonder Gazans Are Angry. The Red Cross Can't Protect Them," press release, July 25, 2014, https://www.icrc.org/eng/resources/documents/article/editorial /07-24-gaza-israel-palestine-maio.htm.

97. Israeli Defense Force, *Decisions of the IDF Military Advocate General Regarding Exceptional Incidents That Allegedly Occurred During Operation 'Protective Edge'— Update No. 6*, August 15, 2018, allegation 16, https://www.idf.il/en/minisites/military-advocate -generals-corps/releases-idf-military-advocate-general/mag-corps-press-release -update-6/.

98. Israeli Defense Force, *Decisions of the IDF Military Advocate General.*

99. B'Tselem, *Whitewash Protocol—The So-Called Investigation of Operation Protective Edge* (Jerusalem: B'Tselem, 2016), https://www.btselem.org/download/201609_whitewash _protocol_eng.pdf.

100. Ambrogio Manenti, Claude de Ville de Goyet, Corinna Reinicke, John Macdonald, and Julian Donald, *Report of a Field Assessment of Health Conditions in the Occupied Palestinian Territory* (World Health Organization, 2016), http://apps.who.int/gb/Statements /Report_Palestinian_territory/Report_Palestinian_territory-en.pdf.

101. *PRCS Operational Reports*, Palestinian Red Crescent Society, https://www.palestinercs .org/index.php?page=search&langid=1.

102. MSF, "Gazans Injuries Risk Permanently Shattering Lises," press release, November 28, 2018, https://www.msf.org/gazans'-injuries-risk-permanently-shattering-lives-palestine.

103. World Health Organization, *Occupied Palestinian Territory, Monthly Report*, January 2020, http://www.emro.who.int/images/stories/palestine/documents/Jan_2020_Monthly .pdf?ua=1.

104. Human Rights Council, *Report of the Independent International Commission of Inquiry on the Protests in the Occupied Palestinian Territory* A/HRC/40/74 2019, 150, https://www .ohchr.org/EN/HRBodies/HRC/CoIOPT/Pages/Report2018OPT.aspx.

## 7. ARMED GROUPS

1. Thérése Pettersson and Magnus Öberg, "Organized Violence, 1989–2019," *Journal of Peace Research* 57, no. 4 (2020): 597–613.

2. Mariya Nikolova, Statement in "Non-State Armed Groups, People, Power, Polices on Armed Groups," webinar, ICRC, October 7, 2020, https://www.icrc.org/en/event/non -state-armed-groups-people-power-policies.

3. Fiona Terry and Brian McQuinn, *Roots of Restraint in War* (Geneva: International Committee of the Red Cross, 2018), 13.

4. Mark Lowcock, "Saving Lives in a Time of Crisis: Why the Global Humanitarian System Matters," Center for Strategic and International Studies, February 5, 2019, https://www.csis.org/analysis/saving-lives-time-crisis-why-global-humanitarian-system-matters.

5. Fédération Internationale des Ligues des Droits de l'Homme (FIDH), "Massacres au Kasaï: Des Crimes Contre l'humanité au Service d'un Chaos Organisé," press release, December 20, 2017, https://www.fidh.org/fr/regions/afrique/rdc/massacres-au-kasai-des-crimes-contre-l-humanite-au-service-d-un-chaos.

6. George Klay Kieh, Jr., "Civilians and Wars in Africa: The Cases of Liberia, Sierra Leone, and Cote D'Ivoire," *Peace Research* 48, no. 1/2 (2016): 203–28.

7. Republic of Liberia, Truth and Reconciliation Commission, *Final Report*, 2009, vol. 2, 174, http://www.pul.org.lr/doc/trc-of-liberia-final-report-volume-ii.pdf.

8. Interview with Walter T. Gwenigale, *International Review of the Red Cross* 95, no. 889 (2013): 13–21, https://international-review.icrc.org/sites/default/files/irrc-889-interview-gwenigale.pdf.

9. International Monetary Fund, *Liberia: Interim Poverty Reduction Strategy* (Washington, DC: International Monetary Fund, 2007), https://www.imf.org/external/pubs/ft/scr/2007/cr0760.pdf.

10. Margaret E. Kruk, Peter C. Rockers, Elizabeth H. Williams, S. Tornorlah Varpilah, Rose Macauley, Geetor Saydee, and Sandro Galea, "Availability of Essential Health Services in Post-Conflict Liberia," *Bulletin of the World Health Organization* 88, no. 7 (2010): 527.

11. Primus Che Chi, Patience Bulage, Henrik Urdal, and Johanne Sundby, "Perceptions of the Effects of Armed Conflict on Maternal and Reproductive Health Services and Outcomes in Burundi and Northern Uganda: A Qualitative Study," *BMC International Health and Human Rights* 15, no. 7 (2015): 1–15; Adanna Chukwuma and Uche Eseosa Ekhator-Mobayode, "Armed Conflict and Maternal Health Care Utilization: Evidence from the Boko Haram Insurgency in Nigeria," *Social Science and Medicine* 226 (2019): 104.

12. Leonard Rubenstein, *Post-Conflict Health Reconstruction: New Foundations for U.S. Policy* (Washington, DC: United States Institute of Peace, 2009), https://www.usip.org/sites/default/files/post-conflict_health_reconstruction_0.pdf.

13. Patrick T. Lee, Gina R. Kruse, Brian T. Chan, Moses BF Massaquoi, Rajesh R. Panjabi, Bernice T. Dahn, and Walter T. Gwenigale, "An Analysis of Liberia's 2007 National Health Policy: Lessons for Health Systems Strengthening and Chronic Disease Care in Poor, Post-Conflict Countries," *Globalization and Health* 7 (2011): Article no. 37.

14. Reed M. Wood, "Intrastate Violence and Civilian Victimization," in *Oxford Encyclopedia of Politics* (Oxford: Oxford University Press, 2016); Hugo Slim, *Killing Civilians* (New York: Columbia University Press, 2008); Stathis N. Kalyvas, *The Logic of Violence in Civil War* (New York: Cambridge University Press, 2006).

15. Fazal Tanisha, *Wars of Law: Unintended Consequences in the Regulation of Armed Conflict* (Ithaca, NY: Cornell University Press, 2018).

16. Jeremy Weinstein, *Inside Rebellion: The Politics of Insurgent Violence* (Cambridge: Cambridge University Press, 2012).

17. Wood, "Intrastate Violence"; Kalyvas, *The Logic of Violence*.

18. Terry and McQuinn, *Roots of Restraint in War*.

19. Kalyvas, *The Logic of Violence*.

20. Jessica A. Stanton, *Violence and Restraint in Civil Wars: Civilian Targeting in the Shadow of International Law* (New York: Cambridge University Press, 2016).

21. Christine Monaghan, *"Everything and Everyone Is a Target": The Impact on Children of Attacks on Health Care and Humanitarian Access in South Sudan* (New York: Watchlist on Children in Armed Conflict, 2018), https://watchlist.org/wp-content/uploads/watchlist -field_report-southsudan-web.pdf.

22. Jason Cone and Françoise Duroch, "Don't Shoot the Ambulance," *World Policy Journal* 30, no. 3 (2013): 66.

23. Abby Stoddard, *Necessary Risks: Professional Humanitarian and Violence Against Aid Workers* (New York: Palgrave MacMillan, 2020); Abby Stoddard, Adele Harmer, and Monica Czwarno, *Aid Worker Security Report 2017, Behind the Attacks: A Look at the Perpetrators of Violence Against Aid Workers* (Humanitarian Outcomes, 2017), 12–15, https:// www.humanitarianoutcomes.org/sites/default/files/publications/awsr_2017.pdf.

24. Scott Gates, Håvard Mokleiv Nygård, and Karim Bahgat, "Patterns of Attacks on Medical Personnel and Facilities: SDG 3 Meets SDG 16," *Conflict Trends* 4 (Oslo: PRIO, 2017).

25. Louis Lillywhite, *Roundtable Summary, Non-State Armed Groups, Health, and Health Care* (London: Chatham House, 2015), https://www.chathamhouse.org/sites/default /files/events/special/NSAGs%20Meeting%20Summary%20in%20template%20-%20 final%20edit%20from%20Jo%20-%20ER-%20PKA%2027.10.15.pdf.

26. ICRC, *Safeguarding the Provision of Health Care: Operational Practices and Relevant International Humanitarian Law Concerning Armed Groups* (Geneva: ICRC, 2015), https:// healthcareindanger.org/wp-content/uploads/2015/09/icrc-002-4243-safeguarding-the -provision-of-health-care.pdf.

27. Chi et al., "Perceptions of the Effects of Armed Conflict"; Justine Namakula and Sophie Witter, "Living Through Conflict and Post-Conflict: Experiences of Health Workers in Northern Uganda and Lessons for People-Centred Health Systems," *Health Policy and Planning* 29, Supp. 2 (2014): ii-6–ii14; Archit Baskaran, "The Islamic State (Daesh) Healthcare Paradox: A Caliphate in Crisis," *Journal of Global Health* 5, no. 2 (2015): 34–38.

28. Personal communication.

29. Ashley Jackson, *In Their Words: Perceptions of Armed Non-State Actors on Humanitarian Action* (Geneva: Geneva Call, 2016), https://www.genevacall.org/wp-content /uploads/dlm_uploads/2016/09/WHS_Report_2016_web.pdf; ICRC, *Safeguarding the Provision of Health Care: Operational Practices and Relevant International*

*Humanitarian Law Concerning Armed Groups* (Geneva: ICRC, 2015), https://healthcareindanger.org/wp-content/uploads/2015/09/icrc-002-4243-safeguarding-the-provision-of-health-care.pdf.

30. "How We Work," Geneva Call, www.genevacall.org/how-we-work/.

31. "Deed of Commitment Under Geneva Call for the Protection of Health Care in Conflict," Geneva Call, 2018, https://www.genevacall.org/wp-content/uploads/2019/07/Deed-of-Commitment-for-the-protection-of-health-care-in-armed-conflict-final-version-4.pdf.

32. Terry and McQuinn, *Roots of Restraint in War*, 39–41.

33. Joe Cropp, *The Humanitarian Fix: Navigating Civilian Protection in Contemporary Wars* (London: Routledge, 2021).

34. Fiona Terry, "The International Committee of the Red Cross in Afghanistan," *International Review of the Red Cross* 93, no. 881 (2011): 174.

35. International Committee of the Red Cross, "Afghanistan: Ambulance Used in Attack on Police Training Compound," press release, April 4, 2011, https://www.icrc.org/en/doc/resources/documents/news-release/2011/afghanistan-news-2011-04-07.htm.

36. "Taliban Rue Ambulance Attack," *New Humanitarian*, April 12, 2011, http://www.thenewhumanitarian.org/news/2011/04/12/taliban-rue-ambulance-attack.

37. Michael Neuman and Fabrice Weissman, eds., *Saving Lives and Staying Alive: Humanitarian Security in the Age of Risk Management* (London: Hurst, 2016); Claire Magone, Michaël Neuman, and Fabrice Weissman, eds., *Humanitarian Negotiations Revealed: The MSF Experience* (London: Hurst, 2011).

38. See details of the training center, called Centre of Competence on Frontline Negotiation, at https://frontline-negotiations.org/.

39. William Carter and Katherine Have, *Humanitarian Access Negotiations with Non-State Actors: Internal Guidance Gaps and Good Practice* (Secure Access in Volatile Environments Research Program Resource Paper, 2016), https://www.gppi.net/media/SAVE__2016__Humanitarian_access_negotiations_with_non-state_armed_groups.pdf.

40. Antonio Giustozzi, *The Military Cohesion of the Taliban* (Washington Center for Research and Policy Analysis, 2017); Yoshinobu Nagamine, *The Legitimization Strategy of the Taliban's Code of Conduct: Through the One-Way Mirror* (New York: Palgrave MacMillan, 2015); Thomas H. Johnson and Matthew C. DuPee, "Analysing the New Taliban Code of Conduct (Layeha): An Assessment of Changing Perspectives and Strategies of the Afghan Taliban," *Central Asian Survey* 31, no. 1 (2012): 77; Kate Clark, *The Layha: Calling the Taleban to Account* (Kabul: Afghanistan Analysts Network, 2011).

41. United Nations Mission in Afghanistan, *Afghanistan: Protection of Civilians in Armed Conflict, Annual Report 2019*, 9, https://unama.unmissions.org/sites/default/files/afghanistan_protection_of_civilians_annual_report_2019_-_22_february.pdf.

42. Theo Farrell and Antonio Giustozzi, "The Taliban at War: Inside the Helmand Insurgency, 2004–2012," *International Affairs* 89, no. 4 (2013): 845–71.

43. Ashley Jackson, "Negotiation Perceptions: Al-Shabaab and Taliban Views of Aid Agencies," *Humanitarian Policy Group Policy Brief 61* (2014), https://www.odi.org/sites /odi.org.uk/files/odi-assets/publications-opinion-files/9104.pdf.

44. Clark, *The Layha*.

45. David Zucchino and Fatima Faizi, "Taliban Attack Aid Group Office in Kabul, in Setback for U.S. Peace Talks," *New York Times*, May 8, 2019, https://www.nytimes.com /2019/05/08/world/asia/kabul-afghanistan-bombing.html.

46. Clark, *The Layha*; Muhammad Munir, "The Layha for the Mujahideen: An Analysis of the Code of Conduct for the Taliban Fighters Under Islamic Law," *International Review of the Red Cross* 93, no. 881 (2011): 81–102.

47. Craig Nelson and Ehsanullah Amiri, "Kabul Bombing: Death Toll Passes 100 in Suicide Attack with Ambulance," *Wall Street Journal*, January 28, 2018, https://www.wsj .com/articles/kabul-bombing-suicide-attacker-kills-dozens-in-afghanistan-1517054456.

48. UNAMA Human Rights Service, *Quarterly Report on the Protection of Civilians in Armed Conflict, 1 January 2019 to 30 September 2019*, October 19, 2019, https://unama.unmissions .org/sites/default/files/unama_protection_of_civilians_in_armed_conflict_-_3rd_quarter _update_2019.pdf; Patty Grossman, *"They've Shot Many Like This": Abusive Raids by CIA-Backed Afghan Strike Forces* (New York: Human Rights Watch, 2019).

49. "Afghanistan War: Deadly Taliban Attack 'Destroys' Hospital," *BBC News*, September 19, 2019, https://www.bbc.com/news/world-asia-49751370.

50. Ashley Jackson and Rahmatullah Amiri, *Insurgent Bureaucracy: How the Taliban Makes Policy*, Peaceworks no. 143 (Washington, DC: United States Institute of Peace, 2010), https://www.usip.org/index.php/publications/2019/11/insurgent-bureaucracy-how -taliban-makes-policy.

51. Leonard Rubenstein, *Defying Expectation: Polio Vaccination Programs Amid Political and Armed Conflict* (Washington, DC: United States Institute of Peace, 2010), https://www .usip.org/sites/default/files/PB%2064%20-%20Polio%20Vaccination%20Programs%20 Amid%20Political%20and%20Armed%20Conflict.pdf.

52. Rubenstein, *Defying Expectations*.

53. Jackson and Amiri, *Insurgent Bureaucracy*.

54. Ashley Jackson, "The Taliban's Fight for Hearts and Minds," *Foreign Policy*, Fall 2018, https://foreignpolicy.com/2018/09/12/the-talibans-fight-for-hearts-and-minds -aghanistan/.

55. Jackson and Amiri, *Insurgent Bureaucracy*.

56. Jackson and Amiri, *Insurgent Bureaucracy*.

57. United Nations Assistance Mission in Afghanistan, *Quarterly Report on Protection of Civilians in Armed Conflict: 1 January 2019–31 March 2019*, https://unama.unmissions.org /sites/default/files/unama_protection_of_civilians_in_armed_conflict_-_first_quarter _report_2019_english_.pdf.

58. "Attacks on Health Care in 2019 as of 22 October," infographic, World Health Organization, https://www.humanitarianresponse.info/sites/www.humanitarianresponse.

info/files/documents/files/afghanistan_attacks_on_health_care_in_2019_20191022
.pdf.

59. Kate Clark, *Clinics Under Fire? Health Workers Caught Up in the Afghan Conflict* (Kabul: Afghanistan Analysts Network, 2016).

60. Ashley Jackson, *Life Under the Taliban Shadow Government* (London: Overseas Development Institute, 2018), https://www.odi.org/sites/odi.org.uk/files/resource-documents /12269.pdf.

61. Ben Farmer, "Taliban 'Will No Longer Protect Red Cross Staff in Afghanistan, Amid Rising Attacks on Health Workers," *Daily Telegraph*, August 15, 2018, https://www .telegraph.co.uk/global-health/terror-and-security/taliban-will-no-longer-protect-red -cross-staff-afghanistan-amid/.

62. United Nations Assistance Mission in Afghanistan and United Nations Human Rights, Afghanistan: Protection of Civilians in Armed Conflict, Annual Report 2018–2019, https://unama.unmissions.org/sites/default/files/unama_annual_protection_of_civilians _report_2018_-_23_feb_2019_-_english.pdf.

63. United Nations Assistance Mission in Afghanistan, *Afghanistan: Protection of Civilians in Armed Conflict, Midyear Update 2018* (2018), https://unama.unmissions.org/sites /default/files/unama_poc_midyear_update_2018_15_july_english.pdf.

64. Nagamine, *The Legitimization Strategy of the Taliban.*

65. United Nations Mission in Afghanistan, *Afghanistan: Protection of Civilians in Armed Conflict, Annual Report 2018* (2019), https://unama.unmissions.org/sites/default/files /unama_annual_protection_of_civilians_report_2018_-_23_feb_2019_-_english.pdf.

66. Jackson and Amiri, *Insurgent Bureaucracy.*

67. Stephen W. Smith, "CAR's History: The Past of a Tense Present," in *Making Sense of the Central African Republic*, ed. Tatiana Carayannis and Louisa Lombard (London: Zed, 2015), 23.

68. Adam Hochschild, *King Leopold's Ghost* (New York: Houghton Mifflin, 1998).

69. Tatiana Carayannis and Louisa Lombard, "Making Sense of CAR, An Introduction," in *Making Sense of the Central African Republic*, 3; Smith, "CAR's History," 20.

70. Smith, "CAR's History," 32

71. International Coalition for the Responsibility to Protect, "Crisis in the Central African Republic," http://www.responsibilitytoprotect.org/index.php/crises/crisis-in-the-central -african-republic.

72. Liesl Louw-Vaudran, "Thousands of Muslims Are Fleeing the CAR, but the Problem Started with the Collapse of the State," Institute for Security Studies, February 26, 2014, https://issafrica.org/iss-today/conflict-in-the-central-african-republic-its-not-just -about-religion; Smith, "CAR's History," 43–44.

73. Nathalia Dukhan, *Splintered Warfare II: How Foreign Interference Is Fueling Kleptocracy, Warlordism, and an Escalating Conflict in the Central African Republic* (Enough Project, 2018), https://enoughproject.org/reports/splintered-warfare-ii-central-african -republic.

74. Liesl Louw-Vaudran, "Conflict in the Central African Republic: It's Not Just About Religion," Institute for Security Studies, February 26, 2014, https://issafrica.org/iss -today/conflict-in-the-central-african-republic-its-not-just-about-religion.

75. International Crisis Group, *Avoiding the Worst in Central African Republic*, Africa Report no. 253 (Brussels: International Crisis Group, 2017), https://d2071andvipowj.cloudfront .net/253-avoiding-the-worst-in-central-african-republic.pdf; Veronique Barbelet, *Central African Republic: Addressing the Protection Crisis*, HPG Working Paper (London: Overseas Development Institute, 2015), https://www.odi.org/sites/odi.org.uk/files/odi -assets/publications-opinion-files/10000.pdf.

76. UN Security Council Resolution 2121 (2013) S/Res/2121, http://www.globalr2p.org /media/files/resolution-2121-car-1.pdf.

77. International Crisis Group, *Avoiding the Worst*; Global Centre for the Responsibility to Protect, *Ongoing Violence by Armed Groups Leave Populations in the Central African Republic at Risk of Recurring Mass Atrocity Crimes*, updated September 2019, http://www .globalr2p.org/regions/central_african_republic.

78. MSF, "Project Update, Suffering Mounts as Armed Groups Return to Bambari," 2018, https://www.msf.org/suffering-mounts-armed-groups-return-bambari.

79. UN Security Council, Letter Dated 23 July 2018 from the Panel of Experts on the Central African Republic Extended Pursuant to Resolution 2399 (2018) Addressed to the President of the Security Council, S/2018/729 (2018), 21–22, https://www.securitycouncilreport .org/atf/cf/%7B65BFCF9B-6D27-4E9C-8CD3-CF6E4FF96FF9%7D/s_2018_729.pdf; MSF, "Suffering Mounts."

80. MSF, "Project Update."

81. Safeguarding Health in Conflict Coalition, *Violence on the Front Line: Attacks on Health Care in 2017* (2018), https://www.safeguardinghealth.org/sites/shcc/files /SHCC2018final.pdf.

82. Ashley Jackson, "Gaining Acceptance: Lessons from Engagement with Armed Groups in Afghanistan and Somalia," *Humanitarian Exchange* no. 62 (September 2014): 37–38, https://odihpn.org/magazine/gaining-acceptance-lessons-from-engagement-with -armed-groups-in-afghanistan-and-somalia/; Barbelet, *Central African Republic*; Larissa Fast and Michael O'Neill, "A Closer Look at Acceptance," *Humanitarian Exchange Magazine* 47 (2010), https://odihpn.org/magazine/humanitarian-security -management/.

83. Barbelet, *Central African Republic*; Fast and O'Neill, "A Closer Look."

84. MSF, *Unprotected: Summary of Internal Review of the October 31st Events in Batangafo, Central African Republic* (Barcelona: MSF, 2019), https://www.msf.org/unprotected -report-violence-and-lack-protection-civilians-car-central-african-republic.

85. MSF, *Unprotected*.

86. MSF, *Unprotected*.

87. UN Human Rights Council, *Report of the Independent Expert on the Situation of Human Rights in the Central African Republic*, A/HRC/36/65 (2017), https://documents-dds-ny .un.org/doc/UNDOC/GEN/G17/226/95/PDF/G1722695.pdf?OpenElement.

88. Human Rights Council, *Report of the Independent Expert on the Situation of Human Rights in the Central African Republic*, A/HRC/33/63 (2016), https://documents-dds-ny .un.org/doc/UNDOC/GEN/G16/164/08/PDF/G1616408.pdf?OpenElement.

89. MSF, "Voice from the Field, Ongoing Fears of Outbursts of Violence in Bambari Hamper Access to Healthcare," June 26, 2018, https://www.msf.org/central-african-republic -ongoing-fears-outbursts-violence-bambari-hamper-access-healthcare.

90. UN Office of the High Committee on Human Rights, *Committee on Economic, Social and Cultural Rights Examines Initial Report of the Central African Republic*, 20 March 2018, https://www.ohchr.org/EN/NewsEvents/Pages/DisplayNews.aspx?NewsID=22864 &LangID=E.

91. Humanitarian Exchange, *Special Feature: The Crisis in the Central African Republic* (London: Overseas Development Institute, 2014); Abby Stoddard, *Necessary Risks*; Gerard McHugh and Manuel Bessler, *Humanitarian Negotiations with Armed Groups: A Manual for Practitioners* (New York: UN Office for Coordination of Humanitarian Assistance, 2006); Magone, Neuman, and Weissman, eds., *Humanitarian Negotiations Revealed*.

92. UN Security Council, "Arria Formula Meeting on Protecting Humanitarian and Medical Personnel," UN Web TV, April 1, 2019, http://webtv.un.org/search/protecting -humanitarian-and-medical-personnel-arria-formula-meeting-of-the-security-council /6021305176001/.

93. ICRC, *Changing Behavior: Tackling Violence Against Health Care in Niger, the Central African Republic, and Nigeria* (Geneva: International Committee of the Red Cross, 2018), https://shop.icrc.org/changing-behaviour-tackling-violence-against-health-care -in-the-central-african-republic-niger-and-nigeria-pdf-en.

94. Rachel Sweet, "Bureaucrats at War: The Resilient State in the Congo," *African Affairs* 119, no. 475 (2020): 224.

95. Safeguarding Health in Conflict Coalition, *Impunity Remains* dataset, https://data .humdata.org/dataset/shcchealthcare-dataset.

96. UN Human Rights Council, *Report of the Independent Expert on the Situation of Human Rights in the Central African Republic*, A/HRC/39/70 (2018), https://documents-dds-ny .un.org/doc/UNDOC/GEN/G18/247/50/PDF/G1824750.pdf.

97. Human Rights Watch, *Looking for Justice: The Special Criminal Court, a New Opportunity for Victims in the Central African Republic* (New York: Human Rights Watch, 2018), https://www.hrw.org/sites/default/files/report_pdf/car0518_web.pdf.

98. Seth Jones, Charles Vallee, Danika Newlee, Nicholas Harrington, Clayton Sharb, and Hannah Byrne, *The Evolution of the Jihadist Threat: Current and Future Challenges from the Islamic State, Al-Qaeda, and Other Groups* (Washington, DC: Center for Strategic and International Studies, 2018), https://csis-website-prod.s3.amazonaws.com/s3fs -public/publication/181221_EvolvingTerroristThreat.pdf.

99. Fawaz A. Gerges, *Isis: A History* (Princeton, NJ: Princeton University Press, 2012).

100. UN Independent International Commission of Inquiry on the Syrian Arab Republic, *Rule of Terror: Living Under ISIS in Syria* (2014), A/HRC/27/CRP.3, https://www.ohchr .org/EN/HRBodies/HRC/IICISyria/Pages/Documentation.aspx.

101. Heba Aly, "Jihadi Jurisprudence? Militant Interpretations of Islamic Rules of War," *New Humanitarian*, April 24, 2014, https://www.thenewhumanitarian.org/analysis /2014/04/24/jihadi-jurisprudence-militant-interpretations-islamic-rules-war.

102. Roy Gutman, "In Recent Months, ISIS Targeted Hospitals, Doctors, Journalists," *McClatchy*, February 11, 2014, https://www.mcclatchydc.com/news/nation-world/world /article24763324.html.

103. Office of Intelligence and Analysis, FBI Directorate of Intelligence, and National Counterterrorism Center, *Fire Line*, February 8, 2017, http://www.arkhospitals.org /Misc.%20Files/AttacksHospitalsHCFacilities.pdf.

104. Carolyn Ho and Archit Baskaran, "The Islamic State (Daesh) Healthcare Paradox: A Caliphate in Crisis," Field Notes, *Global Health Journal*, November 2015, https://www .ghjournal.org/the-islamic-state-daesh-healthcare-paradox-a-caliphate-in-crisis/.

105. Ho and Baskaran, "The Islamic State (Daesh) Healthcare Paradox."

106. John M. Quinn, Omar F. Amouri, and Pete Reed, "Notes from a Field Hospital South of Mosul," *Globalization and Health* 14 (2018): Article 27.

107. Ghaith Abdul-Ahad, "How the People of Mosul Subverted Isis 'Apartheid,'" *Guardian*, January 30, 2018, https://www.theguardian.com/cities/2018/jan/30/mosul-isis-apartheid.

108. Erin Cunningham, "Islamic State Imposes a Reign of Fear in Iraqi Hospitals," *Washington Post*, November 25, 2014, https://www.washingtonpost.com/world/middle_east /islamic-state-imposes-a-reign-of-fear-in-iraqi-hospitals/2014/11/25/94476f3e-6382-11e4 -ab86-46000e1d0035_story.html.

109. Amir Abdallah, "ISIS Executes Four Doctors in Nineveh," *Iraqi News*, July 12, 2016, https://www.iraqinews.com/iraq-war/isis-executes-four-doctors-nineveh/; Loaa Adel, "Source: ISIS Girl Executes 5 Women Including a Doctor in Western Nineveh," *Iraqi News*, March 3, 2016, https://www.iraqinews.com/iraq-war/local-source-isis-girl -executes-5-women-including-doctor-in-western-nineveh/.

110. Amnesty International, *At Any Cost: The Civilian Catastrophe in West Mosul, Iraq* (London: Amnesty International, 2017), 22, https://www.amnesty.org/download/Documents /MDE1466102017ENGLISH.PDF.

111. Shaimaa Ibrahim, Sara Al-Dahir, Taha Al Mulla, Farris Lami, S. M. Moazzem Hossain, Abdullah Baqui, and Gilbert Burnham, "Resilience of Health Systems in Conflict Affected Governorates of Iraq, 2014–2018" (unpublished paper in review, February 26, 2021), Microsoft Word file.

112. Jonathan Kennedy and Domna Michailidou, "Civil War, Contested Sovereignty, and the Limits of Global Health Partnerships: A Case Study of the Syrian Polio Outbreak of 2013," *Health Policy and Planning* 32, no. 5 (2017): 690–98; Spenta Kakalia and Hasan Karrar, "Polio, Public Health, and the New Pathologies of Militancy in Pakistan," *Critical Public Health* 26, no. 4 (2015): 446–54; Ryoko Sato, "Effect of Armed Conflict on Vaccination: Evidence from the Boko Haram Insurgency in Northeastern Nigeria," *Conflict and Health* 13 (2019): Article no. 49.

113. Cunningham, "Islamic State Imposes a Reign of Fear in Iraqi Hospitals."

114. Georgia J. Michlig, Riyadh Lafta, Maha Al-Nuaimi, and Gilbert Burnham, "Providing Healthcare Under ISIS: A Qualitative Analysis of Healthcare Worker Experiences in Mosul, Iraq Between June 2014 and June 2017," *Global Public Health* 14, no. 10 (2019): 1414.

115. Ibrahim et al., "Resilience of Health Systems."

116. Judith Soussan, "Qabassin, Syria: Security Issues and Practices in an MSF Mission in the Land of Jihad," in Michael Neuman and Fabrice Weissman, eds., *Saving Lives and Staying Alive: Humanitarian Security in the Age of Risk Management* (London: Hurst, 2016), 112.

117. Soussan, "Qabassin, Syria."

118. Soussan, "Qabassin, Syria."

119. Stephen Townsend, "Reports of Civilian Casualties in the War Against ISIS Are Vastly Inflated," *Foreign Policy*, September 15, 2017, https://foreignpolicy.com/2017/09/15/reports-of-civilian-casualties-from-coalition-strikes-on-isis-are-vastly-inflated-lt-gen-townsend-cjtf-oir/.

120. Townsend, "Reports of Civilian Casualties."

121. Airwars, *Credibility Gap: United Kingdom Civilian Harm for the Battles of Mosul and Raqqa* (2018), https://airwars.org/wp-content/uploads/2018/09/Credibility-Gap-Airwars-submission-to-UK-Parlt-Defence-Select-Committee-Sept-2018.pdf; Amnesty International, *At Any Cost.*

122. Azmat Khan and Anand Gopal, "The Uncounted," *New York Times Magazine*, November 16, 2017, https://www.nytimes.com/interactive/2017/11/16/magazine/uncounted-civilian-casualties-iraq-airstrikes.html.

123. World Health Organization, *WHO Special Situation Report, Mosul Crisis, Iraq, Issue No. 18: 8–15 May 2017*, https://reliefweb.int/sites/reliefweb.int/files/resources/WHO%20Special%20Situation%20Report%20%2318_%208-15%20May%202017_final.%20%282%29.pdf.

124. "Interview with James Mattis," *Face the Nation*, May 28, 2017, https://www.cbsnews.com/news/face-the-nation-may-28-2017-transcript-secretary-mattis/.

125. "Interview with James Mattis," *Face the Nation.*

126. Anand Gopal, "America's War on Syria's Civilians," *New Yorker*, December 14, 2020, https://www.newyorker.com/magazine/2020/12/21/americas-war-on-syrian-civilians.

127. Alex Hopkins, "Airwars Annual Assessment 2017: Civilians Paid a High Price for Major Coalition Gains," *Airwars*, January 2018, https://airwars.org/report/airwars-annual-assessment-2017/.

128. Elias Groll and Robbie Gramer, "How the U.S. Miscounted the Dead in Syria," *Foreign Policy*, April 25, 2019, https://foreignpolicy.com/2019/04/25/how-the-u-s-miscounted-the-dead-in-syria-raqqa-civilian-casualties-middle-east-isis-fight-islamic-state/.

129. Luke Mogelson, "Dark Victory in Raqqa," *New Yorker*, October 17, 2017, https://www.newyorker.com/magazine/2017/11/06/dark-victory-in-raqqa.

130. Mogelson, "Dark Victory in Raqqa."

131. Shawn Snow, "Marine Artillery Barrage of Raqqa Was So Intense Two Howitzers Burned Out," *Marine Times*, November 2, 2017, https://www.marinecorpstimes.com /flashpoints/2017/11/02/marine-artillery-barrage-of-raqqa-was-so-intense-two -howitzers-burned-out/.

132. Luke Mogelson, "America's Abandonment of Syria," *New Yorker*, April 20, 2020, https://www.newyorker.com/magazine/2020/04/27/americas-abandonment-of-syria.

133. Mogelson, "America's Abandonment of Syria."

134. Amnesty International, "Unprecedented Investigation Reveals U.S.-led Coalition Killed More Than 1,600 Civilians in Raqqa 'Death Trap,'" April 25, 2019, https://www .amnesty.org/en/latest/news/2019/04/syria-unprecedented-investigation-reveals-us-led -coalition-killed-more-than-1600-civilians-in-raqqa-death-trap/; Amnesty International, War in Raqqa: Rhetoric vs. Reality (website), https://raqqa.amnesty.org.

135. Human Rights Watch, Iraq, "In Mosul Battle, ISIS Used Hospital Base," February 8, 2017, https://www.hrw.org/news/2017/02/08/iraq-mosul-battle-isis-used-hospital-base.

136. Médecins Sans Frontières, "Mosul: Hospital Beds Available Still Down 70%, a Year After Battle Ended," July 9, 2018, https://reliefweb.int/report/iraq/mosul-hospital-beds -available-still-down-70-year-after-battle-ended.

137. Department of Defense, "Press Briefing by Colonel Dillon via Teleconference from Baghdad, Iraq, September 17, 2017," https://www.defense.gov/Newsroom/Transcripts /Transcript/Article/1320504/department-of-defense-press-briefing-by-colonel-dillon -via-teleconference-from/.

138. UN Office for the Coordination of Humanitarian Affairs, "Joint Statement on Civilian Casualties Due to Coalition Airstrikes in Ar-Raqqa City, August 22, 2017," https:// reliefweb.int/sites/reliefweb.int/files/resources/joint_statement_on_ar_raqqa_air- strikes_final_version.pdf.

139. Mogelson, "America's Abandonment of Syria."

140. Physicians for Human Rights, "Raqqa Offensive Has Destroyed the City's Health Care System," September 8, 2017, https://phr.org/news/raqqa-offensive-has-destroyed-citys -health-care-system/.

141. Jones et al., *The Evolution of the Jihadist Threat.*

142. Therése Pettersson and Magnus Öberg, "Organized Violence, 1989–2019," *Journal of Peace Research* 57, no. 4 (2020): 597–613.

143. Syrians for Truth and Justice, "Sawa'id Al-Khair" and "Committee of Promotion of Virtue and Prevention of Vice," New Security Arms of Hayat Tahrir al-Sham in Idlib and Arihah, March 16, 2018, https://stj-sy.org/en/465/.

144. Sahar Atrache, *Losing Their Last Refuge: Inside Idlib's Humanitarian Nightmare* (Washington, DC: Refugees International 2019), https://reliefweb.int/sites/reliefweb.int/files /resources/Syria%2BIdlib%2BReport%2B-%2BSeptember%2B2019%2B-%2B1.0.pdf.

145. Al-Hadji Kudra Maliro and Cara Anna, "Attackers Kill Doctor at Hospital in Congo's Ebola Epicenter," APNews, April 19, 2019, https://apnews.com/3b99e6c8b646404288dc 4a288b402044.

146. Tedros Adhanom Ghebreyesus (@DrTedros), "The death of Dr Mouzoko also underscores that when health workers are targeted and attacked, it has huge ripple effects that are felt by the people they served, the communities in need, and of course their loved ones, friends & co-workers. It's a loss for everyone, everywhere," Twitter, April 19, 2019, 6:38 p.m., https://twitter.com/DrTedros/status/1119369646879203328.

147. Helen Branswell, "Modern Science Has Delivered the World Powerful Tools to Defeat Ebola. It Is Not Enough," *Stat News*, August 14, 2019, https://www.statnews.com/2019/08/14/modern-science-has-delivered-the-world-powerful-tools-to-defeat-ebola-it-is-not-enough/.

148. Ebola Gbalo Research Group, "Responding to the Ebola Virus Disease Outbreak in DR Congo: When Will We Learn from Sierra Leone?" *Lancet* 393, no. 10191 (2019): 2647; Independent Oversight and Advisory Committee for the WHO Emergencies Programme, *From Never Again to the New Normal: What Does the 2018–2019 Ebola Outbreak Tell Us About the State of Global Epidemic and Pandemic Preparedness and Response* (2019), 27–28, https://www.who.int/about/who_reform/emergency-capacities/oversight-committee/IOACGPMBEBOLA06.pdf?ua=18.

149. UN High Commissioner for Human Rights, *Human Rights Situation and the Activities of the United Nations Joint Human Rights Office in the Democratic Republic of the Congo*, A/HRC/42/32 (2019), https://daccess-ods.un.org/TMP/2483024.44815636.html; Vinh-Kim Nguyen, "An Epidemic of Suspicion—Ebola and Violence in the DRC," *New England Journal of Medicine* 380 (2019): 1298; World Health Organization Independent Oversight and Advisory Committee for the WHO Health Emergencies Programme, *IOAC Mission Report Democratic Republic of the Congo 24 April–2 May 2019*, https://www.who.int/about/who_reform/emergency-capacities/Mission-Report(English).pdf?ua=1.

150. Congo Research Group, *Congo, Forgotten: The Numbers Behind Africa's Longest Humanitarian Crisis* (2019), https://kivusecurity.nyc3.digitaloceanspaces.com/reports/28/KST%20biannual%20report%20August%2012%20%281%29.pdf.

151. Juliet Bedford, *Key Considerations: The Context of North Kivu Province, DRC* (Social Science in Humanitarian Action, 2018), https://reliefweb.int/sites/reliefweb.int/files/resources/SSHAP_North_Kivu_context.pdf.

152. Letter Dated 8 August 2017 from the Group of Experts on the Democratic Republic of the Congo Extended Pursuant to Security Council Resolution 2293 (2016) Addressed to the President of the Security Council, S/2017/672/Rev.1, https://undocs.org/S/2017/672/Rev.1; Rachel Sweet, "Militarizing the Peace, UN Intervention Against Congo's 'Terrorist' Rebels," Lawfare Blog, June 2, 2019, https://www.lawfareblog.com/militarizing-peace-un-intervention-against-congos-terrorist-rebels.

153. Letter Dated 8 August 2017 from the Group of Experts on the Democratic Republic of the Congo.

154. UN High Commissioner for Human Rights, *Human Rights Situation*; Nguyen, "An Epidemic of Suspicion"; Independent Oversight and Advisory Committee, *IOAC Mission Report*, 52.

155. Hana Rohan and Gillian McKay, "The Ebola Outbreak in the Democratic Republic of Congo: Why There Is No 'Silver Bullet,'" *Nature Immunology* 21 (2020): 591; Hyppolite Kalambay Ntembwa and Wim Van Lerberghe, *Improving Aid Coordination in the Health Sector: Democratic Republic of the Congo Case Study* (Geneva: World Health Organization, 2015), https://www.who.int/health_financing/documents/Efficiency_health _systems_Congo/en/.

156. Ntembwa and Van Lerberghe, *Improving Aid Coordination*, 6, 7.

157. Ntembwa and Van Lerberghe, *Improving Aid Coordination*, 7.

158. J. Stephen Morrison, "The Ebola Virus Is Winning in Eastern Democratic Republic of Congo," Center for Strategic and International Studies Commission on Strengthening America's Health Security, September 12, 2019, https://healthsecurity.csis .org/articles/the-ebola-virus-is-winning-in-eastern-democratic-republic-of-the -congo/.

159. Tanja Ducomble and Etiene Gignoux, "Learning from a Massive Epidemic: Measles in DRC," *Lancet Infectious Diseases* 20, no. 5 (2020): P542.

160. Patrick Vinck, Phuong N. Pham, Kenedy K. Bindu, Juliet Bedford, and Eric J. Nilles, "Institutional Trust and Misinformation in the Response to the 2018–19 Ebola Outbreak in North Kivu, DR Congo: A Population-Based Survey," *Lancet Infectious Diseases* 19, no. 5 (2019): P529.

161. Anne-Lise Dewulf, Antoine Mushagalusa Ciza, Léon Irenge, Emmanuel Kandate, and Véronique Barbelet, *Collective Approaches to Risk Communication and Community Engagement in the Ebola Response in North Kivu, Democratic Republic of Congo* (London: Overseas Development Institute 2020), https://www.odi.org/sites/odi.org.uk/files /resource-documents/unicef_cce_drc_web.pdf.

162. Adelicia Fairbanks, "Security and Access in the DRC: Implementing an Acceptance Strategy in the Ebola Response," *Humanitarian Exchange* 70 (2020), https://odihpn.org /magazine/security-and-access-in-the-drc-implementing-an-acceptance-strategy-in -the-ebola-response/.

163. Philip Kleinfeld and Paisley Dodds, "Exclusive: Leaked Review Exposes Scale of Aid Corruption and Abuse in Congo," *New Humanitarian*, June 12, 2020, https://www .thenewhumanitarian.org/investigation/2020/06/12/Congo-aid-corruption-abuse -DFID-DRC-UN-NGOs.

164. Amy Daffe, "We Can't Stop Congo's Ebola Outbreak Until Communities Lead the Response," *New Humanitarian*, August 2, 2019, https://www.thenewhumanitarian.org /opinion/2019/08/01/Ebola-outbreak-community-response-Congo; Nguyen, "An Epidemic of Suspicion."

165. Rachel Sweet and Juliet Bedford, *Whatsapp and Local Media (Grand Nord) 9–18 September* (Social Science in Humanitarian Action Platform, 2018), https://opendocs.ids.ac.uk /opendocs/bitstream/handle/20.500.12413/14063/SSHAP_WhatsApp_and_local _media_NKivu_180919.pdf?sequence=1&isAllowed=y.

166. Independent Oversight and Advisory Committee, *From Never Again*, 19.

167. Rachel Sweet and Juliet Bedford, *Media and Local Messages on Ebola in the Grand Nord, DRC, November–December* (Social Science in Humanitarian Action, 2018), https://opendocs.ids.ac.uk/opendocs/bitstream/handle/20.500.12413/14270/SSHAP_media_%20local_messages_Grand_Nord_December_2018.pdf?sequence=1&isAllowed=y.

168. Nurith Aizenman, "An Urgent Mystery: Who's Attacking Ebola Responders in Congo—And Why," *NPR Goats and Soda*, June 4, 2019, https://www.npr.org/sections/goatsandsoda/2019/06/04/726139304/an-urgent-mystery-whos-attacking-ebola-responders-in-congo-and-why.

169. Independent Oversight and Advisory Committee, *From Never Again.*

170. Aizenman, "An Urgent Mystery."

171. Independent Oversight and Advisory Committee, *From Never Again*, 19.

172. Rachel Sweet, *Politics, Factions, and Violence: Listening to Local Voices on Ebola, Local Media Update #3 (February–April 2019)* (Social Science in Humanitarian Action, 2019), 3, https://reliefweb.int/sites/reliefweb.int/files/resources/SSHAP%20Local%20and%20social%20media%20brief%203%20-%20February-April%202019.pdf.

173. Sweet, *Politics, Factions, and Violence*, 4–6.

174. Chad R. Wells, Abhishek Pandey, Martial L. Ndeffo Mbah, Bernard-A Gaüzère, Denis Malvy, Burton H. Singer, and Alison P. Galvani, "The Exacerbation of Ebola Outbreaks by Conflict in the Democratic Republic of the Congo," *Proceedings of the National Academy of Sciences* 116, no. 48 (2019): 24366.

175. Sweet, *Politics, Factions, and Violence*, 3.

176. Wells et al., "The Exacerbation of Ebola Outbreaks."

177. Sweet, *Politics, Factions, and Violence*, 7.

178. S. Rae Wannier, Lee Worden, Nicole A. Hoff, Eduardo Amezcua, Bernice Selo, Cyrus Sinai, and Mathias Mossoko et al., "Estimating the Impact of Violent Events on Transmission in Ebola Virus Disease Outbreak, Democratic Republic of the Congo, 2018–2019," *Epidemics* 28 (2019): 100353.

179. Independent Oversight and Advisory Committee, *IOAC Mission Report*, 26.

180. Wells et al., "The Exacerbation of Ebola Outbreaks"; Oly Ilunga Kalenga, Matshidiso Moeti, Annie Sparrow, Vinh-Kim Nguyen, Daniel Lucey, and Tedros A. Ghebreyesus, "The Ongoing Ebola Epidemic in the Democratic Republic of Congo, 2018–2019," *New England Journal of Medicine* 381 (2019): 373.

181. John Daniel Kelly, Sarah Rae Wannier, Cyrus Sinai, Caitlin A Moe, Nicole A Hoff, Seth Blumberg, and Bernice Selo et al., "The Impact of Different Types of Violence on Ebola Virus Transmission During the 2018–2020 Outbreak in the Democratic Republic of the Congo," *Journal of Infectious Diseases* 22, no. 12 (2020): 2021–29.

182. Wells et al., "The Exacerbation of Ebola Outbreaks"; Kalenga et al., "The Ongoing Ebola Epidemic"; Gbalo Research Group, "Responding to the Ebola Virus", UN High Commissioner for Human Rights, *Human Rights Situation*; Vinh-Kim Nguyen, "An Epidemic of Suspicion"; Sweet, *Politics, Factions, and Violence*, 2; "Statement by

Mr. Andrew Gilmour, Assistant Secretary-General for Human Rights," 41st Human Rights Council Session—Item 10, Enhanced Interactive Dialogue on the Situation of Human Rights in the Democratic Republic of the Congo, July 9, 2019, https://www.ohchr.org/EN/NewsEvents/Pages/DisplayNews.aspx?NewsID=24808&LangID=E.

183. Tom Miles, "Battle Against Ebola Being Lost Amid Militarized Response, MSF Says," *Reuters*, March 7, 2019, https://www.reuters.com/article/us-health-ebola-congo/battle-against-ebola-being-lost-amid-militarized-response-msf-says-idUSKCN1QO1F1.

184. Emmanuel Freudenthal, "In Congo, a 'Militarized' Ebola Response Has Fueled Community Resistance," *New Humanitarian*, October 2, 2019, https://www.thenewhumanitarian.org/news-feature/2019/10/02/Congo-militarised-Ebola-response-community-resistance.

185. Sweet, *Politics, Factions, and Violence*, 2.

186. Associated Press, "Ebola Response Workers Killed in Congo," *New York Times*, November 28, 2019, https://www.nytimes.com/2019/11/28/world/africa/ebola-congo.html.

187. Colin Dwyer, "'It Was Unmistakably a Directed Attack': 4 Ebola Workers Killed in Congo," *NPR*, November 28, 2019, https://www.npr.org/2019/11/28/783582331/it-was-unmistakably-a-directed-attack-4-ebola-workers-killed-in-congo.

188. Dewulf et al., *Collective Approaches*.

189. Independent Oversight and Advisory Committee, *IOAC Mission Report*, 40; Nguyen, "An Epidemic of Suspicion"; Wells et al., "The Exacerbation of Ebola Outbreaks."

190. Tolbert Nyenswah, Cyrus Engineer, and David H. Peters, "Leadership in Times of Crisis: The Example of Ebola Virus Disease in Liberia," *Health Systems and Reform* 2, no. 3 (2016): 194.

191. Adam Kamradt-Scott, Sophie Harman, Clare Wenham, and Frank Smith III, "Civil–Military Cooperation in Ebola and Beyond," *Lancet* 387, no. 10014 (2016): P104–05.

192. ICRC, *Protecting Health Care, Key Recommendations* (Geneva: ICRC, 2016), https://shop.icrc.org/protecting-health-care-key-recommendations.html?___store=en.

193. Luke Taylor, "COVID-19 Misinformation Sparks Threats and Violence Against Doctors in Latin America," *British Medical Journal 370* (2020): m3088; Shamila Devi, "COVID-19 Exacerbates Violence Against Health Workers," *Lancet* 396, no. 10252 (2020): P658; Paola Forgione, "New Patterns of Violence Against Healthcare in the COVID-19 Pandemic," blog, *British Medical Journal*, May 15, 2020, https://blogs.bmj.com/bmj/2020/05/15/new-patterns-of-violence-against-healthcare-in-the-covid-19-pandemic/; Russell Seth Martins, Omaima Anis Bhatti, and Asad I. Mian, "Violence Against Health Care Workers in Pakistan During the COVID-19 Pandemic," *JAMA Health Forum* 1, no. 10 (2020): E201263.

194. Remarks of Ellen Watson-Stryker, panel, "Navigating the DRC Ebola Outbreak," CSIS Global Health Policy Center, September 19, 2019, https://www.csis.org/events/access-hot-zone-navigating-drc-ebola-outbreak.

## 8. CHALLENGES IN MAKING NORMS MATTER

1. Rony Brauman, *Humanitarian Wars? Lies and Brainwashing, in Conversation with Regis Meyran* (London: Hurst, 2019), 104–5.

2. World Health Organization, "WHO Condemns Rising Violence Against Health Care Workers, Patients," *World Health Organization*, September 25, 2014, http://www.who .int/hac/events/HCWviolence/en/.

3. David Miliband, President, International Rescue Committee, "Welcome to the Age of Impunity: David Miliband's World Economic Forum Speech, January 24, 2020," https://www.rescue.org/press-release/welcome-age-impunity-david-milibands-world -economic-forum-speech.

4. Matthew Evangelista and Nina Tannenwald, eds., *Do the Geneva Conventions Matter?* (New York: Oxford University Press, 2017).

5. Peter Maurer, "Changing World, Unchanged Protection? 70 Years of the Geneva Conventions," President's Address at the Graduate Institute, Geneva, March 13, 2019, https://www.icrc.org/en/document/changing-world-unchanged-protection-70-years -geneva-conventions.

6. Kathryn Sikkink, *Evidence for Hope: Making Human Rights Work in the 21st Century* (Princeton, NJ: Princeton University Press, 2017), 157–61.

7. Jessica A. Stanton, *Violence and Restraint in Civil Wars: Civilian Targeting in the Shadow of International Law* (New York: Cambridge University Press, 2016).

8. Neta C. Crawford, "Targeting Civilians and U.S. Strategic Bombing Norms," in *The American Way of Bombing: Changing Ethics and Legal Norms, from Flying Fortresses to Drones*, ed. Matthew Evangelista and Henry Shue (Ithaca, NY: Cornell University Press, 2014).

9 Hugo Slim, *Killing Civilians: Method, Morality, and Madness in War* (Oxford: Oxford University Press, 2010), 151–55.

10. John Fabian Witt, "Two Conceptions of Suffering in War," in *Knowing the Suffering of Others: Legal Perspectives on Pain and Its Meaning*, ed. Austin Sarat, Montre D. Carodine, Cathy Caruth, Alan Durham, and Brian Fair (Tuscaloosa: University of Alabama Press, 2014), 129, 140–41.

11. Witt, "Two Conceptions of Suffering," 148–49.

12. Witt, "Two Conceptions of Suffering," 140.

13. Witt, "Two Conceptions of Suffering," 144.

14. Paul C. Ney, "Remarks by Defense Dept. General Counsel Paul C. Ney on the Law of War," *Just Security*, May 28, 2019, https://www.justsecurity.org/64313/remarks-by-defense -dept-general-counsel-paul-c-ney-jr-on-the-law-of-war/.

15. Ney, "Remarks."

16. David Luban, "Book Review, *Lincoln's Code*," *Just Security*, October 3, 2013, https://www .justsecurity.org/1609/book-review-lincolns-code.

17. Department of Defense, "Assistant Secretary of Defense for Public Affairs Jonathan R. Hoffman Press Briefing," transcript, February 3, 2020, https://www.defense

.gov/Newsroom/Transcripts/Transcript/Article/2073437/assistant-to-the-secretary-of
-defense-for-public-affairs-jonathan-r-hoffman-pre/.

18. *Statement of Alexandra Boivin, Head of Regional Delegation for the U.S. and Canada Before U.S. Congress, Tom Lantos Commission on Human Rights*, October 31, 2019, https:// humanrightscommission.house.gov/sites/humanrightscommission.house.gov/files /documents/Protecting%20Health%20Care_Testimony_ICRC.pdf.

19. Anthony Pfaff and Patrick Granfield, "The Moral Peril of Proxy Wars," *Foreign Policy*, April 5, 2019, https://foreignpolicy.com/2019/04/05/proxy-wars-are-never-moral/; Daniel Bynum, "Why Engage in a Proxy War? A State's Perspective," *Lawfare*, blog, May 21, 2018, https://www.lawfareblog.com/why-engage-proxy-war-states-perspective.

20. ICRC, "Commentary of 2016 on Convention (I) for the Amelioration of the Condition of the Wounded and Sick in Armed Forces in the Field, Geneva, 12 August 1949," Article 1: Respect for the Convention, paragraphs 164–73, https://ihl-databases.icrc.org /applic/ihl/ihl.nsf/Treaty.xsp?action=openDocument&documentId=4825657B0C7E6 BF0C12563CD002D6B0B.

21. ICRC, "Commentary," article 1, paragraph 171.

22. ICRC, "Commentary," article 1, paragraph 162.

23. Ryan Goodman, "Two U.S. Positions on the Duty to Ensure Respect for the Geneva Conventions," *Just Security*, blog, September 2, 2016, https://www.justsecurity.org/33166 /u-s-positions-duty-ensure-respect-geneva-conventions/.

24. Ney, "Remarks."

25. Diederik Lohman, Matthew Parsons, and Courtney Tran, "Lack of Accountability for War Crimes," in *Impunity Must End: Attacks on Health in 23 Countries in Conflict in 2016* (Safeguarding Health in Conflict Coalition, 2017), 51–60, https://www.safeguardinghealth .org/sites/shcc/files/SHCC2017final.pdf.

26. Anna Khalfaoui, Daniel Mahanty, Alex Moorehead, and Priyanka Motaparthy, *In Search of Answers: U.S. Military Investigations and Civilian Harm* (Washington, DC: Center for Civilians in Conflict, 2019), https://civiliansinconflict.org/wp-content /uploads/2020/02/PDF-Report-for-Website.pdf.

27. B'Tselem, *Occupation's Fig Leaf: Israel's Military Law Enforcement System as a Whitewash Mechanism* (2016), https://www.btselem.org/sites/default/files/sites/default/files2/201609_ whitewash_protocol_eng.pdf.

28. ICRC, *Health Care in Danger: A Sixteen Country Study* (Geneva: ICRC, 2011), https:// www.icrc.org/en/doc/assets/files/reports/report-hcid-16-country-study-2011-08-10.pdf.

29. Leonard Rubenstein and Melanie Bittle, "Responsibility for Protection of Medical Workers and Facilities in Armed Conflict," *Lancet* 375, no. 9711 (2010): 329–40.

30. Leonard Rubenstein, "Transforming the WHO's Role in Advancing the Right to Health in Conflict," *Global Health Governance* 12, no. 1 (Spring 2018): 11–16.

31. Sixty-Fifth World Health Assembly, Resolution 65.20, WHO's Response, and Role as Health Cluster Lead, in Meeting the Growing Demands of Health in Humanitarian Emergencies (2012), https://apps.who.int/iris/bitstream/handle/10665/80494/A65_R20 -en.pdf?sequence=1&isAllowed=y.

32. World Health Organization, Surveillance System for Attacks on Health Care website, https://publicspace.who.int/sites/ssa/SitePages/PublicDashboard.aspx.

33. Mohamad Elamein, Hilary Bower, Camilo Valderrama, Daher Zedan, Hazem Rihawi, Khaled Almilaji, Nabil Tabbal, Naser Almhawish, Sophie Maes, and Alaa AbouZeid, "Attacks Against Health Care in Syria, 2015–16: Results from a Real-Time Reporting Tool," *Lancet* 390, no. 10109 (2017): 2278; Rohini J. Haar, Casey B. Risko, Sonal Singh, Diana Rayes, Ahmad Albaik, Mohammed Alnajar, Mazen Kewara, Emily Clouse, Elise Baker, and Leonard Rubenstein, "Determining the Scope of Attacks on Health in Four Governorates of Syria in 2016: Results of a Field Surveillance Program," *PLOS Medicine* 15, no. 4 (2018): e1002559; Rohini J. Haar, Katherine H. A. Footer, Sonal Singh, Susan G. Sherman, Casey Branchini, Joshua Sclar, Emily Clouse, and Leonard S. Rubenstein, "Measurement of Attacks and Interferences with Health Care in Conflict: Validation of an Incident Reporting Tool for Attacks on and Interferences with Health Care in Eastern Burma," *Conflict and Health* 8 (2014): Article no. 23; "Methodology," n.d., Physicians for Human Rights (website), https://syriamap.phr.org/#/en/methodology; Swedish Red Cross, *Examining Violence Against Health from a Gender Perspective* (Stockholm: Swedish Red Cross, 2015), https://www.rodakorset.se/globalassets/rodakorset.se/dokument/krigets-lagar /cadesky-examining-violence-against-health-care-from-a-gender-perspective.pdf; "Attacks on Health Care," n.d., Insecurity Insight (website), http://insecurityinsight .org/projects/healthcare; ICRC, *Health Care in Danger: Violent Incidents Affecting the Delivery of Health Care, January 2012–December 2013* (2014), https://shop.icrc.org/health -care-in-danger-violent-incidents-affecting-the-delivery-of-health-care-january-2012 -to-december-2013-pdf-en.

34. ICRC, *Protecting Health Care, Key Recommendations* (Geneva: ICRC, 2016).

35. UN Security Council Resolution 2286, S/Res/2286 (2016), http://unscr.com/en /resolutions/doc/2286.

36. Letter Dated 18 August 2016 from the Secretary-General Addressed to the President of the Security Council, S/2016/722, https://reliefweb.int/sites/reliefweb.int/files/resources /N1626255.pdf.

37. Els Debuf, *Evaluating Mechanisms for Investigating Attacks on Healthcare* (New York: International Peace Institute, 2017).

38. Peter J. Hoffman and Thomas G. Weiss, *Humanitarianism, War, and Politics: Solferino to Syria and Beyond* (Lanham, MD: Rowman & Littlefield, 2017), 161–63.

39. Melissa Dalton et al., *The Protection of Civilians in Partnered Operations* (Center for Strategic and International Studies, Center for Civilians in Conflict, and InterAction, 2018), https://civiliansinconflict.org/wp-content/uploads/2018/10/USProgram_Partnered Operations.pdf.

40. Leonard Rubenstein, "Security Council Can Do More to Protect Health Care in Conflict" (Blog), *Global Health Now*, September 28, 2019, https://www .globalhealthnow.org/2016-09/security-council-can-do-more-protect-health-care -conflict.

41. UN Security Council, 7779th meeting, 28 September 2016, S/PV.7779, http://www
.securitycouncilreport.org/atf/cf/%7B65BFCF9B-6D27-4E9C-8CD3-CF6E4FF96
FF9%7D/s_pv_7779.pdf.

42. UN Security Council, 7779th meeting.

43. Peter Maurer, "Amid COVID-19, We Must Not Lose Focus on Violations and Abuses
in War, Statement to UN Security Council Open Debate: Protection of Civilians in
Armed Conflict," ICRC, May 27, 2020, https://www.icrc.org/en/document/amid-covid
-we-must-not-lose-focus-violations-and-abuses-war.

44. "Memorandum from Secretary of Defense," Department of Defense, October 3,
2016, https://dod.defense.gov/Portals/1/Documents/pubs/Principle-Promulgation
-Memo.pdf.

45. UN Security Council, *Children and Armed Conflict, Report of the Secretary-General*,
A/74/845-S/2020/525 (2020), https://reliefweb.int/sites/reliefweb.int/files/resources/15
-June-2020_Secretary-General_Report_on_CAAC_Eng.pdf.

## CONCLUSION

1. William M. (Mac) Thornberry National Defense Authorization Act for Fiscal Year
2021, Pub. L NO. 116-283, Section 1299J.

2. National Emergency Operations Center for Polio Eradication, *National Emergency
Action Plan for Polio Eradication, 1 July 2018–30 June 2019*, http://polioeradication.org/wp
-content/uploads/2016/07/Pakistan-NEAP-2018-2019.pdf.

3. World Health Organization, *Attacks on Health Care Initiative 2019–2022*, https://www
.who.int/publications-detail/attacks-on-health-care-initiative-2019-2022.

4. Henri Dunant, *A Memory of Solferino* (Geneva: International Committee of the Red
Cross, 1959), 118.

# INDEX

# ABOUT THE AUTHOR

Leonard Rubenstein is Professor of the Practice and director of the Program on Human Rights and Health in Conflict at the Johns Hopkins Bloomberg School of Public Health. A graduate of Wesleyan University and Harvard Law School, he previously served as executive director and president of Physicians for Human Rights and in a Jennings Randolph Senior Fellowship at the United States Institute of Peace. He is a member of the Council of Foreign Relations and is a recipient of the American Public Health Association's Sidel-Levy Award for Peace.

Milton Keynes UK
Ingram Content Group UK Ltd.
UKHW031622061224
451878UK00002B/18/J

9 780231 192460